The biophysical basis of excitability

The biophysical basis of
excitability

HUGO GIL FERREIRA

Laboratorio de Fisiologia, Instituto Gulbenkian de Ciência, Oeiras, Portugal

MICHAEL W. MARSHALL

Senior Lecturer in Physiology, University of Newcastle upon Tyne

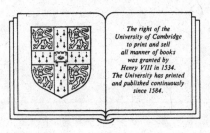

The right of the
University of Cambridge
to print and sell
all manner of books
was granted by
Henry VIII in 1534.
The University has printed
and published continuously
since 1584.

CAMBRIDGE UNIVERSITY PRESS

Cambridge

London New York New Rochelle

Melbourne Sydney

CAMBRIDGE UNIVERSITY PRESS
Cambridge, New York, Melbourne, Madrid, Cape Town, Singapore, São Paulo

Cambridge University Press
The Edinburgh Building, Cambridge CB2 8RU, UK

Published in the United States of America by Cambridge University Press, New York

www.cambridge.org
Information on this title: www.cambridge.org/9780521301510

© Cambridge University Press 1985

First published 1985
This digitally printed version 2008

A catalogue record for this publication is available from the British Library

Library of Congress Catalogue Card Number: 85-3741

ISBN 978-0-521-30151-0 hardback
ISBN 978-0-521-06727-0 paperback

For Karin, Claudia, Paula and Pedro
For Eliska, Jennifer, Joan, Dylan and Emily
For Freedom

CONTENTS

Acknowledgements xiv
Definitions, abbreviations and conventions xv

1 Introduction and overview 1

2 Ions in solution 5

Introduction 5
Formation of ions 5
Electron affinity 6
Equilibrium at the electrode/solution interphase 7
The chemical potential and the electrochemical potential 8
Electrode potentials 9
Junction potentials 10
Standard reference 11
Standard electrode potentials 11
Tables of electrode potentials 12
Measurement of biological potentials 12
The need for salt bridges 14
Silver/silver chloride electrodes 14
Diffusion potentials across a barrier 15
The Nernst equation 17
I/V curve of a slab of solution 18
Conductance of a solution 20
Conductivity and resistivity 20
Molar conductances: the effect of concentration on conductance 21
Concentration dependence of molar conductance 21
Concentration dependence of molar conductances of strong electrolytes 22
Ion flux densities and ion velocities 22
Ion velocities and the electrical field 24
Electrical potential gradient 25
Balance between electrical and frictional forces 25
Ion mobilities 25
Relationship between the flux density and the local potential gradient: the driving force 26
Relationship between ion mobilities and ion conductances 26
The measurement of ionic conductances 28
Transfer or transport numbers 28
Concentration dependence of ion mobilities 28
The activity coefficient 29
The activity of an ion 29
The measurement of ion activities 29

3 Diffusion in free solution   31

Diffusion of non-electrolytes in solution   31
Fick's First Law   31
The diffusion coefficient   32
Driving forces   32
Mobility and the diffusion coefficient: Einstein's equation   34
The relationship between the diffusion coefficient and the ionic (molar) conductance   35
Diffusion across a slab: transient conditions   35
Diffusion across a slab: steady state   37
The permeability constant   37
The Second Law of Fick: transient solution   37
Solution of Fick's Second Law: boundary conditions   39
The speed of diffusional processes   39
Diffusion times for certain molecules   42
Diffusion of electrolytes   43
Diffusional currents   44
The equivalent circuit of a slab of solution   44
Ionic conductances   44
The equivalent circuit for more than one ion   47
Lumped and non-lumped equivalent circuits   48
Diffusion potentials   49

4 Diffusion within a membrane   51

The constant-field assumption   53
Integration of the Nernst–Planck equation   53
The partition coefficient at the membrane–solution interphase   54
The membrane permeability   55
The Goldman–Hodgkin–Katz (constant-field) equation for the membrane current density   55
Assumptions made in the derivation of the constant-field equation   55
The constant-field I/V curve   57
Constant-field rectification   57
Anomalous rectification   57
Characteristics of constant-field rectification   58
The maximum value of a constant-field rectification   59
When the constant-field equation becomes linear   59
The constant-field equation at zero transmembrane potential   60
The constant-field equation at zero current   60
The constant-field equation for more than one ion current: the independence principle   61
The resting membrane potential   62
The G-H-K equation for the potential   62
The slope conductance   63
The full formula for the slope conductance   64
The slope conductance when $V=0$ 64
The slope conductance for V positive and very large   65
The slope conductance for V negative and very large   65
The chord conductance   66
Current flow at two different ion concentrations: scaling of the constant-field equation   66
The independence principle   67
Computation of the membrane permeability   68

5 Membranes, channels, carriers and pumps   70

Regulation of composition and volume of biological compartments   70
Coupling mechanisms in membrane transport   70
Chemical composition of biological membranes   71

Interaction between phospholipids and water   71
Forms of aggregation of phospholipids in water: monolayers   72
Micelles   73
Bilayers – liposomes and microsomes   73
Gorter and Grundel's experiment   73
Phase transitions: surface pressure   73
Temperature-dependence of phase transitions   75
Lipid bilayers as experimental models of biological membranes: liposomes and BLMs   75
Permeability of lipid bilayers: fluidity   76
Cholesterol in lipid bilayers   77
Flip-flopping of phospholipids in lipid bilayers   77
The mechanism of permeation in lipid bilayers: the partition–diffusion model   78
The limiting case when diffusion within the membrane is rate-limiting   80
Permeability of lipid bilayers   80
Ion permeabilities of lipid bilayers   80
Ionophores   81
The relationship between permeability and conductance channels   82
The kinetics of pore formation   83
Pore selectivity   84
Fluctuations in membrane conductance   84
Membrane noise   84
Voltage-dependent conductances   85
Voltage-dependent channels in excitable membranes   85
Carriers and pores in natural membranes   87
Uphill transport   87
Pumps   88
Flux-coupling mechanisms   88
The operation of an ion pump   89
The Na/K pump: a thermodynamical description   92
The maximum electrochemical gradient that can be generated by Na/K pump   94
The membrane potential   94
The relationship between pumping and the membrane potential   95
The contribution of the rate of pumping to the membrane potential   96
Stoichiometry of the pump and the membrane potential   97
Electrogenicity of the pump   98

6 Membrane equivalent circuits   99

The equilibrium potentials for K, Na and Cl   99
The equivalent circuit of a membrane   100
Membrane resistance and conductance   103
The membrane equilibrium potential for an ion   105
The relationship between chord and slope conductance   106
The full equivalent circuit of a membrane   107
The open-circuit potential   107
The membrane capacitance   108
Charge separation across a membrane   108
The capacitance current   111
The membrane voltage in response to a current step   111
The membrane time constant   112
The computation of the capacitative currents   114
The voltage-clamp techniques   114

7 Voltage-sensitive channels: the membrane action potential   117

Introduction   117
Propagated and local action potentials   117
The action potential and the membrane current   119
Voltage and current clamps   119

The squid axon as an idealized experimental model 119
Lumped electrical equivalent circuit of the membrane 120
Current sign convention 121
Membrane potential transients under current clamp 122
The full equation for a voltage transient 124
Conductance changes in excitable membranes 125
The independence of the membrane conductances: ion substitutions and the use of inhibitors 126
Elimination of sodium conductance 128
I/V curves 128
The capacitative current 130
Removal of capacitative current by voltage clamp 131
Potassium conductance as a function of time and voltage 132
Potassium channels 134
The formation or opening of potassium channels 134
The maximum potassium conductance 135
The Hodgkin–Huxley model of channel opening (formation) 136
Charge movements inside the membranes of excitable cells: displacement currents 138
Voltage-dependence of the rate constants 141
Potassium channels are ohmic: instantaneous *I/V* curves 143
The potassium equilibrium potential 144
The sodium current 145
The sodium conductance 145
Sodium inactivation 147
Voltage-dependence of inactivation 148
Time-dependence of the inactivation 150
The voltage- and time-dependence of *m* 152
Four-particle models of the sodium channel 154
The full analytical expression for the voltage- and time-dependence of the sodium channel 155
The sodium channels are ohmic conductors 156
Voltage-dependence of the rate constants 157
The leak conductance 157
Action potential generation 158
The Hodgkin cycle 158
The membrane action potential 160
Sodium and potassium channels 162
Evidence that channels are pores 162
Patch-clamp technique 163
Membrane noise 163
Basic properties of the unit conductance 164
Unit conductances 165
Effective pore diameters 165
Channel selectivity 167
Activation energy of ion permeation 167

8 The propagated action potential 168

Non-uniform distribution of currents and voltages along the axon 168
Three-dimensional analysis of current distribution along the axon 168
The equivalent circuit of an axon 172
Derivation of the cable equation 178
Solutions of the cable equation 180
  Steady-state solution 180
  The space constant 181
  Non-steady-state solution 181
  The input resistance 182
  The membrane time constant 183
  Non-infinite cables 183

Current injection in the middle of the fibre   184
Current input at one end of the fibre   184
Space-clamping   185
Point-clamp techniques   186
End of the fibre voltage-clamp technique   187
Middle of the fibre voltage-clamp   188
Calculation of the propagated action potential: derivation of the wave equation   189
The one-dimensional wave equation   191
Solution of the wave equation: the propagated action potential   192
Distributed model of the axon to solve the propagating action potential   192
Conduction velocity   194
Saltatory conduction   194

9 Synaptic potentials   195

Introduction   195
The neuromuscular junction   195
The synapse   195
The end-plate potential (EPP)   196
The miniature end-plate potential (MEPP)   197
Amplitude distribution of EPPs: the Poisson distribution   198
Presynaptic depolarization   199
Synaptic delay   200
The release of acetylcholine (Ach)   200
Effect of curare   200
Competitive inhibition   201
Inhibitors of Ach release   201
Postsynaptic inhibitors: depolarizing blockers   201
Synaptic vesicles and the role of calcium   201
Synaptic delay: diffusion over the synaptic cleft   202
Number of Ach molecules that interact with a receptor site   202
Depolarization induced by 1–2 molecules of Ach   202
Number of Ach molecules per vesicle   202
Number of vesicles required to trigger an action potential   203
Conductance changes in the postsynaptic membrane   203
The reversal potential of the postsynaptic membrane in the presence of Ach   204
Ach-gated channels   204
The electrical equivalent circuit of the postsynaptic membrane   204
A simple cable model for the end-plate region: transient analysis   205
The shape of the EPP   210
Attenuation of the EPP with distance   210
Spatial summation   211
Temporal summation   212
Other synapses   213
Other transmitter substances   213
Depolarizing and hyperpolarizing transmitters: EPSPs and IPSPs   213
Combined effect of EPSPs and IPSPs   214
The flow of current in the synaptic region   214
Kinetics of the transmitter–receptor interaction   215
The kinetic scheme   217
The mathematical model   217
The solution of the mathematical model   218
The postsynaptic conductance transient   221
The voltage dependence of the conductance change   221
Sensory receptors   223
Generator and receptor potentials   223
Tonic and phasic receptors   224
Changes in conductance in receptors   224

Biological transducers   224
Frequency coding   225
Electrical synapses   225
Gap junctions   225

10 Membrane noise   227

Introduction   227
A probabilistic model of quantal release   227
Setting up the model   228
Analytical solution of the model   232
Amplitude distribution of MEPPs   234
Postsynaptic membrane noise   235
Measurement of synaptic noise   236
Variance and time average of a time signal   236
Signal averaging, noise reduction   238
Analysis of noise   239
Relationship between postsynaptic membrane noise and postsynaptic membrane depolarization   239
Relationship between synaptic noise and the molecular events of synaptic transmission   240
Model dependency of the analysis   243
A model encoding the receptor-transmitter interaction   243
An expression for the concentration of transmitter–receptor complex   243
Probabilities of the closing and opening of the transmitter–receptor complex   245
The concentration of transmitter as a delta function   247
The solution   248
Fluctuations of conductance at the end-plate region   248
The end-plate current   249
Postsynaptic current noise under voltage-clamp and continuous perfusion with Ach   249
The conductance of a channel   251
The autocovariance of the channel current   254
The power density spectrum of the synaptic noise   257

Appendices   259

1 Units and numbers   259
2 Algebra and calculus – a review   268
3 Trigonometric functions   307
4 The Taylor series   323
5 Stirling's formula   324
6 The Wallis's formula – the recurrence formula for integration   329
7 Introduction to probability theory   333
8 Partial fractions   348
9 Integration of differential equations: the separation of variables technique   350
10 Integration of differential equations by the integrating factor   353
11 The Fourier expansion   354
12 The Fourier integral   365
13 Harmonic analysis of non-periodic signals   375
14 The Laplace transform   386
15 Fundamental circuit equations   390
16 Solution of linear differential equations by the Laplace transform   399
17 The application of Laplace transforms to circuit theory: the concept of complex impedance   400
18 Partial differentiation: the gradient and divergence   402
19 Partial differential equations: integration of the diffusion equation   410
20 Solution of the cable equation for different boundary conditions   417
21 The Boltzmann factor   425
22 The Poisson equation   431

23 Coulomb's Law and the dielectric constant 435
24 Membrane capacitance and charge movements 438
25 Free energy 440
26 The temperature dependence of rate constants 449
27 Junction potentials 451
28 Competitive inhibition kinetics 455
29 Acetylcholine–receptor interaction 457
30 Measurement of membrane permeability with radioisotopes 458
31 Voltage- and current-clamp techniques 461
32 Tables of constants for axons and muscles 465
33 Work, energy and potential energy 467

Suggested further reading 469

Index 478

ACKNOWLEDGEMENTS

We would like to thank the following for many valuable discussions and for their time spend reading some of the original draft manuscripts: Professor R. H. Adrian, Professor E. L. Blair, Dr F. Costa, Dr P. Fernandes, Dr G. Green, Dr A. Hill, Dr S. Hollingworth, Dr V. Lew, Mr N. Pedro, Ms J. Peachey, Mr S. M. Smith and Mr R. Zorec.

We would like to thank the Gulbenkian Foundation for financial support and our special thanks are due to Mr U. Santos for his invaluable work in preparing the illustrations. We are grateful to the secretarial assistance given to us by Mrs E. Hill, Mrs C. Wood, Mrs L. Santos and Mrs A. Speed and we would like to thank Dr A. O. Smith for seeing the book through the press.

Finally we would like to thank our colleagues, families and friends who have encouraged us to produce this book. Special thanks must go to Karin, Jennifer and Peter, whose good humour, enthusiasm and tolerance were greatly appreciated.

DEFINITIONS, ABBREVIATIONS AND CONVENTIONS

Symbol

a radius of a cell; chemical activity in solution; $= ZFV/RT\delta$; ratio between the numerical values of a concentration expressed in two different units (g/l and mol/l for example); $= 4Dt$; mathematical coefficient

$a_{M^+(aq)}$ activity of metal ion M^+ in aqueous solution

a_n, b_n real and imaginary amplitudes of the nth harmonic in a fourier series

A, A ampere, unit of electric current; area; gain of an electronic amplifier; symbol for a channel-forming antibiotic in aqueous solution

A^- anion

Ach   acetylcholine

A_m channel-forming antibiotic dissolved in the membrane

b $= \bar{J}/D$; mathematical coefficient

c concentration; mathematical coefficient

c_m capacitance of a small area element (in farads); complex amplitude of the mth harmonic in a complex fourier series; capacitance per unit length (farad $\cdot$ cm^{-1})

cm   symbol of centimetre, unit of length

$c_{m,1}$ concentration in membrane on side 1

c_{In} concentration inside a cell or a compartment

c_{Na} concentration of sodium

$c_{Na.In}$ concentration of sodium inside a cell or a compartment

$c_{Na.o}$ concentration of sodium outside a cell or a compartment

$c(x)$ concentration at point or a plane located at coordinate x

$c(x, t)$ concentration at point or a plane located at coordinate t

c_K^* concentration of radioactive potassium

c_m^* membrane capacitance per sector of axon, per unit length $(\text{farad}\cdot\text{cm}^{-1})$

$c_{(1)}$ concentration in compartment (1)

[ch]   concentration of channels

C   symbol for a capacitor in an electrical circuit; coulomb, unit of charge

C_m membrane capacitance (farads)

$\bar{C}_m$ membrane capacitance per unit area $(\text{farad}\cdot\text{cm}^{-2})$

$C(\tau)$ autocovariance function

$C_1(\tau)$ autocovariance function (of voltage, current or conductance) of channel 1

Cu   chemical symbol for copper

$Cu_{(s)}$ chemical symbol for metal copper: (s) means solid metal

Cu^{2+} chemical symbol for ionic copper

$Cu_{(aq)}^{2+}$ chemical symbol for ionic copper in aqueous solution

dyn   symbol for dyne, unit of force in c.g.s. system

D diffusion coefficient, as defined from 1st Law of Fick. Has the dimensions $\text{cm}^2\cdot\text{s}^{-1}$

D_i diffusion coefficient of ion i (example D_{Na}, for sodium ion)

D_m diffusion coefficient of a given molecular species within the membrane

$e, (e^-)$ base of natural logarithms (2.71828); electronic charge $(1.602\times10^{-19}\ \text{C})$

E energy (joules or calories); electromotive force; electrical potential difference $(V_{(2)}-V_{(1)})$

$\vec{E}$ activation energy for the transition of a particle from the $\bar{n}$ state into the n state

$\bar{E}$ electrical field strength (in volts)

E_{eq} equilibrium potential across an Ach-gated channel

E_i equilibrium potential for ion i (for example, E_{Na} is the Nernst or equilibrium potential for sodium across a membrane)

E_i' overall diffusion potential across a slab of solution of thickness l and unit cross-sectional area. It is given by the expression

$$E_i' = RT/ZF\ \ln(c_i(l)/c_i(0))$$

where $c_i(l)$ and $c_i(0)$ are the concentrations at $x=1$ and $x=0$

EPP   end-plate potential (for muscle)

EPSP   excitatory postsynaptic potential (for nerve cells)

erf(x)   error function, defined as

$$\text{erf}(x) = (2/\sqrt{\pi})\int_0^x e^{-n^2}\,dn$$

E_s electromotive force of a voltage source; reversal potential of an Ach channel

$E[x_i]$	expected value or average $(\bar{x})$ of a discrete random value (x_i)
E^0	standard electrode potential
E_{Cu}	electrical potential difference between a copper electrode (wire) and a copper solution in which it is dipped (half cell)
E_{Cu}^0	standard electrode potential of copper
$E_{H_2^+}$	electrode potential of a hydrogen half cell
E_j	junction potential
E_M	electrode potential of a half cell of metal M
f	symbol for frequency (in Hz); driving force (volt $\cdot$ cm^{-1})
f'	driving force per mole (J $\cdot$ mol^{-1})
$\bar{f}$	average value of a function
f_q	frictional coefficient exerted on charge q (dyn $\cdot$ cm^{-1} $\cdot$ s)
f_q'	frictional coefficient per unit charge (dyn $\cdot$ cm^{-1} $\cdot$ C^{-1})
F	symbol of farad, unit of capacitance; faraday (9.648456×10^4C $\cdot$ mol^{-1})
F_e	electrical force, or force executed by an electrical field on a charge q
F_f	frictional force
$F(\omega)$	Fourier integral of time function $f(t)$
g, g	symbol for gram; slope conductance, defined as dI/dV
gr-eq	quantity of a substance whose mass in grams is equal to its equivalent weight. The equivalent weight is the atomic weight divided by the charge number or valence. A gram-equivalent of calcium corresponds to 20 grams of calcium
g_i	internal conductance (cytoplasmic conductance) per unit length (S $\cdot$ cm)
$g_i^*(P)$	internal conductance of a sector (P) of cytoplasm per unit length (e.g. 8.35)
g_{Na}^*	membrane sodium conductance per unit length of a sector of squid axon
G	symbol for a conductance in an electrical circuit (siemens, S)
G_A	conductance of a conductor of cross-sectional area A
$\bar{G}$	conductance per unit area (S $\cdot$ cm^{-2})
$\bar{G}_+$	cation conductance per unit area of solution
G_i'	conductance per unit length (S $\cdot$ cm^{-1}) of ion i in solution
$\bar{G}_i$	conductance per unit area (S $\cdot$ cm^{-2}) of an ion i
G_{Na}	membrane sodium conductance (S)
G_t	total membrane conductance
G_t'	total membrane conductance per unit length
$\bar{G}_b$	backward conductance per unit area (in Goldman rectification)
$\bar{G}_f$	forward conductance per unit area (in Goldman rectification)
$\bar{G}_m$	membrane conductance (S)

G_p — conductance of a pore (S)

G_g — conductance of a Gramicydin-induced channel (S)

ΔG_{Na} — free energy change due to the movement of m moles of sodium from compartment (1) to compartment (2) (joules)

ΔG_t — total change in free energy in a given process (J)

$\bar{G}_m$ — membrane conductance per unit area ($S \cdot cm^{-2}$)

G_{Kch} — conductance of a potassium channel (S)

$\bar{G}_K$ — potassium conductance per unit area of membrane at maximum potassium activation

$\bar{G}_{Na}$ — sodium conductance per unit area of membrane at maximum sodium activation

$\tilde{G}_{Na}$ — sodium conductance per unit area of membrane when inactivation is removed ($h = 1$). Given by
$$\tilde{G}_{Na} = \bar{G}_{Na} m^a$$
or
$$\tilde{G}_{Na} = \bar{G}_{Na}/h$$

G_{Na}^* — sodium conductance of a membrane area element (S) (units S)

$\dot{G}_{ch}(t)$ — mean conductance of population of channels at time t (S)

G_s — conductance of an Ach channel (S)

G_{sK} — potassium conductance of an Ach channel

G_{sNa} — sodium conductance of an Ach channel

$h, \bar{h}, h(t)$ — sodium inactivation parameters of H. H model of squid axon

H_2 — symbol for molecular hydrogen

$H_{(aq)}^+$ — protons (or hydrogen ions) in aqueous solution

H — enthalpy

H_σ — enthalpy of a system

Hz — unit of frequency (s^{-1})

i_m — membrane current per unit length

$i_m(j)$ — membrane current per unit length at port j in a multiport axon

$i_t^*(p)$ — total membrane current per unit length and for sector p of axon

I — symbol for electric current (measured in amperes, A)

$\bar{I}$ — current density ($A \cdot cm^{-2}$)

I_+ — current due to the flow of a cation (A)

$\bar{I}_+$ — current density due to the flow of a cation ($A \cdot cm^{-2}$)

$\bar{I}_c$ — capacitative current density ($A \cdot cm^{-2}$)

$\dot{I}_{ch}(t)$ — average current of a population of channels at time t (A)

$\bar{I}_i$ — ionic current density ($A \cdot cm^{-2}$)

$\bar{I}_{Na,0}$ — sodium current density at time zero ($A \cdot cm^{-2}$)

$\bar{I}_{Na,t}$ — sodium current density at time t

IPSP	inhibitory postsynaptic potential
I_s	synaptic current
$\bar{I}_t$	total current density at time t
j,j	$\sqrt{-1}$; activity coefficient
j′	$RT \ln(j)$
J	symbol for joule, unit of energy; flux $(mol \cdot s^{-1})$
J	flux of a cation $(mol \cdot s^{-1})$
$\bar{J}$	flux density $(mol \cdot s^{-1} \cdot cm^{-2})$
$\vec{J}$	flux density from left to right $(mol \cdot s^{-1} \cdot cm^{-2})$
$\bar{J}_{DNa}$	diffusional flux density of sodium
$\bar{J}_K^*$	flux density of radioactive potassium $(mol \cdot s^{-1} \cdot cm^{-2})$
J_K^*	flux of radioactive potassium $(mol \cdot s^{-1})$
$\bar{J}_{Na}$	Abbreviation for
	$P_{Na} U c_{Na,o}/(\exp(U)-1)$
	where $U = ZFV/RT$
J_{Na}	flux of sodium $(mol \cdot s^{-1})$
$J(x)$	flux along x direction and at point x
J_{21}	flux from compartment 2 to compartment 1
k	Boltzmann constant $(1.380662 \times 10^{-23} \, J \cdot K^{-1})$; decay constant (s^{-1}); conductivity $(S \cdot cm^{-1})$; dielectric constant
k_f, k_b	rate constants in the forward and backward directions; dimensions depend on molarity of reaction
k_D	rate constant of diffusion of transmitter away from synapse. Defined by
	$J_D = k_D[T]$
k_E	rate constant of enzymatic breakdown of Ach
$k_{m,s}, k_{s,m}$	rate constants of release and uptake of a substance by membrane $cm \cdot s^{-1}$ or $cm^3 \cdot s^{-1}$ (according to method of expressing flux)
k_1, k_{-1}	rate constants of a reaction in the forward and backward directions
k_+	conductivity of an electrolyte solution due to the cation
K	degree Kelvin
K	equilibrium constant
l	distance (cm); symbol for litre, unit of volume
L_D	Debye length, given by
	$L_D = 1/(8c_{NaCl}\pi F(1/\varepsilon)(F/RT))$
m	symbol for metre
$m, \bar{m}, m(t)$	sodium activation parameters of H.H model of squid axon
mol	abbreviation for mole
M	molar concentration $(1 \, M = 1 \, mol/l)$

M	symbol for a metal in solid form
$M_{(aq)}^{2+}$	divalent ionic metal in aqueous solution
$M_{(S)}$	metal in solid form
MEPP	miniature end-plate potential
n	number of moles
$n, \bar{n}, n(t)$	potassium activation parameters of H.H model of squid axon
n_0, n_∞	value of n at $t=$ zero and $t \to \infty$ respectively
N	abbreviation for newton, unit of force
$\bar{N}, N$	potassium activation parameters of H.H model of squid axon related to n and $\bar{n}$ by the expressions

$$n = N/(N+\bar{N}) \quad \text{and} \quad \bar{n} = \bar{N}/(N+N)$$

N_A	Avogadro's number (6.022045×10^{23} mol^{-1})
N_{ch}	number of open channels per unit area of membrane
N_{ch_T}	total number of channels per unit area of membrane
N_T	maximum number of particles per unit membrane
p	correction factor in equation (8.92); see Laplace variable
$p(x)$	probability density of occurrence of value x where x is a random variable
P	permeability (cm·s^{-1}); pressure
$P(A1/A2)$	probability of occurrence of event A1 once event A2 has taken place (in a conceptual random experiment)
$P(A1, A2)$	probability of the simultaneous occurrence of events A1 and A2 (in a conceptual random experiment)
$P(A)$	probability of occurrence of event A (in a conceptual random experiment)
$\bar{P}_c(t)$	probability of not closing one channel during time t
$P_c(t)$	probability of closing one channel during time t
$P_o(t)$	probability that a channel is open at time t
P_K^E	permeability to potassium due to an exchange process (measured with radioisotopes)
P_K^D	diffusional permeability to potassium
$P_n(t)$	probability of releasing n quanta during time t
$P_n(x)$	probability of obtaining outcome x in a conceptual random experiment performed n times
P_{Na}	sodium permeability (cm·s^{-1})
$\bar{P}_o(t)$	probability of not opening a channel during time t
$P_o(t)$	probability of opening a channel during time t
$P_o(0/t)$	probability of finding a channel open at time t when it was open at time zero

$P_o(c/t)$ probability of finding a channel open at time t when it was closed at time zero

q quantity of electricity (C)

Q quantity of electricity or charge in the plates of a capacitor; amount of a solute in moles

Q_{cy} total amount of charge in the cytoplasm of a cell due to its anions (or its cations) (C)

Q_t total charge stored in a capacitor with plates of surface areas (C)

Q_0 amount of charge injected across a membrane at time zero

Q_{10} change in the rate of a reaction (expressed as a ratio) when the temperature is increased by $10\,°C$

r stoichiometry of the sodium pump

r_i resistance of cytoplasm (internal resistance) per unit length ($\Omega \cdot cm^{-1}$)

r_i^* internal resistance of sector of axon per unit length ($\Omega \cdot cm^{-1}$)

R_m membrane resistance per unit length

R resistance (Ω); symbol for a resistor; gas constant ($8.31441\ J \cdot K^{-1} \cdot mol^{-1}$)

$[IR]$ concentration of transmitter–receptor

$\bar{R}_i$ resistance $\cdot$ unit area ($\Omega \cdot cm^2$) of a solution due to ion i

R_i resistance of a solution, due to ion i (Ω)

R_i^* longitudinal resistance of a volume element (see (8.15))

R_{In} input resistance (see (8.74))

$\bar{R}_m$ membrane resistance $\cdot$ unit area ($\Omega \cdot cm^2$)

R_s source resistance (Ω)

$[R_t]$ total concentration of transmitter receptor

$[RT]$ concentration of transmitter–receptor complex

s, s symbol for second; Laplace variable

s^2 variance of a random variable

S, S entropy ($J \cdot K^{-1} \cdot mol^{-1}$); surface area of a cell membrane; symbol for Siemens, unit of conductance

$S(t)$ time-varying signal

t_y decay constant of function $y(t)$ (see e.g. (7.45)), s^{-1}

t_+, t_- transport numbers

T, T absolute temperature (in K); period of a function $= 1/f$ (units, s); normalized time given by $T = t/\tau_m$

$[T]$ concentration of transmitter

T_i transmitter in inactive form

TTX   tetrodotoxin

u_+ mobility of cation ($cm^2 \cdot s^{-1} \cdot V^{-1}$)

u'_{Na} mobility of sodium defined as
$u'_{Na} = u_{Na}/ZF$ $(cm \cdot s^{-1} \cdot N^{-1} \cdot mol)$

U a quantity defined as
ZFV/RT; or as $(X^2 + 4(T - \Delta T)^2)/4(T - \Delta T)$

v velocity $(cm \cdot s^{-1})$

$\bar{v}$ average velocity (of a particle in a random walk)

v_b, v_f velocity of a reaction $(mol \cdot s^{-1})$ in the backward (b) and forward (f) reactions

v_+ velocity of a cation $(cm \cdot s^{-1})$

v_1, v_{-1} similar to v_b, v_f

V, V symbol of volt, unit of electrical potential; symbol of voltmeter in electrical circuit; voltage

$\bar{V}$ average value of a time-varying voltage

$V_{(aq),1}$ voltage at aqueous compartment (1)

$V_{(aq)}$ voltage in aqueous phase

$\bar{V}_{EPP}$ average value of end-plate potential

$\bar{V}_h, \bar{V}_n, \bar{V}_m$ parameters of functions which give the voltage dependence of the rate constants $\alpha_h, \beta_h, \alpha_n, \beta_n$ and α_m, β_m in H.H model of squid axon

V_m voltage in the cytoplasm

$\bar{V}_{MEPP}$ average voltage of miniature end-plate potentials

V_j $V(j)$ voltage at station (j)

V_m voltage inside the membrane

$V_{m,1}$ voltage inside the membrane at the interphase with compartment (1)

V_0 voltage at $t = 0$ or at $x = 0$ according to definition in text

V_{oc} open-circuit voltage (when $I_t =$ zero)

$V_{(\delta)}$ voltage at point δ

V_s source voltage

$V_{(x)}$ voltage at x

$V(x, t)$ voltage at x and t

$V_{(1)}$ voltage in compartment (1)

$V(\infty)$ or V_∞ voltage at $t \to \infty$ or at $x \to \infty$ according to definitions in text

V' $= -V$

v volume (cm^3); velocity

W_1 energy, work (J); also expressed as $J \cdot mol^{-1} \cdot K^{-1}$ (Boltzmann's formula)

x distance (cm)

x_i discrete random variable

$\bar{x}$ average value of a discrete random variable

X normalized distance defined as

$$X = x/\lambda$$

in which λ is a space constant as defined below; term defined as

$$X = P_{Na}c_{Na,1} + P_K c_{K,1} + P_{Cl}c_{Cl,2}$$

Y term defined as

$$Y = P_{Na}c_{Na,2} + P_K c_{K,2} + P_{Cl}c_{Cl,1}$$

Z, Z_i valence or charge number $(gr\text{-}eq \cdot mol^{-1})$; length of the arc expressed in radians

α, β rates of closing and opening the transmitter–receptor complex

$\alpha_n, \alpha_m, \alpha_h, \bar{\alpha}_n, \bar{\alpha}_m, \bar{\alpha}_h, \beta_n, \beta_m, \beta_h, \bar{\beta}_n, \bar{\beta}_m, \bar{\beta}_h$ rate constants in H.H model of squid axon

α_1 ratio P_K/P_{Na}

β partition coefficient given by

$$\beta = c_{(0)}/c_{(1)} = c_{(\delta)}/c_{(2)}$$

γ' activity coefficient

δ thickness of a membrane (cm)

$\delta(t), \delta(t-t_0)$ delta function

$\delta_\tau(t)$ periodic delta function (period τ)

ε permittivity of a dielectric; mean of Poisson and normal distributions

ε_0 permittivity of vacuum

θ probability of getting a favourable outcome in a conceptual random experiment with only two possible outcomes

λ space constant (cm) defined as

$$\lambda = \sqrt{(r_m/r_i)}$$

λ_i molar conductivity of ion i in solution $(S \cdot cm^2 \cdot mol^{-1})$

λ_0 limiting conductivity $(S \cdot cm^2 \cdot mol^{-1})$

μ electrochemical potential $(J \cdot mol^{-1})$

μ^0 standard electrochemical potential $(J \cdot mol^{-1})$

$\mu_{Na,m}$ electrochemical potential of sodium in membrane

$\mu^0_{1(aq)}$ standard electrochemical potential in aqueous compartment (1)

$\mu^0_{i(m)}$ standard electrochemical potential of component i in membrane

π 3.14159 ...

ρ charge density $(C \cdot cm^{-3})$

ρ_{In} resistivity of cytoplasm $(\Omega \cdot cm)$

$\rho(t)$ rate of production of transmitter $(mol \cdot s^{-1} \cdot cm^{-3})$

σ standard deviation

τ_m membrane time constant

τ_h, τ_m, τ_n time constants of, respectively, sodium inactivation, sodium activation and potassium activation

ϕ angle in degrees

Ψ electrical potential (V)

$\Psi_{tt}(\tau)$ autocorrelation function

Ω symbol for ohm, unit of resistance

ω angular velocity (radians $\cdot$ s^{-1})

Please note that

$$(\mathrm{d}/\mathrm{d}t)(x) \equiv \mathrm{d}x/\mathrm{d}t \equiv \frac{\mathrm{d}x}{\mathrm{d}t}$$

and

$$(\mathrm{d}/\mathrm{d}t)^2(x) \equiv \mathrm{d}^2x/\mathrm{d}t^2 \equiv \frac{\mathrm{d}^2x}{\mathrm{d}t^2}$$

Other symbols are defined as they are introduced.

1

Introduction and overview

This book is not a textbook of biophysics, cell biology or the electro-physiology of excitable cells, as there are already a number of excellent books available which deal with these subjects. The book instead is an attempt to describe the origins and derivations of the principles upon which these other books are based.

To understand and apply the principles of excitability requires a knowledge of subjects as diverse as physiology, physics, mathematics, statistics, signal and system analysis. It is a difficult task to obtain this knowledge because the jargon in other fields is often obscure, mathematical proofs are frequently abstruse and generally many original manuscripts have to be consulted. We can both testify to the frustrations that accompany such efforts and this has therefore been written in an attempt to enable the reader to acquire more easily this knowledge. Half of the book is appendices which deal with many of the key concepts from a fairly basic level.

We have assumed that the reader has only a modest mathematical background (about G.C.E. 'O' level) and most formulae are derived from first principles. For people with mathematical ability this approach may be somewhat tedious but we make no apologies for this. We consider it necessary that most of the steps in the derivation of an important equation are left in. Far too often have we struggled to follow mathematical proofs that are presented by an author in two lines which in reality take pages to derive.

The title of the book should not be taken too literally. The principles of excitability apply to many other biological fields. For example, Chapters 2–6, which deal with the movements of ions in solution and across barriers, could be useful to those who study ion transport in non-excitable cells. Chapters 7–9 give a good basis for research workers interested in a more analytical study of excitability. Chapters 7–9 should also provide a good basis for those wishing to study more advanced electrophysiological texts (such as Jack, Nobel and Tsien's *Electric Current Flow in Excitable Cells*).

The book is intended to be as self-contained as possible and it is for this reason that there are extensive appendices. In the appendices we have attempted to lay out most of the fundamental concepts in a simple way and by separating them from the remainder of the text to avoid interrupting the flow of the main text with derivations.

The appendices can be broadly categorized into three groups. These are mathematics, signal analysis (harmonic analysis) and physical chemistry. The mathematical appendices cover calculus (differential and integral), number theory, probability, solutions of differential equations and some special mathematical relationships such as Stirling's formula and Wallis's product. In the appendices on signal analysis the aim is to introduce the harmonic analysis of stochastic signals. Physical chemistry covers some key concepts such as free energy and Debye layers.

At all times we have tried to develop the theory presented in the appendices in a semi-intuitive way, and this is often at the expense of mathematical rigour. The reader approaching the book for the first time should realize that the appendices tend to build on one another so that there is a gradual increase in both mathematical and conceptual difficulty This occurs throughout the book. Conceptually the content of Chapters 2–6, which deals with the principles of excitability, is easier to understand than the content of Chapters 7–10 which deals with the applications. This is not surprising, since Chapters 7–10 integrate and extend the ideas and theory developed in the previous chapters.

There are a large number of diagrams and figures and, rathor than borrowing from original experimental records, journals or books, we have presented almost exclusively our own computed curves.

When we think of the long-term usefulness of this book we are aware that not all the basic principles presented here will still obtain in some years' time. We believe that concepts developed in the earlier chapters (like chemical potential, free energy, the Nernst–Planck equation and Fick's Laws) will remain of value for some time. Chapters 6–9 deal with more recent mid-twentieth-century advances that have survived more or less intact to this day. Chapter 10 deals with some of the most recent additions to the field of excitability and these have yet to withstand the test of time. This chapter was included as it is about an exciting, rapidly expanding subject and also because we think some of the concepts it develops are rather difficult. We have tried to present our analysis as clearly as possible, but some of the ideas are not easy to comprehend and we can only hope we have succeeded.

Dimensional arguments are often used in the book, not only to show that the derivations are correct, but also to derive some equations. It is our experience that dimensional analysis can be an excellent way of checking equations that set out to describe the physical world.

It may be helpful to provide a more detailed overview of the book. Chapter 2 sets out to show how to solve the problem of establishing electrical continuity between measuring equipment and biological compartments, which are aqueous solutions. Such continuity is achieved by means of metal electrodes. The chapter then develops such concepts as electrochemical potentials, standard electrode potentials and molar conductances of solutions.

Chapter 3 presents the two Laws of Fick along with the general flux equation and the concept of a driving force. The Nernst–Planck equation is derived from first principles, and (based upon the treatment used by Finchelstein & Mauro) the equation is integrated in such a way as to allow the representation of an electrodiffusional process by electrical equivalent circuits. This approach, using electrical equivalent circuits to model biophysical processes, is a powerful technique often used by electrophysiologists and we use it extensively in the later part of the book.

Chapter 4 deals with a special case of the integration of the Nernst–Planck equation. This is when the electric field is constant throughout the membrane and this constant-field assumption leads to the derivation of the Goldman–Hodgkin–Katz equation. This equation is then analysed in some detail. Membrane permeability and membrane conductance are also presented along with the idea of rectification in membranes. In Appendix 27 (which can be thought of as an extension of this chapter) liquid junction potentials are discussed.

Chapter 5 provides an introduction to the lipid component of biological membranes and to specialized transport systems that are important for setting up membrane potentials.

Our development of electrical equivalent circuits for membranes is presented in Chapter 6 where membrane capacitance is also discussed. A more detailed discussion of membrane capacitance can be found in Appendix 24.

Chapter 7 is entirely devoted to the development of the Hodgkin–Huxley model of excitable membranes. This chapter draws extensively on material given in the previous chapters and shows how action potentials can be modelled using digital computers.

Chapter 8 is an extension of Chapter 7 and deals with the so-called 'cable properties' of cells. The propagated action potential is introduced at this point.

Chapter 9 describes in a semi-quantitative way the events that take place at synapses. In this chapter the probabilistic behaviour of synaptic transmission is examined and used as a starting point for an analysis of membrane noise.

Chapter 10 is a more formal treatment of membrane noise and should be read in connection with the appendices on signal analysis.

In conclusion, the aim of the book is not to set out to derive any new fundamental physical laws or propose any new physiological models. Rather, our intention is to present existing knowledge in a way that clearly explains the basic principles underlying excitability in biological tissues.

2

Ions in solution

Introduction

A living organism consists of a very large number of inter-dependent fluid compartments. These compartments are bounded by lipid barriers (membranes) and they contain mainly water and exist in an environment that is mostly water. Communication and exchanges between these compartments are carried out by molecules or ions that are able to move through the water and the lipid phases. In order to study these compartmental exchanges it is thus necessary to examine the way in which molecules and ions move through homogeneous liquid phases. We shall consider homogeneous liquid phases because the membrane lipids are in a liquid state and can be treated in the same way as water – that is, as a homogeneous liquid phase (see Chapter 5). Let us first start by an examination of the way in which ions are formed and then go on to analyse the way in which they move through aqueous solutions under the influence of an electric field.

Formation of ions

Ions are formed when neutral molecules are dissociated or when salts are dissolved. To dissolve a salt, or dissociate a molecule, requires a medium with a high dielectric constant (see Appendix 24 where dielectric constants are discussed) which is then able to weaken ionic bonds. An example of an ionic bond is the bond that holds Na^+ and Cl ions together in a NaCl crystal. Methane, for example (CH_4), is held together by covalent bonds. Ionic and covalent bonds are extreme cases; most chemical bonds are a mixture of the two types. These ionic bonds arise from the coulombic attraction that exists between charged particles and, as shown in Appendix 23, these forces depend on the dielectric coefficient of the medium. The larger the dielectric coefficient of the medium the smaller the attraction.

Water, which is a good solvent for electrolytes, has a large dielectric coefficient (around 80).

Ions can also be formed at an interphase between a metal and a salt solution. If, for example, we immerse a solid plate of metal zinc ($Zn_{(s)}$) in a copper sulphate solution a spontaneous reaction occurs where zinc ions are passed into the solution and copper ions ($Cu^{2+}_{(aq)}$) are deposited as solid metal copper ($Cu_{(s)}$) in place of the zinc. The reaction can be described by the chemical equation:

$$Zn_{(s)} + Cu^{2+}_{(aq)} \rightarrow Zn^{2+}_{(aq)} + Cu_{(s)} \tag{2.1}$$

which can be split into two partial reactions

$$Zn_{(s)} \rightarrow Zn^{2+}_{(aq)} + 2e^- \quad \text{(oxidation)} \tag{2.2}$$

$$Cu^{2+}_{(aq)} + 2e^- \rightarrow Cu_{(s)} \quad \text{(reduction)} \tag{2.3}$$

Electron affinity

Chemical equation (2.1) tells us that the affinity of zinc for electrons (e^-) is less than that of copper. We can set up an experiment in which we are able to compare quantitatively the attraction of any two metals for electrons. An example is shown in Figure 2.1. Here the zinc ($Zn_{(s)}$) and the

Fig.2.1

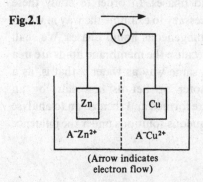

(Arrow indicates
electron flow)

copper ($Cu_{(s)}$) plates are placed in their respective equimolar salt solutions (Figure 2.1). The zinc and the copper plates (called electrodes) and their salt solutions have to be separated by a porous barrier. If it were not for this barrier the zinc electrode would give its electrons directly to the copper ions in the solution and there would not be a net flow of electrons through the wire that connects the two electrodes, and we would be unable to measure a voltage between the two cells. It is necessary for the barrier to be porous so that there is a flow of ions, and thus of current, through the solution. We should emphasize here that in solution current is carried by mobile ions; this is because, unlike metals, solutions do not contain free electrons. At both metal–solution interphases the following reaction takes place

$$M_{(s)} = M^{2+}_{(aq)} + 2e^-$$ (2.4)

When an atom of metal (M) loses two electrons and goes into solution it goes from energy state $M_{(s)}$ into energy state $M^{2+}_{(aq)}$, this is because the energy (W_1) required to remove a metal atom from the metal is different from the energy (W_2) required to remove its ion (M^{2+}) from the solution.

Equilibrium at the electrode/solution interphase

When equilibrium is reached we should be able to relate the number of particles in energy state $M_{(s)}$ (atoms of the metal) to the number of particles in energy state $M^{2+}_{(aq)}$ (ions in solution). This is done by considering the 'concentration' of metal atoms ($[M_{(s)}]$) in the metal. In a pure metal the atoms are bound to each other by sharing electrons. These electrons are responsible for the electrical conductivity of metals and can be thought of as a sea (gas) of electrons that link together the metal atoms. We can think of $[M_{(s)}]$ as the number of atoms per unit volume of metal. However, this definition is not used and later on in this chapter we will describe the convention that is now widely accepted. Through the Boltzmann's factor (see Appendix 21) we can relate the concentration of atoms in state $[M_{(S)}]$ to the concentration of ions $[M^{2+}_{(aq)}]$ by the equation

$$[M^{2+}_{(aq)}]/[M_{(s)}] = \exp(-(W_2 - W_1)/RT)$$ (2.5)

where W_1 and W_2 are the potential energies of a metal atom and the metal ion respectively (see Appendix 33, where the relationship between potential energy and work is discussed).

By taking logarithms we obtain

$$(W_1 - W_2)/RT = \ln([M^{2+}_{(aq)}]/[M_{(s)}])$$ (2.6)

or

$$(W_1 - W_2)/RT = \ln([M^{2+}_{(aq)}]) - \ln([M_{(s)}])$$ (2.7)

As we are taking logarithms the concentration terms in equation (2.7) have to be defined as dimensionless quantities. This is because if $c = b^x$ from the definition of a logarithm $x = \log_b(c)$. Since b is dimensionless (because it is a base) and an exponent is always dimensionless, we can think of c as a dimensionless quantity, that is, the number of concentration units. This number can be obtained by dividing the concentration $[M_{(s)}]$ (or $[M^{2+}_{(aq)}]$) by the corresponding unit concentrations. Rearranging and collecting terms for the metal and the aqueous phases, equation (2.6) becomes

metal aqueous

$$W_1 + RT \ln([M_{(s)}]) = W_2 + RT \ln([M^{2+}_{(aq)}])$$ (2.8)

Equation (2.8) was derived from the Boltzmann factor, which requires that the system be in equilibrium. An electrode/solution system is in equilibrium when no current passes through the electrode. This is when the rate at which the metal goes into the solution as metal ions is equal to the rate of deposition of metal at the electrode.

The chemical potential and the electrochemical potential

Since we are dealing with collected terms and an equilibrium situation, we should be able to write an expression based upon equation (2.8) for two-state equilibrium situations in general. From equation (2.8) the expression which applies to a single compartment can be written as follows

$$\mu = W + RT \ln(c) \qquad (2.9)$$

Since the meaning of the concentration term c is different for different phases (that is, a gas, liquid or solid) we must adopt some convention for the expression of c. Since it is a rule that any two different conventions can be related by multiplying one of the conventions by a constant (a),

$$c' = ac''$$

where c' is one convention and c'' is a different convention. For example, c' may be expressed in grams per litre and c'' in moles per litre. If this were the case a will be the molecular weight of the solute.

Equation (2.9) can be written more generally as

$$\mu = W + RT \ln(ac)$$
$$= W + RT \ln(a) + RT \ln(c) \qquad (2.10)$$

If we define

$$\mu^0 = RT \ln(a) \qquad (2.11)$$

then

$$\mu = \mu^0 + RT \ln(c) + W \qquad (2.12)$$

In expression (2.12), μ^0 is a constant which takes into account the definition of c; that is, if we define c differently equation (2.12) will still be valid but with a different μ^0. The ease with which a metal goes into solution as an ion depends upon its concentration in the solution and the electrical potential that exists between the solution and the metal. This means that in expression (2.12) W represents the work that has to be done against the electrical potential. To express this work term (W) in terms of an electrical potential V we write

$$W = ZFV \qquad (2.13)$$

This relationship comes from the definition of the electrical potential. The electrical potential (in volts) at a point in an electrical field, is the amount of work (i.e. number of joules) required to bring 1 coulomb of charge from outside the electrical field (i.e. zero potential) to that point. Since W is the work in joule/mole, F is the charge in faraday (in coulomb per gr-eq) and Z is the valence (gr-eq $\cdot$ mol^{-1}).

Equation (2.13) is dimensionally correct because

$$\text{joule/mol} = (\text{gr-eq/mol}) \cdot (\text{coul./gr-eq}) \cdot (\text{joule/coul.})$$

From this definition an electrical potential difference can be defined. Thus one volt electrical potential difference between two points in an electrical field exists when a joule of work is required to transfer one coulomb of charge between those two points within the electrical field. Substituting (2.13) in (2.12)

$$\mu = \mu^0 + RT\ln(c) + ZFV \tag{2.14}$$

At unit concentration ($c = 1$) and $V = 0$, then

$$\mu = \mu^0 \tag{2.15}$$

μ is called the electrochemical potential and μ^0 is the standard electrochemical potential. The standard electrochemical potential μ^0 of an ion is its electrochemical potential when the electrical potential is zero and its concentration is 1. We can now substitute equation (2.14) into equation (2.8) and obtain

$$\underbrace{\mu_{(1)}^0 + RT\ln([M_{(s)}]) + ZFV_{(1)}}_{\mu_{M(1)}} = \underbrace{\mu_{(2)}^0 + RT\ln([M_{(aq)}^{2+}]) + ZFV_{(2)}}_{\mu_{M(2)}} \tag{2.16a}$$

where the left side refers to the electrode and the right-hand side to the solution. Equation (2.16a) states that at equilibrium the electrochemical potential of a substance in phase 1, $\mu_{M(1)}$, is equal to the electrochemical potential of the same substance in phase 2, $\mu_{M(2)}$. Thus, at equilibrium,

$$\mu_{M(1)} = \mu_{M(2)} \tag{2.16b}$$

The adopted convention is that the concentration of a pure metal in its natural state is 1, which means that the term

$$RT\ln([M_{(s)}])$$

in equation (2.16a) becomes zero and the equation can now be written as

$$\mu_{(1)}^0 + ZFV_{(1)} = \mu_{(2)}^0 + RT\ln([M_{(aq)}^{2+}]) + ZFV_{(2)} \tag{2.17}$$

Electrode potentials

The electrical potential difference ($V_2 - V_1$) between the two phases can be expressed as

$$V_{(2)} - V_{(1)} = (\mu_{(1)}^0 - \mu_{(2)}^0)/(ZF) - (RT/ZF)\ln([M_{(aq)}^{2+}]) \tag{2.18}$$

If we define

$$E = V_{(2)} - V_{(1)}$$

and
$$E^0 = (\mu_{(1)}^0 - \mu_{(2)}^0)/(ZF)$$
where E^0 is the electrical potential difference between the solution and the electrode when the ion concentration ($[M_{(aq)}^{2+}]$) is one unit, then
$$V_{(2)} - V_{(1)} = E = E^\circ - (RT/ZF)\ln([M_{(aq)}^{2+}]) \qquad (2.19)$$
We can write an equation like (2.19) for each of two electrodes (Cu and Zn). If we substitute 2 for Z we obtain
$$E_{Zn} = (V_{(2)} - V_{(1)})_{Zn} = E_{Zn}^0 - (RT/2F)\ln([Zn_{(aq)}^{2+}]) \qquad (2.20)$$
$$E_{Cu} = (V_{(2)} - V_{(1)})_{Cu} = E_{Cu}^0 - (RT/2F)\ln([Cu_{(aq)}^{2+}]) \qquad (2.21)$$

Junction potentials

In practice if we want to measure the potential difference between the zinc and the copper electrodes dipped in their respective salt solutions, an electrical continuity between the two solutions has to be established but at the same time mixing of the solutions must be prevented. Experimentally this is achieved by separating the solutions by a porous barrier. However, since the ionic concentrations of the two solutions will be, in general, different, ions will migrate across the porous barrier at different speeds until an electrical potential (diffusion potential) E_j reaches a value which prevents a further net charge movement across the barrier. In order to compute the potential difference that exists, for example, between the zinc electrode and the copper electrode equation (2.21) is subtracted from equation (2.20) and a term corresponding to E_j is included. So
$$E_{Zn} - E_{Cu} = (E_{Zn}^0 - E_{Cu}^0) - (RT/2F)\ln([Zn_{(aq)}^{2+}]/[Cu_{(aq)}^{2+}]) + E_j \qquad (2.22)$$
Equation (2.22) tells us that the electrical potential difference between the two electrodes is the sum of three terms. These are the difference between the two standard potentials ($E_{Cu}^0 - E_{Zn}^0$), the electrical potential difference across the porous barrier (E_j) and a term which depends on the concentrations of $[Zn_{(aq)}^{2+}]$ and $[Cu_{(aq)}^{2+}]$.

We can *measure* the potential difference between the electrodes ($E_{Zn} - E_{Cu}$) with a voltmeter. If the compartments are big enough the concentrations of the ions (Zn^{2+} and Cu^{2+}) will be fixed and so be known. But it is not possible to *compute* the absolute values of $Z_{Zn} - E_{Cu}$ since we are unable to measure or compute independently the diffusion potential E_j. This is because in order to measure the electrical potential across the porous barrier we require another electrode to be inserted into the solution. But this electrode would have its own unknown E^0. E_j is known as the junction potential. E_j is in this case the electrical potential difference across the porous barrier. Since the barrier allows the flow of ions across it, in time both solutions will mix completely and there will be no concentration gradients. However, if both compartments are made very large this will take a very long time and E_j will be constant. It is possible to design systems where E_j is very small, for example by replacing the barrier with a concentrated potassium chloride salt bridge. The reason E_j is small in this case is discussed in Appendix 27.

Standard reference

Even if the E_j term can be ignored it is more useful to measure electrode potentials against a common standard reference electrode rather than against one another. The standard reference that is chosen is the hydrogen electrode. It is not possible, of course, to make a 'solid-gas' hydrogen electrode but the same effect is achieved when hydrogen is bubbled over an inert substance such as platinum.

Under these conditions hydrogen gas dissociates according to the electrode equation

$$H_{2(g)} = 2H^+_{(aq)} + 2e^- \tag{2.23}$$

and electrons will flow through the platinum and the connection to the other electrode.

Standard electrode potentials

If we use the hydrogen electrode instead of the copper electrode equation (2.22) becomes

$$E_{Zn} - E_{H_2} = (E^0_{Zn} - E^0_{H_2}) + E_j - (RT/ZF)\ln([Zn^{2+}_{(aq)}]/[H^+_{(aq)}]^2) \tag{2.24}$$

When both $[Zn^{2+}_{(aq)}]$ and $[H^+_{(aq)}]$ are set at unit concentrations equation (2.24) reduces to

$$E_{Zn} - E_{H_2} = (E^0_{Zn} - E^0_{H_2}) + E_j \tag{2.25}$$

If E_j can be made negligible and, by convention, $E^0_{H_2}$ is set to zero, (2.25) then simplifies to

$$E_{Zn} - E_{H_2} = E^0_{Zn} \tag{2.26}$$

The measured potential $(E_{Zn} - E_{H_2})$ under these conditions is called the standard electrode potential (E^0_{Zn}). The adopted convention is that the metal ion (Zn^{2+} in this case) and hydrogen are at a concentration of 1 M (1 mole/litre) and hydrogen gas is bubbling at one atmosphere of pressure (Figure 2.2). Equation (2.24) can thus be written for the case in which the hydrogen electrode is used as the reference electrode ($E_{H_2,ref}$). In the hydrogen electrode $[H^+_{(aq)}] = 1$ M and the partial pressure of H_2 is one atmosphere. So

$$E = E_{Zn} - E_{H_2,ref} = E^0_{Zn} - (RT/ZF)\ln([Zn^{2+}_{(aq)}]) \tag{2.25a}$$

Equation (2.25a) relates the electrode potential E (with reference to a hydrogen electrode) to the concentration of the corresponding ion in solution.

Tables of electrode potentials

In this way we can set up a table of standard electrode potentials (E_{ion}^0) relative to the hydrogen electrode. If electrons flow through the wire from the test electrode to the hydrogen electrode (or vice versa) the sign of the potential is negative (or positive). The size of the potential is a measure of the ease with which the test electrode loses (or gains, for opposite current flow) electrons.

Fig.2.2

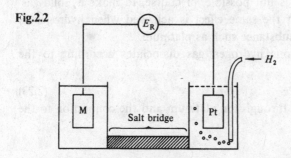

With equation (2.25a) we are now in a position to calculate the potential of an electrode placed in a known solution of one of its salts. This is because E_{ion}^0 can be obtained from tables and we know the concentration of the ion in the solution.

Measurement of biological potentials

If we want to measure a bioelectrical potential that exists between two different compartments (Figure 2.3b) it is unfortunately necessary to consider these electrode potentials (E_{Zn} in Figure 2.3a) in addition to the bioelectrical potential we wish to measure (V_m).

Electrophysiologists attempt to minimize the complication due to these electrode potentials by making their bioelectrical measurements with two matched electrodes, so that the electrode potentials cancel each other out (Figure 2.3c). However, there are two further problems associated with the measurement of bioelectric potentials in solution and these are demonstrated in Figure 2.3c and d. One is that in order to have electrical continuity with the solutions the electrodes (zinc metal/ion solution) themselves must make contact with the solutions in the two compartments. But as soon as contact is made, zinc ions will start to diffuse away from the electrode (Figure 2.3c) with the result that the zinc concentration $[Zn_{(aq)}^{2+}]$

around the electrode becomes undefined (see equation (2.25), $[Zn^{2+}_{(aq)}]$-dependent term). This causes the two-electrode system to become unbalanced and the electrode potentials now no longer cancel one another.

The second problem is that the potential difference between the two

Fig.2.3

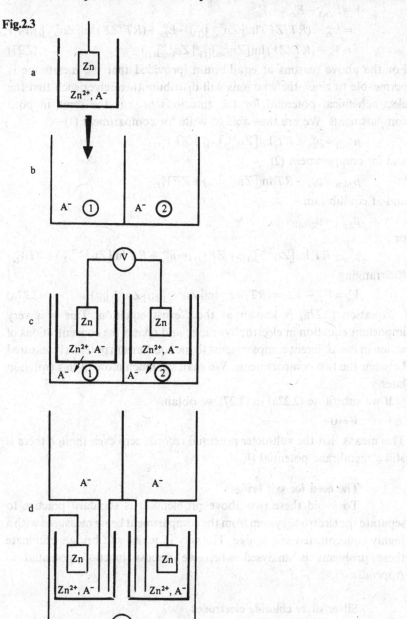

electrodes (measured by the voltmeter) is the sum of the bioelectrical potential (V_m) and the difference of the zinc electrochemical potentials in the two compartments $(E_{Zn,1} - E_{Zn,2})$. Thus in Figure 2.3c the measured potential difference (V) is given by

$$V = E_{Zn,1} - E_{Zn,2} + V_m$$
$$= E_{Zn}^0 - (RT/ZF)\ln([Zn_{(aq)}^{2+}]_{(1)}) - E_{Zn}^0 + (RT/ZF)\ln([Zn_{(aq)}^{2+}]_{(2)}) + V_m$$
$$= V_m - (RT/ZF)\ln([Zn_{(aq)}^{2+}]_{(1)}/[Zn_{(aq)}^{2+}]_{(2)}) \tag{2.27}$$

For the above reasons at equilibrium (provided that the membrane is permeable to zinc), the zinc ions will distribute themselves such that the electrochemical potential for the zinc ions (μ_{Zn}) is the same in both compartments. We are thus able to write for compartment (1)

$$\mu_{Zn(1)} = \mu_{Zn}^0 + RT\ln([Zn_{(aq)}^{2+}]_{(1)}) + ZFV_{(1)}$$

and for compartment (2)

$$\mu_{Zn(2)} = \mu_{Zn}^0 + RT\ln([Zn_{(aq)}^{2+}]_{(2)}) + ZFV_{(2)}$$

and at equilibrium

$$\mu_{Zn(1)} = \mu_{Zn(2)}$$

or

$$\mu_{Zn}^0 + RT\ln([Zn^{2+}]_{(1)}) + ZFV_{(1)} = \mu_{Zn}^0 + RT\ln([Zn^{2+}]_{(2)}) + ZFV_{(2)}$$

Rearranging

$$V_m = V_{(2)} - V_{(1)} = (RT/ZF)\ln([Zn^{2+}]_{(2)}/[Zn^{2+}]_{(1)}) \tag{2.27a}$$

Equation (2.27a) is known as the Nernst equation. This is a very important equation in electrophysiology and relates the concentrations of an ion in two different compartments to the equilibrium potential measured between the two compartments. We shall see much more of this equation later.

If we substitute (2.27a) in (2.27) we obtain

$$V = 0$$

This means that the voltmeter potential records zero even though there is still a membrane potential (V_m)!

The need for salt bridges

To avoid these two above problems it is standard practice to separate the electrode system from the compartment being measured with a highly concentrated salt bridge. The way in which salt bridges eliminate these problems is analysed when we discuss junction potential in Appendix 27.

Silver/silver chloride electrodes

In practice, electrophysiologists choose silver rather than zinc electrodes because silver electrodes are reasonably inert, non-toxic and very stable. The silver electrode is known as a silver/silver chloride electrode (Ag/AgCl). This is because the solubility of AgCl is very low and as soon as Ag^+ goes into solution it combines with Cl^- and is deposited as AgCl. The reactions that take place at the electrode/solution interphase are as follows:

$$Ag_{(s)} \rightleftharpoons Ag^+_{(aq)} + e^- \qquad (2.28)$$

$$Cl^-_{(aq)} + Ag^+_{(aq)} \rightleftharpoons AgCl_{(s)} \qquad (2.29)$$

The overall chemical reaction can be obtained if these two equations are summed

$$Cl^-_{(aq)} + Ag^+_{(aq)} + Ag_{(s)} \rightleftharpoons Ag^+_{(aq)} + AgCl_{(s)} + e^- \qquad (2.30)$$

to obtain

$$Cl^-_{(aq)} + Ag_{(s)} \rightleftharpoons AgCl_{(s)} + e^- \qquad (2.31)$$

One of the advantages of this Ag/AgCl electrode is that it is a reversible electrode. That is, in a system like the one shown in Figure 2.3d (in which $Ag_{(s)}$ replaces $Zn_{(s)}$) current can be passed through the electrodes in either direction. The reversibility of the Ag/AgCl electrode can be seen if equation (2.31) is examined in detail. If electrons leave the electrode through the external circuit AgCl is deposited (right-hand side of equation (2.31)). If electrons enter the electrode, silver metal is deposited (left-hand side of equation (2.31)). The Ag/AgCl electrode can thus be used either to measure potentials in biological compartments or to inject current of either polarity into these compartments. In both of these applications there will be an electrical potential difference between the electrode and the solution (E from the equation (2.25)) due to the electrochemical potential gradient at the metal–metal–ion solution interphase. We also saw (equations (2.26) and (2.27)) that an electrical potential (V_m) could produce a concentration gradient of ions $[Zn^{2+}]$ in the case of equations (2.26) and (2.27). So obviously a concentration gradient across a permeable barrier must be able to produce an electrical potential difference.

Diffusion potentials across a barrier

In the same way as we obtained equation (2.16) the electrochemical potential also allows us to calculate the electrical potential difference that results from a concentration gradient across a barrier and between two solutions. It is important that the barrier is permeable to only one ion species. Because if the barrier is permeable to more than one ion species, the concentration gradient will run down since there will be a net flow of salt (positive and negative ions) in order to preserve electroneutrality in the solutions. The rate at which the gradient is dissipated depends upon how permeable the membrane is to the ion species and the relative ionic concentrations. In order to understand the genesis of this potential we can imagine that at time zero ($t = 0$; see Figure 2.4a), when the system was first set up, both solutions were electroneutral. That is, the number of positive ions is equal to the number of negative ions in each compartment.

Because the concentration of ion A^- is greater on side 2, there will be a net flow of negative ions from this compartment. This continues until the electrical potential generated across the barrier is sufficiently large so as to stop the flow. The potential generated is the result of a separation of charge across the barrier (see Figure 2.4b and c). At equilibrium ($t \rightarrow \infty$) there has been a net loss of negative charge from compartment (2) which results in an excess of positive charge.

In side 1 there is now a net excess of negative charge (see Figure 2.4c: this figure shows the net charge as a function of x and time $t \rightarrow \infty$, that is, at a steady state). We can calculate the concentration profiles of charge separation on both sides of the membrane by Poisson's equation (see Appendix 22).

The Poisson equation predicts that at a certain distance (λ) from both

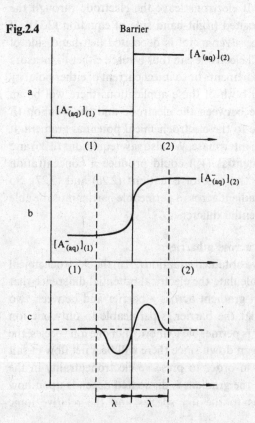

Fig.2.4

sides of the membrane electroneutrality applies again (Figure 2.4c). The size of λ depends on many factors which might be, for example, the concentration of the ions around the membrane, the dielectric constant and viscosity of the solvent, the degree of stirring of the solutions on either side of the membrane. But since our main interest is in the genesis of the potential across the barrier we will concern ourselves only with the relationship that exists between the two compartmental concentrations of A^- and the potential difference that can be measured between them. At equilibrium the electrochemical potential (equation (2.16a, b)) of A^- is the same in compartments 1 and 2, so, equating the electrochemical potentials, we write that

$$\mu_{A^-(1)} = \mu_{A^-(2)} \quad \text{(from 2.16b)} \tag{2.32}$$

where

$$\mu_{A^-(1)} = \mu^0_{A(1)} + RT \ln([A^-_{(aq)}]_{(1)}) + ZFV_{(1)}$$

and $\tag{2.33}$

$$\mu_{A^-(2)} = \mu^0_{A(2)} + RT \ln([A^-_{(aq)}]_{(2)}) + ZFV_{(2)}$$

The Nernst equation

$\mu^0_{A(1)}$ may be different from $\mu^0_{A(2)}$ if the concentrations of $[A^-_{(aq)}]_{(1)}$ and $[A^-_{(aq)}]_{(2)}$ are very different but that is not usually the case in biological systems. If a strong electrolytic solution is very concentrated, ions tend to interact with each other because they feel each other's respective field. These effects should be taken into account when writing equations (2.33). When this is done we use activities instead of concentrations (see page 29 for a discussion of activities). It is usually assumed that the standard potentials ($\mu^0_{A(1)}$ and $\mu^0_{A(2)}$) are the same because the solutions are made up in the same solvent (water) and are dilute. If we substitute equations (2.33) in equation (2.32) we obtain

$$\mu^0_{A(1)} + RT \ln([A^-_{(aq)}]_{(1)}) + ZFV_{(1)} = \mu^0_{A(2)} + RT \ln([A^-_{(aq)}]_{(2)}) + ZFV_{(2)}$$
$$\tag{2.34}$$

In order to obtain the electrical potential difference $(E_1 - E_2)$ across the barrier, we rearrange (2.34) to obtain

$$E_A = V_{(1)} - V_{(2)} = (RT/ZF) \ln([A^-_{(aq)}]_{(2)}/[A^-_{(aq)}]_{(1)}) \tag{2.35}$$

E_A obtained from equation (2.35) is the equilibrium potential or the potential of ion A^- across the barrier. This equation, which was first derived by Nernst, is one of the cornerstones of electrophysiology and, as we shall show later (Chapters 6–8), is used extensively to calculate membrane potentials from ionic concentration gradients in order to describe the movements of ions across membranes.

So far we have analysed ion formation and the events that take place at a metal–metal ion interphase and at a permeable barrier that separates two different ionic concentrations. Both systems were examined in their equilibrium state but, although there are some quasi-equilibrium situations in biology that can be treated as if they were in equilibrium, most biological systems are not in equilibrium (strictly speaking, these electrode potentials are not true electrode potentials as a current always flows through them and so the system is not at equilibrium). A good example of a non-equilibrium system is when a net movement of ions, or of molecules, takes place between two biological compartments or alternatively within one compartment. The second part of this chapter will deal with this non-equilibrium movement of ions in an aqueous solution.

The passage of an electrical current through a solution involves a movement of ions. One way in which this ion movement can easily be studied is to inject an external current into an electrolyte solution by means of electrodes. One apparatus which uses this technique is shown in Figure 2.5. The two metal electrodes (M) pass a current I (measured at A) through the solution and this current is driven by a variable source of potential (battery, Figure 2.5). The potentials that we discussed above that occur at the interphase of the metal electrodes and the solution are ignored as the electrodes are used only to inject current. Two more identical electrodes are placed in the solution l cm apart and both are connected to a voltmeter. As both these electrodes are dipped in the same solution their electrode potentials are equal and so cancel one another. Furthermore, because they are in series with a voltmeter (which has a high internal resistance), the injected current that flows into them is very small and so can be neglected. This means that the electrodes are almost at equilibrium and, as there are no concentration gradients, the electrode potentials will be stable.

I/V curve of a slab of solution

The voltage measured across these two electrodes is the potential difference that occurs across a volume of solution of length l and cross-sectional area A. This potential difference can be set at different values by passing different amounts of current through the system. Figure 2.5b shows a typical current/voltage relationship (I/V curve) obtained, and we see that it is linear. If the voltage is very large this linear relationship will break down. This non-linearity can arise from a number of different causes; for example, electrode polarization – that is, when there is a breakdown of equilibrium conditions in the electrolyte/electrode interphase. However, we will concern ourselves only with the linear part of the curve.

Fig.2.5

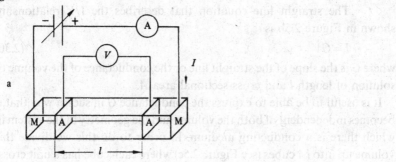

a

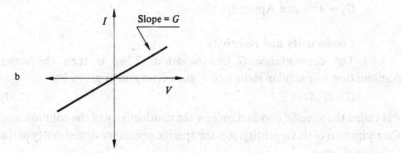

b

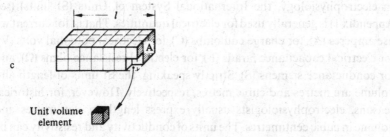

c

Unit volume
element

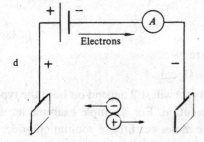

d

Electrons

Conductance of a solution

The straight line equation that describes the I/V relationship shown in Figure 2.5b is

$$I = GV \tag{2.36}$$

where G is the slope of the straight line or the conductance of the volume of solution of length l and cross-sectional area A.

It is useful to be able to express the conductance G in such a way that it becomes independent of both the volume and the geometry of the system in which there is a conducting medium. In order to do this we divide this volume up into lA cubes (see Figure 2.5c) where each cube has a unit cross-sectional area, a unit length and a conductance k. The conductance G_A of a slab (that is, the shaded slab in Figure 2.5c) of cross-sectional area A is

$$G_A = Ak \quad \text{(see Appendix 15)}$$

Conductivity and resistivity

The conductance G (see equation (2.36)) is then the series combination of l similar slabs (see Figure 2.5c) and is given by

$$G = G_A/l = kA/l \tag{2.37}$$

k is called the specific conductance or the conductivity of the solution and the reciprocal of this quantity, ρ, is the specific resistance or resistivity of the solution. That is,

$$\rho = 1/k \tag{2.37a}$$

In electrophysiology, the International System of Units (SI units) (see Appendix 1) is generally used for electrical quantities. That is, for current we use amperes (A), for charge coulombs (C), for electrical potential volts (V), for electrical capacitance farads (F), for electrical resistance ohms (Ω), and for conductance siemens (S). Strictly speaking, the SI units of length and volume are metres and cubic metres, respectively. However, for historical reasons, electrophysiologists usually express length in centimetres and volume in cubic centimetres. The units of conductivity and resistivity can be derived from equations (2.36) and (2.37). If we rearrange (2.37) we obtain

$$k = Gl/A \tag{2.38}$$

dimensionally

$$k = S \cdot cm/cm^2 = S \cdot cm^{-1} \tag{2.38a}$$

From (2.38a) the dimensions of ρ are

$$\rho = 1/(S \cdot cm^{-1}) = (1/S) \cdot cm = \Omega \cdot cm$$

The conductivity (k) or the resistivity (ρ) will still depend on both the type and concentration of the ions in solution. For a simple example let us consider an electrolyte solution of c moles per litre of sodium chloride.

Molar conductances: the effect of concentration on conductance

The conductivity of a solution containing a concentration (c) of salt depends upon the number of ions per unit volume and also on the ability of the ions to move (mobility). The ability of the ions to move is itself dependent on concentration, since the more ions there are per unit volume the larger the interaction between the ions and so the mobility is lower. By dividing the conductivity of a solution by its concentration we define a quantity (Λ) which is independent of the number of ions in the solution. This leaves us free to analyse the effect of mobility on conductance. If we do this we obtain the molar conductance (Λ)

$$\Lambda = k/c \qquad (2.39)$$

The dimensions of molar conductance are

$$\Lambda = (S \cdot cm^{-1})/(mol \cdot litre^{-1}) = S \cdot cm^{-1} \cdot litre \cdot mol^{-1}$$

To express concentration in terms of $mol \cdot cm^{-3}$ we multiply the above equation by 10^3 cm^3 and divide it by a litre (10^3 cm^3), so that we obtain the units of

$$\Lambda = (S \cdot cm^{-1} \cdot litre/mol) \cdot (10^3 \ cm^3/litre) = 10^3 \ S \cdot cm^2 \cdot mol^{-1}$$

Concentration dependence of molar conductance

Although for any one electrolyte Λ ought to be independent of c, in practice different values of Λ are obtained at different concentrations. This concentration dependence is shown in Figure 2.6 and means that the molar conductance is not a useful quantity for comparing the conductance of different electrolytes. If the curve in Figure 2.6a is extrapolated back to zero concentration (that is, infinite dilution) we obtain the theoretical conductivity at infinite dilution (known as Λ_0) which, by definition, is a conductivity that is independent of c. Thus Λ_0 can be used to compare different electrolyte conductivities. If a weak electrolyte is used instead of a strong electrolyte a curve similar to that shown in Figure 2.6b is obtained.

Fig.2.6

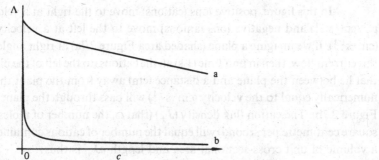

Compared with a, curve b is shifted down the axis and as the concentration is reduced increases more rapidly at low concentrations. The two curves are different and emphasize that the concentration dependence of the conductivity is markedly different for strong and weak electrolytes. For weak electrolytes (such as acetic acid), at high concentrations most of the electrolyte will be in the associated form.

Thus the chemical equilibrium

$$CH_3COOH \rightleftharpoons CH_3COO^- + H^+ \tag{2.40}$$

is driven to the left. In dilute solutions the reaction is driven to the right, which means that dissociation increases so that the number of ions in solution will increase. Since the number of ions becomes larger, a larger fraction of the dissolved acid is now available for carrying current and so the conductivity increases. This explanation will not apply to strong electrolytes because they are completely dissociated at any dilution.

Concentration dependence of molar conductances of strong electrolytes

In order to understand why the molar conductivity of strong electrolytes increases with dilution we need to analyse the way in which current is carried by each of the ions in a solution. Figure 2.7 shows a dissociated electrolyte sitting in solution between two plate electrodes that are connected to a battery. The electrode connected to the positive terminal of the battery is called the *anode* and the electrode connected to the negative terminal is called the *cathode*. In the solution, negative ions move towards the anode and are known as *anions*, while positive ions move towards the cathode and are known as *cations*. The current through the solution, which is equal to the current (electron-flow) through the external circuit, is due to the flow of both positive and negative ions in the directions indicated in Figure 2.7a.

Ion flux densities and ion velocities

In this figure, positive ions (cations) move to the right at a velocity v_+ (cm·s^{-1}) and negative ions (anions) move to the left at a velocity v_- (cm·s^{-1}). If we imagine a plane (shaded area Figure 2.7a) at right angles to this current flow, then in unit time (1 s) all the cations (to the left of the plane) that lie between the plane and a distance (cm) away from the plant that is numerically equal to the velocity (cm·s^{-1}) will pass through the plane (see Figure 2.7b). The cation flux density ($\bar{J}_+$) (that is, the number of moles per square centimetre per second) will equal the number of cations contained in a volume of unit cross-sectional area and length $v\bar{J}_+$ is thus:

$$\bar{J}_+ = v_+ c \tag{2.41}$$

Since each mole of positive ions carried Z faradays of charge (where Z is the valence of the ions and one faraday is equal to 96 458 coulombs·gr-eq^{-1}), the flux of positive ions is equivalent to a current density ($\bar{I}_+$) of

$$\bar{J}_+ Z^+ F = \bar{I}_+ = Z^+ F v_+ c \tag{2.42}$$

Fig.2.7

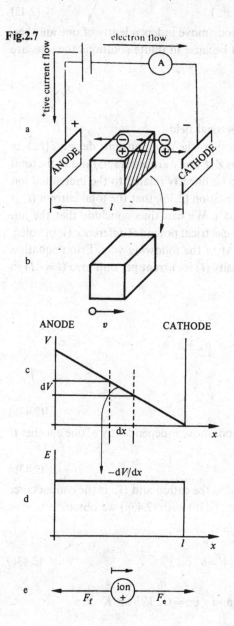

Dimensionally the current density is $amp \cdot cm^{-2}$. Equation (2.42) does have the correct dimensions, as:

$$\bar{I}_+ = \bar{J}_+ Z^+ F = (mol \cdot cm^{-2} \cdot s^{-1})(gr\text{-}eq \cdot mol^{-1})(coul \cdot gr\text{-}eq^{-1})$$
$$= coul \cdot cm^{-2} \cdot s^{-1} = amp \cdot cm^{-2}$$

The total current density through the solution $(\bar{I})$ is

$$\bar{I}_- + \bar{I}_+ = Fc(Z^+ v_+ + Z^- v_-) \tag{2.43}$$

This equation assumes that the ions move independently of one another. This is a reasonable assumption because in dilute solutions the ions are dissociated and widely spaced.

Ion velocities and the electrical field

Equation (2.42) shows that the ion current density $(\bar{I}_+)$ is proportional to the ion velocity (as Z, F and c are constants) and so the total current density $(\bar{I})$ (2.43) will also be linearly related to the individual ion velocities. We also know, from equation (2.36), that the total current (I) is linearly related to voltage $(I = GV)$. We can thus conclude that the ion velocities are proportional to the electrical potential difference (V in volts). This conclusion can be arrived at in the following way. From equation (2.36) $I = GV$, but the current density $(\bar{I})$ is current per unit area $(I = A\bar{I})$ so $A\bar{I} = GV$, or

$$\bar{I} = (G/A)V = \bar{G}V$$

From equation (2.43)

$$\bar{I} = FcZ^+ v_+ + FcZ^- v_- = b_+ v_+ + b_- v_-$$

where

$$b_{\pm} = FcZ^{\pm}$$

so

$$\bar{G}V = b_+ v_+ + b_- v_- \tag{2.43a}$$

Since we have assumed that the ions move independently of one another $\bar{G}$ is the sum of two conductances

$$\bar{G} = \bar{G}_+ + \bar{G}_- \tag{2.43b}$$

where $\bar{G}_+$ is the conductance due to the cation and $\bar{G}_-$ is the conductance due to the anion. If we compare (2.43b) with (2.43a) we obtain

$$\bar{G}_+ V + \bar{G}_- V = b_+ v_+ + b_- v_-$$

or

$$\bar{G}_+ V = b_+ v_+ \quad \text{and} \quad \bar{G}_- V = b_- v_- \tag{2.43c}$$

If we rearrange (2.43c)

$$v_+ = \bar{G}_+ V / b_+ = K_+ V \quad \text{and} \quad v_- = \bar{G}_- V / b_- = K_- V$$

Electrical potential gradient

In order to understand equation (2.43) we must remember that the ions move because they are subject to a force which is due to the electrical field that exists between the two electrodes. This field $(\bar{E})$ is shown in Figure 2.7d and is the gradient (Appendix 23) of the electrical potential that exists between the two electrodes. If the ions were in a vacuum, the field $(\bar{E})$ would subject them to a continuous acceleration. But, as they are surrounded by water molecules, collisions between the ions and the water molecules occur, so that the ions lose part of their kinetic energy, their speed is reduced and their velocity reaches a steady value.

Balance between electrical and frictional forces

In this steady state, that is, when the ion velocity is constant, the force per unit charge due to the electrical field $(\bar{E}$, see Appendix 23) is exactly opposed by the frictional force per unit charge (F_q) due to the collisions that occur between the ions and the water molecules. An individual ion has a charge q given by the equation

$$q = ZF/N_A \tag{2.44}$$

where N_A is the Avogadro's number. The ion is subject to an electrical force (F_e) given by the equation

$$F_e = \bar{E}q \tag{2.44a}$$

where $\bar{E}$ (volt $\cdot$ cm^{-1}) is the electrical field strength. The frictional force is proportional to the velocity and opposite in direction (see Figure 2.7e), thus

$$F_f = -f_q v \tag{2.45}$$

where f_q is the frictional coefficient. At constant velocity, force F_e is exactly balanced by the frictional force F_f, so that

$$F_e + F_f = 0 \quad \text{or} \quad F_e = -F_f$$

If we substitute the value of F_e we obtain

$$\bar{E}_q = -F_f = f_q v$$

Dividing both sides of the equation by q

$$\bar{E} = -F_f/q = f_q v/q = f_q' v \tag{2.45a}$$

Ion mobilities

To compute v we rearrange equation (2.45a) and obtain

$$v = \bar{E}/f_q' \tag{2.46}$$

where $(u = 1/f_q')$ is the ion mobility. Equation (2.46) can be written for both ions as

$$v_+ = u_+ \bar{E} \quad \text{and} \quad v_- = u_- \bar{E} \tag{2.47}$$

The current density $\bar{I}$ is obtained if (2.47) and (2.44) are substituted in (2.43)

$$\bar{I} = Fc(Z^+u_+ + Z^-u_-)\bar{E} \tag{2.48}$$

Since $\bar{E}$ (see Appendices 23, 24) is the local gradient of the electrical potential (see Figure 2.7c and d)

$$\bar{E} = -dV/dx \tag{2.49}$$

Then

$$\bar{I} = -Fc(Z^+u_+ + Z^-u_-)(dV/dx) \tag{2.50}$$

Relationship between the flux density and the local potential gradient: the driving force

Equation (2.50) can be rearranged as follows

$$\bar{I} = -Z^+Fcu_+(dV/dx) - Z^+Fcu_-(dV/dx)$$

and then the two terms on the right-hand side of this equation correspond to the flow of positive and negative ions. Thus

$$\bar{I}_+ = -Z^+Fcu_+(dV/dx) \quad \text{and} \quad \bar{I}_- = -Z^+Fcu_-(dV/dx)$$

since

$$dV/dx \equiv (\text{joule} \cdot \text{coul}^{-1} \cdot \text{m}^{-1}) = (\text{newton} \cdot \text{m} \cdot \text{coul}^{-1} \cdot \text{m}^{-1})$$

$$= (\text{newton/coul}) \equiv \text{force/charge}$$

both equations are of the general form

Flux density of charge = conc. of charge · mobility · force/charge

The *force* in the above equation is generally known as the *driving force*. We shall be using this equation in Chapter 3.

Equation (2.50) relates the current density to a point (x) between the two electrodes to the local potential gradient (dV/dx) at that point. At steady state (when v is constant) the $\bar{I}$ is the same at any point between the two electrodes. The potential gradient will also be constant (see Figure 2.7c and d), which means that the potential profile is a straight line. The local potential gradient can thus be computed from the relationship

$$dV/dx = -V/l \tag{2.51}$$

where l is the length of the volume of solution and

$$V = V_{\text{anode}} - V_{\text{cathode}}$$

Relationship between ion mobilities and ion conductances

If we substitute (2.51) in (2.50) we obtain

$$\bar{I} = Fc(Z^+u_+ + Z^-u_-)V/l \tag{2.52}$$

or

$$\bar{I} = (c/l)F(Z^+u_+ + Z^-u_-)V$$
$$= \bar{G}V \tag{2.53}$$

where

$$\bar{G} = (c/l)F(Z^+u_+ + Z^-u_-) \quad \text{(in } S \cdot cm^{-2}) \tag{2.54}$$

By definition (compare equation (2.53) with equation (2.36)) $\bar{G}$ is the conductance per unit area of the electrolyte solution. In order to compute the molar conductance we have to reduce $\bar{G}$ to cm per unit length and divide it by the concentration c. Equation (2.54) becomes

$$\Lambda = F(Z^+u_+ + Z^-u_-)$$
$$= \Lambda_+ + \Lambda_- \tag{2.55}$$

where Λ_+ and Λ_- are the conductances due to the cation and the anion respectively and are defined by the equations

$$\Lambda_+ = FZ^+u_+ \quad \text{and} \quad \Lambda_- = FZ^-u_- \tag{2.56}$$

The units of $\Lambda_\pm$ can be derived from equation (2.54). If we substitute equations (2.56) into (2.54) we obtain

$$\bar{G} = (c/l)(\Lambda_+ + \Lambda_-) \tag{2.56a}$$

At infinite dilution (see Figure 2.5)

$$\Lambda_0 = \Lambda_{0+} + \Lambda_{0-} \tag{2.57}$$

Equation (2.57) is known as the *Law of independent migration of ions* and was formulated by Kohlrausch. From (2.56a)

$$\Lambda_+ + \Lambda_- = \bar{G}l/c = S \cdot cm^{-2} \cdot cm \cdot mol^{-1} \cdot litre$$
$$= S \cdot cm^{-1} \cdot mol^{-1} \cdot litre$$

For continuity of the concentration units we reduce litres to cm^3 by multiplying by

$$10^3 \, cm^3 \cdot litre^{-1}$$

so

$$\Lambda_+ + \Lambda_- = S \cdot cm^{-1} \cdot mol^{-1} \cdot litre \cdot cm^3 \cdot litre^{-1} \cdot 10^3$$
$$= S \cdot cm^2 \cdot mol^{-1} \cdot 10^3$$

The units of mobility ($u_\pm$) can be obtained from equation (2.56). If we arrange this equation in order to find u we obtain

$$u_\pm = \Lambda_\pm/FZ^\pm = (S \cdot cm^2 \cdot mol^{-1})/(coul \cdot gr\text{-}eq^{-1} \cdot gr\text{-}eq \cdot mol^{-1})$$

But

$$S = amp \cdot vol^{-1} = coul \cdot s^{-1} \cdot volt^{-1}$$

so

$$u_\pm = cm^2 \cdot V^{-1} \cdot s^{-1}$$

Since F and Z are constant, the different values of Λ_+ and Λ_- will be due to the effects of dilution on the ionic mobilities (u_+ and u_-). The different values of Λ_0 for ions of the same valence are due to different ionic mobilities at infinite dilution.

The measurement of ionic conductances

In practice, $\Lambda_{0\pm}$ or $u_{0\pm}$ cannot be measured because it is not possible to monitor separately the movement of cations *or* anions. However, the fraction of the current which is carried by either the cations or anions can be computed by measuring the amount of ions accumulated or discharged at each electrode. Since the current in solution is carried only by ions it follows from equations (2.43) and (2.57) that the cationic fraction of the current is

$$\bar{I}_+/\bar{I}=\Lambda_+/\Lambda \qquad\qquad (2.58)$$

and the anionic fraction of the current is

$$\bar{I}_-/\bar{I}=\Lambda_-/\Lambda \qquad\qquad (2.58a)$$

Transfer or transport numbers

The ratios defined by equation (2.58) are usually called the transfer or transport numbers (t_+, t_-). Thus

$$t_+ =\bar{I}_+/I=\Lambda_+/\Lambda \quad \text{and} \quad t_- =\bar{I}_-/\bar{I}=\Lambda_-/\Lambda \qquad (2.59)$$

From equation (2.59) we can see that transfer numbers are dimensionless and have values between 0 and 1.

Also from equation (2.58)

$$\Lambda_+/\Lambda+\Lambda_-/\Lambda=t_+ +t_- =1 \qquad\qquad (2.60)$$

Once we know the transport numbers $(t_+$ and $t_-)$ and the equivalent conductance of the solution (Λ), the ion conductances $(\Lambda_+$ and $\Lambda_-)$ can be computed from equation (2.60). If this equation is rearranged we obtain

$$\Lambda_+ =\Lambda t_+ \quad \text{and} \quad \Lambda_- =\Lambda t_- \qquad\qquad (2.61)$$

If t_+ and t_- and Λ are measured at a variety of concentrations we can use an extrapolation method similar to that used in Figure 2.5 to obtain t_{0+} and t_{0-} from the equations

$$\Lambda_{0+} =\Lambda_0 t_+ \quad \text{and} \quad \Lambda_{0-} =\Lambda_0 t_-$$

Tabulated conductivity data are normally given in terms of

$$\Lambda_{0+} \quad \text{and} \quad \Lambda_{0-}$$

Concentration dependence of ion mobilities

It is possible to quantify the effect of dilution of ion mobilities so that mobilities can be related to ion concentrations.

Equation (2.61) relates the measured quantities Λ, t_+ and t_- to Λ_+ and Λ_-, so that Λ_+ and Λ_- can be used to compute u_+ and u_- from equation (2.56).

As pointed out above, ionic mobilities are related to the number of collisions that occur between the moving ions and the surrounding particles. In dilute solutions the ions will interact only with the solvent molecules because the ions are now so far apart.

As the ion concentration increases, the distances between ions become smaller and so ion interaction increases. This ion interaction can be thought of as an electrostatic interaction that occurs between oppositely charged ions. In the original theory of Debye and Huckel a positive ion was assumed to be surrounded by a cloud of negatively charged ions. (Similarly, negative ions were surrounded by positive ions.) This cloud has two effects: first when a positive (or negative) ion moves, the surrounding cloud will act as a 'drag' and slow down ion movement. The second effect is that the cloud will change the electrochemical potential of the ion so that extra work will be required to remove an ion from or add an ion to the solution. This effect is in addition to the concentration-dependent energy term of the electro-chemical potential equation that was derived on page 9 (equation (2.14)).

The activity coefficient

To take into account this extra work an additional term (j') can be introduced into equation (2.14) to obtain

$$\mu = \mu^0 + RT \ln(c) + ZFV + j' \tag{2.62}$$

j' is conventionally defined as

$$j' = RT \ln(j) \tag{2.63}$$

Equation (2.63) then can be rewritten as

$$\mu = \mu^0 + RT \ln(c) + ZFV + RT \ln(j)$$

so

$$\mu = \mu^0 + RT \ln(cj) + ZFV \tag{2.64}$$

The activity of an ion

j' (and thus j) will be different for different concentrations because the higher the ion concentration the greater the energy required to remove or add an ion to the solution. j is called the activity coefficient and the product jc is known as the activity (a) of the ion. So

$$a = jc$$

Equation (2.64) is more usually written as

$$\mu = \mu^0 + RT \ln(a) + ZFV \tag{2.65}$$

At high dilutions the cloud effect vanishes so $j' = 0$ or $j = 1$ and a becomes equal to the concentration.

The measurement of ion activities

Although it is theoretically possible to calculate j, or a for a number of different ions and solvents, in practice we make use of tabulated values if the activity coefficients are required (see Chapter 5). The tabulated values of these activity coefficients have been obtained from either conductivity measurements or from EMF measurements. EMF measurements have become the standard way of measuring activities (*jc*) in biological compartments.

From equation (2.14) the potential (*E*) of a metal electrode, dipped into a solution that contains the metal ion and related to a standard hydrogen electrode, is

$$V = E^0 - (RT/ZF)\ln([M_{(aq)}^+]) \qquad (2.66)$$

Although in this equation the concentration of ion $[M_{(aq)}^+]$ is used to take into account ionic interactions discussed above, strictly the equation should be written as

$$E = E^0 - (RT/ZF)\ln[a_{M_{(aq)}^+}]$$

where a_{M^+} given by the equation

$$[a_{M_{(aq)}^+}] = j_{M^+}[M_{(aq)}^+]$$

is the activity coefficient. Thus, by measuring *E* (see Figure 2.8) and by using the appropriate value of E_0 we can compute $[a_{M^+}]$.

Fig.2.8

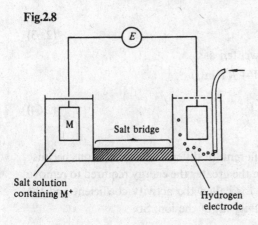

Salt solution
containing M⁺

Salt bridge

Hydrogen
electrode

from neutral molecules where $Z = 0$), can be used to describe the movements of ions under both concentrations and electrical gradients.

The relationship between the diffusion coefficient and the ionic (molar) conductance

The values of D for a large number of molecules and ions are tabulated in a number of reference books (the *Handbook of Chemistry and Physics*, for example) for standard conditions. Since the mobility u' discussed in Chapter 2 depends on concentration, so the u' will also depend on concentration and thus D. From equation (3.12) it can be seen that D depends on temperature. In order to estimate the effects of concentration and temperature on D (for ions), we can use the following relationship that was first derived by Nernst. This equation is derived as follows. From equations (3.12) and (3.8)

$$D_i = u_i'RT = u_iRT/(|Z|F)$$

But from equation (2.56)

$$\Lambda = FZu_i$$
$$= Fu_i \quad \text{where } Z = 1$$

so

$$u_i = \Lambda_i/F \tag{3.14}$$

and

$$D_i = \Lambda_i RT/|Z|F^2$$

the absolute value of Z ($|Z|$) is taken so that D_i does not become negative where Λ_i is the molar conductance of an ion i (see Chapter 2). Molar conductances can be obtained from tables (see Chapter 2), and Z is known, so D_i can be calculated.

Diffusion across a slab: transient conditions

We saw earlier that Fick's First Law of diffusion (equation (3.2)) related the flux density of a neutral solute to its concentration gradient in a solution. This law can also be used to describe the flux density ($\bar{J}$) of a neutral solute across a permeable barrier that separates two solutions at different concentrations (c_1 and c_2, see Figure 3.2). The barrier does not allow the two solutions to intermix but does allow solute and solvent exchange between the two compartments. This barrier might be, for example, filter paper which does not discriminate between solute and solvent but does prevent mixing by convection. The concentration profile inside the filter paper barrier is shown in Figure 3.2b and c. Figure 3.2c shows two different concentration profiles inside the barrier for the same overall concentration difference ($c_1 - c_2$). In curve (2) the profile is a straight line and the local gradient is thus constant. In curve (1) the profile is curved and so the local gradient is different at every point in the membrane. Fick's First Law ($\bar{J} = -D(\mathrm{d}c/\mathrm{d}x)$) describes the local flux densities ($\bar{J}$) for the two curves. In curve (1) the flux density ($\bar{J}$) changes from point to point and since the local concentration gradient ($\mathrm{d}c/\mathrm{d}x$) decreases with x, so does the flux density.

This decrease of the flux density with distance means that an accumulation (or depletion) of solute is taking place at every point so that curve (1) describes a transient (non-steady-state) situation. It is as if the filter paper only recently became permeable to the solute, while previously it had acted as an impermeable barrier separating the two solutions.

Fig.3.2

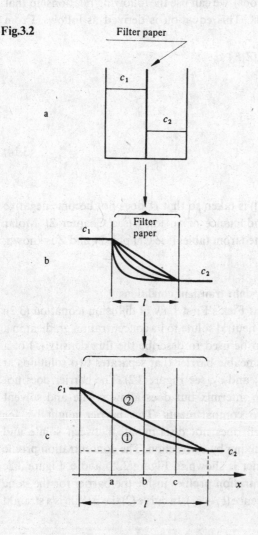

Diffusion across a slab: steady-state

Curve (2) shows the concentration profile obtained after a steady-state has been reached. The time taken to reach this steady-state will depend upon the nature of the barrier and the nature of the solute. A linear profile corresponds, by definition, to a steady-state situation because the local gradient (dc/dx) (and thus the flux density $\bar{J}$) is constant with x. Because the flux density is the same at any point x across the barrier, there is no accumulation of solute. For this steady-state, that is, when the transbarrier flux density is constant $(dc/dx = \text{constant})$ we can write Fick's equation as

$$\bar{J} = -D(d/dx)(c(x)) = -D\,\Delta c(x)/l = +(D/l)(c_1 - c_2) \qquad (3.15)$$

where l is the barrier thickness and $\Delta c = c_2 - c_1$.

The permeability constant

The ratio D/l is conventionally known as the permeability constant (P) and has the units of D/l $(cm^2/s/cm)$ which is $cm \cdot s^{-1}$. The permeability (P) can be computed directly from quantities that can be measured (flux density and concentrations c_1, c_2). Rearranging equation (3.15) we obtain

$$P = (D/l) = \bar{J}/(c_1 - c_2) \qquad (3.16)$$

The permeability constant (P) can be thought of as a measure of the ease with which a solute crosses a barrier. From equation (3.16) it can be seen that the more impermeable the barrier, for a given steady-state flux density, the greater the required concentration difference across the barrier.

The Second Law of Fick: transient solution

Fick's First Law allows the flux to be computed as a function of distance. In order to express concentration as a function of both distance and time we use *Fick's Second Law*. In this law, Fick derived an equation for the rate of change of the local concentration (dc/dt). This rate of change is due to a net influx of solute (influx − outflux) into a volume element. The volume element (Δv) can be thought of as a slab of solution area A and length Δx (Figure 3.3). The influx into the volume element (dn/dt) across the face of area A and position x is given by

$$\text{influx} = A\bar{J}(x) \qquad (3.17)$$

where $\bar{J}(x)$ is the flux density across the same face. Similarly for the face at $x + \Delta x$ the outflux is:

$$\text{outflux} = A\bar{J}(x + \Delta x) \qquad (3.17a)$$

The amount of solute (ΔQ) contained in the slab is given by

$$\Delta Q = c\,\Delta v \qquad (3.18)$$

where c is the concentration of solute in the slab and Δv is given by

$$\Delta v = A \, \Delta x \qquad (3.19)$$

In equation (3.18) we should recall that A in the Δv is the cross-sectional area of the slab and Δx its thickness. The rate of change of ΔQ with time ($\mathrm{d}(\Delta Q)/\mathrm{d}t$) is then given by

$$\mathrm{d}(c \, \Delta v)/\mathrm{d}t = \text{influx} - \text{outflux} \qquad (3.20)$$

If we substitute (3.17), (3.17a), (3.18) and (3.19) in (3.20) we obtain

$$\mathrm{d}(c \, \Delta v)/\mathrm{d}t = \Delta v \, \mathrm{d}c/\mathrm{d}t$$
$$= A \, \Delta x \, \mathrm{d}c/\mathrm{d}t$$
$$= A\bar{J}(x) - A\bar{J}(x + \Delta x)$$

If we rearrange this equation we obtain

$$\mathrm{d}(c(x, t))/\mathrm{d}t = -(A(\bar{J}(x + \Delta x) - \bar{J}(x)))/A \, \Delta x$$
$$= -(\bar{J}(x + \Delta x) - \bar{J}(x))/\Delta x \qquad (3.21)$$

In the limiting case ($\Delta x \to 0$) the right-hand side of equation (3.21) becomes the derivative of the flux density with respect to distance. Equation (3.21) can thus be written

$$\partial(c(x, t))/\partial t = -\partial(\bar{J}(x, t))/\partial x \qquad (3.22)$$

Fig.3.3

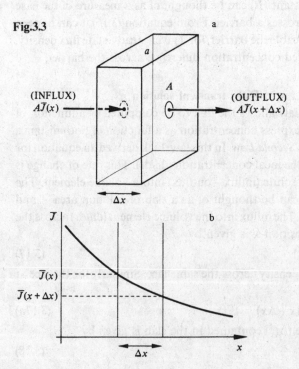

(INFLUX)
$A\bar{J}(x)$

A

(OUTFLUX)
$A\bar{J}(x + \Delta x)$

Δx

J

$\bar{J}(x)$

$\bar{J}(x + \Delta x)$

Δx

x

since quantities c and $\bar{J}$ are functions of x and t. To be mathematically correct we wrote c as $c(x, t)$ and J as $J(x, t)$. Partial derivatives ($\partial/\partial t$ and $\partial/\partial x$) are used to show that we are dealing with both distance (x) and time (t).

From Fick's First Law (equation (3.2)) we can substitute for $\bar{J}$ (where $\bar{J} = -D(\mathrm{d}c/\mathrm{d}x)$ and write

$$\partial(c(x, t))/\partial t = D \,\partial^2(c(x, t))/\partial x^2 \tag{3.23}$$

This equation is Fick's Second Law of Diffusion in one dimension (x). Equation (3.23) is a second-order partial differential equation. The solution of this equation will give the concentration c as a function of time (t) and distance (x). The specific form of this solution will depend upon the conditions under which it is solved.

Solution of Fick's Second Law: boundary conditions

These conditions are known as 'initial' (in time) and 'boundary' (in space) conditions (see Appendix 19). For example, in the experiment described in Figure 3.1 we have a specific set of conditions. These are at time zero ($t = 0$) all the solute is in the slab, so $c(x) = 0$; at any time (t) when x is very large ($x \rightarrow \infty$) the solute concentration $c(x)$ is zero ($c(x) = 0$). One of the solutions of Fick's Second Law is (Appendix 19):

$$c(x, t) = (M/(\sqrt{\pi a})) \exp(-(x/a)^2) \tag{3.24}$$

where $a = 4Dt$.

The conditions for this solution were that at $t = 0$, M moles of solute were placed in a slab of unit cross-sectional area and of negligible thickness. The slab is located at $x = 0$ and separates two infinitely long slabs ($x \rightarrow \pm \infty$) of solvent of unit cross-sectional area. D is the diffusion coefficient of the solute in the solvent, c is the solute concentration in the solvent ($\mathrm{mol \cdot cm^{-3}}$) at any point x and at time t. Equation (3.24) is plotted in Figure 3.4 where c/M is plotted (instead of c) against the distance x for four different times. Figure 3.4 shows how the M moles originally placed at $x = 0$ spread with time along the x axis.

Often it is very important in electrophysiology to calculate the time it takes for particles to diffuse certain distances.

The speed of diffusional processes

Equation (3.24) could be used to quantify the speed of solute spread by calculating a family of concentration profiles at different times. However, this method is cumbersome and a simpler mathematical relationship is preferable. To obtain one let us consider particles in a solution that are undergoing random motions as a result of collisions with other particles. The movements of the individual particles are random (they are said to undertake 'random walks') so that for each instant of time there is an equal probability of a particle moving in any one direction (for the discussion of probability, see Appendix 7). The movements of the particles are assumed to be a sequence of discrete jumps. Diffusion can be considered the overall result (or net movement) of a large number of these particles (or molecules). Diffusion down a concentration gradient occurs because there are more particles in a region of high concentration, so the probability is greater that they will move to a region of lower concentration (Figure 3.4b).

Figure 3.5 shows a cylinder of unit cross-sectional area divided into two equal halves of length $\bar{x}$ by an imaginary plane. The cylinder contains a solution in which the solute concentration decays continuously from left to right. If the average concentrations in the two halves are c_1 and c_2, respectively, for a small distance x across the imaginary plane (see Figure 3.5b) the curve (1) approaches a straight line and so we can write, from the definition of a derivative, that

$$((c_{(2)} - c_{(1)})/x)x \approx (\mathrm{d}(c(x))/\mathrm{d}x)x$$

Fig.3.4

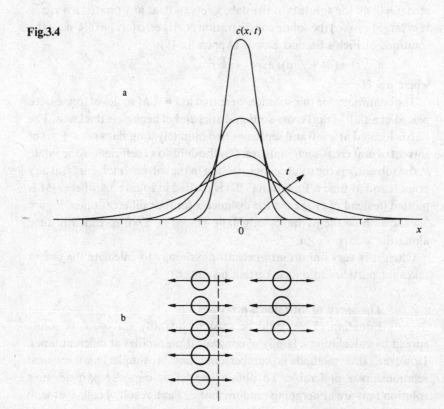

Since

$$c_{(1)} + ((c_{(2)} - c_{(1)})/x) = c_{(1)} + c_{(2)} - c_{(1)} = c_{(2)}$$

then

$$c_{(2)} = c_{(1)} + (dc/dx)x \qquad (3.25)$$

Each particle travels a distance x_i (see Figure 3.5c) in the x direction in time t. The average distance travelled by all the N particles is

$$\bar{x} = \sum_{i=1}^{i=N} (x_i/N)$$

Because diffusion is equally likely in any direction, half of the particles inside a distance $\bar{x}$ on either side of the imaginary plane will pass through this area. The flow from left to right is then

$$\vec{J} = (\tfrac{1}{2})c_{(1)}\bar{x}/t \qquad (3.25a)$$

Equation (3.25a) can be rewritten as

$$\vec{J} = (\tfrac{1}{2})c_{(1)}\bar{v}$$

Fig.3.5

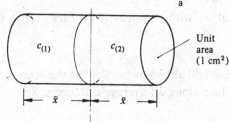

a

$c_{(1)}$ $c_{(2)}$ Unit area (1 cm²)

$\bar{x}$ $\bar{x}$

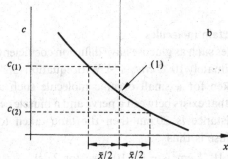

c

b

$c_{(1)}$ (1)

$c_{(2)}$

$\bar{x}/2$ $\bar{x}/2$ x

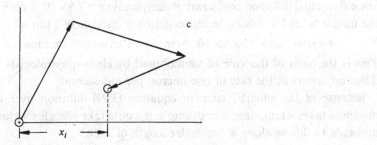

c

x_i

where

$$\bar{v} = \bar{x}/t = cm \cdot s^{-1}$$

so

$$\vec{J} = (mol/cm^3)(cm/s)$$
$$= mol \cdot cm^{-2} \cdot s^{-1}$$

and $\bar{v}$ is the average particle velocity along the x axis. Since movement in any direction is equally probable, only half of the particles have a net displacement to the right. Therefore, the flux is obtained by multiplying the velocity ($\bar{v}$) by $c_{(1)}/2$. The flow from right to left

$$\overleftarrow{J} = (\tfrac{1}{2})c_{(2)}(\bar{x}/t)$$

the net flow ($\bar{J}$) is then given by

$$\bar{J} = \vec{J} - \overleftarrow{J} = (\tfrac{1}{2})(\bar{x}/t)(c_{(1)} - c_{(2)}) \tag{3.26}$$

Using equation (3.25) in equation (3.26) we obtain

$$\bar{J} = (\tfrac{1}{2})(\bar{x}/t)(c_1 - c_1 - (dc/dx)\bar{x})$$
$$= -(\tfrac{1}{2})(\bar{x}^2/t)(dc/dx) \tag{3.27}$$

If we compare this equation with equation (3.2) (Fick's First Law of Diffusion) we see that

$$D = \bar{x}^2/2t \tag{3.28}$$

This is a simple relationship and allows us to calculate the average time (t) taken by a particle to diffuse along an average distance $\bar{x}$. So

$$t = \bar{x}^2/2D \tag{3.29}$$

Diffusion times for certain molecules

Small organic molecules such as glucose have diffusion coefficients in aqueous solutions of approximately 10^{-6} cm$^2 \cdot$ s^{-1}. With equation (3.29) we can calculate the time taken for a small organic molecule such as acetylcholine, to cross the gap that exists between a nerve and a muscle cell (the synaptic cleft). If this distance is 20 nm then the time taken for acetylcholine molecules to diffuse is thus

$$t \approx (2 \times 10^{-6} \text{ cm})^2/(2 \times 10^{-6} \text{ cm}^2/\text{s}) = 2 \times 10^{-6} \text{ s} \quad (\text{or } 2 \text{ μs})$$

Since the actual diffusion coefficient of acetylcholine is 7.6×10^{-6} cm^2 s^{-1}, the time it takes for this molecule to diffuse a distance of 1 μm is

$$t \approx (10^{-4} \text{ cm})^2/(2 \times 8 \times 10^{-6} \text{ cm}^2/\text{s}) \approx 10.6 \times 10^{-3} \text{ s} \approx 1 \text{ ms}$$

This is the basis of the 'rule of thumb' used by electrophysiologists that diffusion occurs at the rate of one micron per millisecond.

Because of the squared term in equation (3.29) diffusion over long distances takes a long time. For example, it would take years for a glucose molecule to diffuse along a one-metre length of axon!

Diffusion of electrolytes

So far we have considered the movement of non-electrolytes down their concentration gradients. In Chapter 2 we considered the movements of ions when they were subjected to electric fields. In the rest of this chapter we will consider the movement of ions subject to the joint effect of a concentration gradient and an electrical field. Equation (3.10) (the Nernst–Planck equation) describes mathematically this joint effect. The relationship between the local flux of an ion and its local electrochemical potential gradient is obtained from equation (3.10).

$$\bar{J} = -u'c[(d/dx)(RT\ln(c)) + ZF(dV/dx)] \tag{3.10}$$

On page 34 this equation was rearranged to give equation (3.13)

$$\bar{J} = -D[dc/dx + (ZF/RT)c(dV/dx)] \tag{3.13}$$

where D is the diffusion coefficient.

In Figure 3.6a we represent a cuboid of solution of unit cross-sectional area and length l. At steady-state the concentration of ion (i) will decay continuously from left to right along the x axis. If we assume that the concentration of ion (i) is constant along both y and z axes, we can consider that the diffusion of the ion occurs only in one dimension (x). Although D, the diffusion constant, was obtained for a three-dimensional process, as is the case now, we assume that there is a net flux of ion only along the x axis even though each ion is free to move in any direction. Figure 3.6a also

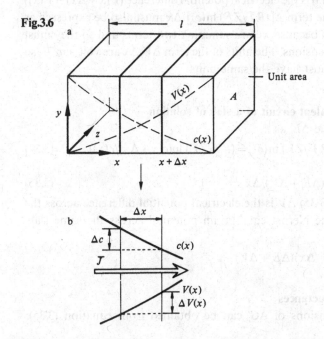

Fig.3.6

shows that the ion is subject to an electrical potential (V) which increases from left to right along the x axis. For this one-dimensional case the electrical potential is also assumed to be constant along the y and the z axes.

Diffusional currents

Figure 3.6b shows a slab of length Δx of solution taken from the cuboid of Figure 3.6a. The flux of ion (i) through this slab is related to the concentration and the electrical potential gradient across it by equation (3.13) provided that Δx is small. Since equations (3.10) and (3.13) describe the flux density of an ion (i) through a slab of solvent and, as ions are charged particles, their movement in a solution is equivalent to a current flow through the solution. The flux density ($\bar{J_i}$) in equation (3.10) becomes a current density when it is multiplied by ZF (see Chapter 2). So

$$\bar{I_i} = ZFJ_i = -ZFu_i'c_i[(\mathrm{d}/\mathrm{d}x)(RT\ln(c)) + ZF(\mathrm{d}V/\mathrm{d}x)] \tag{3.30}$$

Rearranging

$$\bar{I_i} = -(ZF)^2 u_i'c_i[(\mathrm{d}/\mathrm{d}x)(RT\ln(c)/ZF) + \mathrm{d}V/\mathrm{d}x] \tag{3.31}$$

If we call the quantity $-(ZF)^2 u_i'c_i$ the quantity $-(\Delta G_i')$, we obtain

$$\bar{I_i} = -\Delta G_i'[(\mathrm{d}/\mathrm{d}x)(RT\ln(c)/ZF) + \mathrm{d}V/\mathrm{d}x] \tag{3.32}$$

For a small Δx

$$\bar{I_i} \approx \Delta G_i'[\Delta[(RT/ZF)\ln(c)]/\Delta x + \Delta V/\Delta x] \tag{3.33}$$

ΔV in equation (3.33) is the electrical potential difference ($V(x + \Delta x) - V(x)$) across the slab. The term $\Delta[(RT/ZF)\ln(c)]/\Delta x$ must also be expressed as $\mathrm{volt} \cdot \mathrm{cm}^{-1}$. This is because we are summing two terms and so they must have the same dimensions. The units of the term $\Delta V/\Delta x$ are $\mathrm{volt} \cdot \mathrm{cm}^{-1}$, so the second term must have the same units.

The equivalent circuit of a slab of solution

If we define ΔE_i as

$$\Delta E_i = \Delta[(RT/ZF)\ln(c)] = (RT/ZF)\ln(c(x+\Delta x)/c(x)) \tag{3.34}$$

and

$$\bar{I_i} \approx -\Delta G_i'(\Delta E_i + \Delta V)/\Delta x \tag{3.35}$$

then in equation (3.35) ΔV is the electrical potential difference across the slab and ΔE_i is the Nernst equilibrium potential across the same slab. Rearranging (3.35)

$$\bar{I_i} = -(\Delta G_i'/\Delta x)(\Delta E_i + \Delta V)$$

Ionic conductances

The dimensions of $\Delta G_i'$ can be obtained from equation (3.35).

Dimensionally this equation is

$$amp \cdot cm^{-2} = \Delta G_i \cdot volt \cdot cm^{-1}$$

So the dimensions of $\Delta G_i'$ are

$$\Delta G_i' = amp \cdot volt^{-1} \cdot cm^{-1} = S \cdot cm^{-1}$$

Also

$$\Delta G_i' = (ZF)^2 u_i' c_i$$

or dimensionally

$$\Delta G_i' = \underbrace{\frac{(gr\text{-}eq/mol)^2 \cdot (coul/gr\text{-}eq)^2}{(ZF)^2}}$$

$$\underbrace{\cdot (cm^2 \cdot mol \cdot joule^{-1} \cdot s^{-1})}_{u_i'} \cdot \underbrace{(mol/cm^3)}_{c_i}$$

$$= (coul^2 \cdot cm^{-1} \cdot s^{-1} \cdot joule^{-1})$$

or

$$= (coul/s)(coul/joule) \cdot cm^{-1}$$
$$= amp \cdot volt^{-1} \cdot cm^{-1}$$
$$= S \cdot cm^{-1}$$

Equation (3.35) can be rearranged to obtain

$$\bar{I}_i = -\Delta \bar{G}_i(\Delta E_i + \Delta V) \tag{3.36}$$

where

$$\Delta \bar{G}_i = \Delta G_i'/\Delta x$$

and $\Delta \bar{G}_i$ is now a conductance per unit area of a slab of thickness Δx.

Equation (3.36) can be represented by an equivalent circuit of the type shown in Figure 3.7b. The whole cuboid of solution is then the sum of n such elements (as shown in Figure 3.7c). To obtain a simple electrical equivalent circuit of the cuboid of solution shown in Figure 3.7a, we are able to apply Kirchhoff's Laws (see Appendix 15) to the equivalent circuit of Figure 3.7c. So

$$E_i' = \sum_{j=1}^{j=n} \Delta E_i(j) \tag{3.37}$$

where i refers to the ion and j the 'jth' slab. For V' we write

$$V' = \sum_{j=1}^{j=n} \Delta V(j) = V_1 - V_0 \tag{3.38}$$

In order to obtain the overall conductance ($\bar{G}_i$) of the cuboid, we first define the incremental resistance $\Delta \bar{R}_i$ as

$$\Delta \bar{R}_i(j) = 1/\Delta \bar{G}_i(j) \quad \text{(where } \Delta \bar{R}_i \text{ has the dimensions of } \Omega \cdot cm^2) \tag{3.39}$$

From Kirchhoff's Laws (see Appendix 15) the overall resistance R_i is simply the sum of the incremental resistances in series. So

$$\bar{R}_i = \sum_{j=1}^{j=n} \Delta \bar{R}_i(j) \tag{3.40}$$

and as

$$\bar{G}_i = 1/\bar{R}_i \tag{3.41}$$

from the definition of ΔE_i (see equation (3.37)) we can obtain a simple expression for E'_i defined as

$$E'_i = \sum_{j=1}^{j=n} \Delta E_i(j) = \Delta E_{i_{(1)}} + \Delta E_{i_{(2)}} + \cdots + \Delta E_{i_{(n)}}$$

From equation (3.34)

$$\begin{aligned}
E'_i &= (RT/ZF) \ln(c_i(\Delta x)/c_i(0)) + (RT/ZF) \ln(c_i(2\,\Delta x)/c_i(\Delta x)) + \cdots \\
&\quad + (RT/ZF) \ln(c_i(l)/c_i((n-1)\cdot\Delta x)) \\
&= (RT/ZF) \ln(c_i(\Delta x)c_i(2\,\Delta x)\cdots c_i(l)/c_i(0)c_i(\Delta x)\cdots c_i((n-1)\,\Delta x)) \\
&= (RT/ZF) \ln(c_i(l)/c_i(0)) \tag{3.42}
\end{aligned}$$

where $l = n\,\Delta x$.

The equation that relates the current density ($\bar{I}$) through the cuboid to the electrical potential drop across the cuboid can be derived from equation (3.36)

$$\bar{I}_i/\Delta\bar{G}_i(j) = \Delta\bar{R}_i(j)\bar{I}_i = -(\Delta E_i cj + \Delta Vcj)$$

Fig.3.7

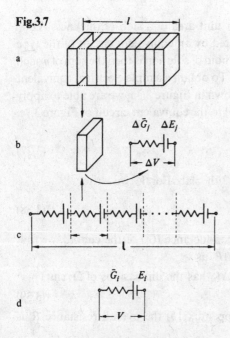

or

$$\sum_{j=1}^{j=n} (\Delta \bar{R}_i(j) I_i) = \bar{I}_i \sum_{j=1}^{j=n} \Delta \bar{R}_i(j) = \bar{I}_i \bar{R}_i = \bar{I}_i / \bar{G}_i$$

and

$$-\sum_{j=1}^{j=n} (\Delta E_i(j) + \Delta V(j)) = -\left(\sum_{j=1}^{j=n} \Delta E_i(j) + \sum_{j=1}^{j=n} \Delta V(j) \right)$$

$$= -(E_i' + V')$$

from (3.37) and (3.38), or

$$\bar{I}_i / \bar{G}_i = -(E_i' + V')$$

so

$$\bar{I}_i = -\bar{G}_i (E_i' + V') \tag{3.43}$$

where $\bar{G}_i$ is the total conductance per unit area. When the current through the cuboid is zero, equation (3.43) becomes

$$0 = -\bar{G}_i (E_i' + V')$$

or, from (3.42),

$$V' = -E_i' = (RT/ZF) \ln(c_{i(0)}/c_{i(l)}) \tag{3.44}$$

where $c_{i(0)}$ is the concentration of ions (i) in the first slab and $c_{i(l)}$ is the concentration of ions (i) in the last slab.

Because the concentration and voltage profiles are fixed (at a steady-state) and because there is no current flow, equation (3.44) gives the voltage across the slab under equilibrium conditions. Equation (3.44) was derived in Chapter 2 (page 17) and is the *Nernst equation*.

The equivalent circuit for more than one ion

In an electrolyte solution that has just been made up the number of positive ions equals the number of negative ions (electroneutrality). This is because under usual conditions it is not possible to add separately to a solution positive or negative ions. Because of this electroneutrality, more than one ion species has to be present in the cuboid of solution. So the overall equivalent circuit of the cuboid of Figure 3.7a can be represented by the parallel combination of two (or more) equivalent circuits of the type shown in Figure 3.7d (see Figure 3.8). These parallel combinations have been used extensively by electrophysiologists to describe the electrical behaviour of biological membranes and in Chapter 7 we will see how the squid axon membrane can be described by a similar circuit with three parallel branches.

If we wish to examine the potentials associated with ion concentration gradients within a solution, the easiest approach is to sum the individual ionic currents so as to get the total current. This approach involves using equation (3.10) to describe the flux of each of the ions in solution. When only Na^+ and Cl^- are present, we write for sodium ions

$$\bar{J}_{Na} = -u'_{Na}c_{Na}[d(RT \ln c_{Na})/dx + F \, dV/dx] \tag{3.45}$$

and for chloride ions

$$\bar{J}_{Cl} = -u'_{Cl}c_{Cl}[d(RT \ln c_{Cl})/dx - F \, dV/dx]$$

The ion current densities corresponding to these flux densities are then

$$\bar{I}_{Na} = FJ_{Na} = -Fu'_{Na}c_{Na}[d(RT \ln c_{Na})/dx + F \, dV/dx]$$
$$\bar{I}_{Cl} = -FJ_{Cl} = +Fu'_{Cl}c_{Cl}[d(RT \ln c_{Cl})/dx - F \, dV/dx] \tag{3.46}$$

and the total current density $(\bar{I}_t)$ is so given as the sum of the individual ionic current densities.

$$\bar{I}_t = \bar{I}_{Na} + \bar{I}_{Cl}$$

or

$$\bar{I}_t = F[u'_{Cl}c_{Cl} \, d(RT \ln c_{Cl})/dx - u'_{Na}c_{Na} \, d(RT \ln c_{Na})/dx]$$
$$- (u'_{Na}c_{Na} + u'_{Cl}c_{Cl})F^2 \, dV/dx \tag{3.47}$$

Lumped and non-lumped equivalent circuits

If the only ions in solution are Na^+ and Cl^-, because of electroneutrality,

$$c_{Na} = c_{Cl} = c \tag{3.48}$$

where c is thus the molar concentration of NaCl; c_{Na} is the number of gram-equivalents of sodium ion per litre, c_{Cl} is the number of gram-equivalents of chloride ion per litre and so c is the number of moles of sodium chloride per

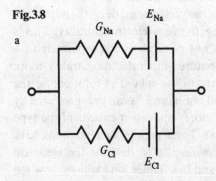

Fig.3.8

a

b

litre. If we substitute (3.48) into (3.47) we obtain

$$\bar{I}_t = F(u'_{Cl}c\, d(RT \ln c)/dx - u'_{Na}c\, d(RT \ln c)/dx)$$
$$- (u'_{Na}c + u'_{Cl}c)F^2\, dV/dx \qquad (3.49)$$

If we rearrange equation (3.49) we obtain

$$\bar{I}_t = (u'_{Cl} - u'_{Na})Fc\, d(RT \ln c)/dx - (u'_{Na} + u'_{Cl})cF^2\, dV/dx \qquad (3.50)$$

This equation can be put into a form similar to equation (3.31) to give

$$\bar{I}_t = (u'_{Na} + u'_{Cl})cF^2$$
$$\times [((u'_{Cl} - u'_{Na})/(u'_{Cl} + u'_{Na}))\, d((RT/F) \ln c)/dx - dV/dx]$$

On rearranging

$$\bar{I}_t = -(u'_{Na} + u'_{Cl})cF^2$$
$$\times [((u'_{Na} - u'_{Cl})/(u'_{Na} + u'_{Cl}))(d/dx)((RT/F) \ln c) + dV/dx] \qquad (3.51)$$

The quantity $(u'_{Na} + u'_{Cl})cF^2$ has the same dimensions ($\text{S} \cdot \text{cm}^{-1}$) as ΔG_i that was used in equation (3.32). So we can write

$$\bar{I}_t = -\Delta G'_t[((u'_{Na} - u'_{Cl})/(u'_{Na} + u'_{Cl}))(d/dx)((RT/F) \ln c) + dV/dx] \qquad (3.52)$$

where

$$\Delta G'_t = (u'_{Na} + u'_{Cl})cF^2 \qquad (3.53)$$

With the same reasoning that was used to derive equations (3.36) to (3.43), we write for the whole cuboid of solution that

$$\bar{I}_t = -\bar{G}_t(E_t + V) \qquad (3.54)$$

where

$$\bar{G}_t = 1 \Big/ \Big(\sum_n (\Delta x/\Delta \bar{G}'_t) \Big) \qquad (3.55)$$

$$V = \sum_{j=1}^{n} \Delta Vj \qquad (3.56)$$

$$\Delta E_t = ((u'_{Na} - u'_{Cl})/(u'_{Na} + u'_{Cl}))(d/dx)((RT/F) \ln c) \qquad (3.57)$$

and

$$E_t = \sum_n \Delta E_t = ((u'_{Na} - u'_{Cl})/(u'_{Na} + u'_{Cl}))(RT/F) \ln(c(l)/c(0)) \qquad (3.58)$$

In equations (3.53) and (3.58) the contributions of sodium and chloride ions to the conductance of a slab and to the potential across it are 'lumped'. By this we mean that we cannot separate out the contribution of the individual ions to the overall parameters of the circuit $\bar{G}_t$ and E_t.

Diffusion potentials

Equation (3.54) has an equivalent circuit of the type shown in Figure 3.8b. Equation (3.57) describes the current flow ($\bar{I}_t$) through the solution in terms of a lumped conductance ($\bar{G}'_t$) and an overall diffusion potential E_t. It can be seen from equations (3.53), (3.55) and (3.58) that both $\bar{G}_t$ and E_t depend on the ion mobilities (u'_{Na} and u'_{Cl}).

From equation (3.57) we can also see that for the same salt concentration gradients the polarity of E_t depends upon the relative ion mobilities. For a salt where both ions (sodium and chloride ions in this case) are univalent, if the mobility of the cation is the same as that of the anion, the diffusion potential E_t is zero. This is the basis of the use of potassium chloride in the salt bridges that were previously described. The mobility of the potassium ions is 7.9×10^{-9} cm$^2 \cdot$joule$^{-1} \cdot$s^{-1} and the mobility of chloride ions is 8.2×10^{-9} cm$^{-2} \cdot$joule$^{-1} \cdot$s^{-1} so the diffusion potential (E_t) is very small. In addition, electrophysiologists use a highly concentrated (3 M) potassium chloride solution in the salt bridges. This is because at such high concentrations the *junction potential* (see Chapter 2) at the salt-bridge/ solution interphase is shunted by the diffusion of potassium chloride. At the interphase between the 3 M KCl salt-bridge and the solution there will be electrochemical gradients for all the ions in the solution. It is possible to derive an equation of the type shown in (3.58) for more than two ions by the technique demonstrated above. With this equation it can be shown that for large concentrations of K and Cl the diffusional potential due to the other ions is negligible (see Appendix 27).

In conclusion, this chapter has dealt with the movement of ions in solution when they are subject to combined electrical and concentration gradients. In the chapters that follow we will consider the movements of solutes across the barriers (membranes) that exist between biological compartments.

4

Diffusion within a membrane

In the previous chapters we dealt with the biophysical basis of solute movement within fluid compartments. In this chapter we will consider the movement of ions through biological membranes which we shall treat, for the moment, as thin homogeneous slabs.

Our starting point is the general equation that describes the flux of ions in free solution. This was derived from first principles in Chapter 3 and is the Nernst–Planck equation. For one ion the flux density ($\bar{J}$) is given by

$$\bar{J} = -D[dc/dx + (ZF/RT)c\, dV/dx] \tag{3.13}$$

As pointed out in Chapter 3 and Figure 3.6, this equation relates the local concentration (c) and electrical (V) gradients (dc/dx and dV/dx) to the local flux density ($\bar{J}$); D is the *diffusion coefficient*. Although the Nernst–Planck equation was derived for diffusion in free solution, we can also apply it to diffusion in a narrow homogeneous slab of membrane (Figure 4.1).

This means that the concentration (c) and potential (V) terms apply also to a slab *within* the membrane and therefore cannot be measured directly. The only values of c and V that can be measured directly are the compartmental values ($c_{(1)}$, $c_{(2)}$ and $V_{(1)}$, $V_{(2)}$). Since equation (3.13) describes only the local flux as a function of the local gradients, if we are to obtain the transmembrane flux we need to integrate equation (3.13) over the width (δ) of the membrane (see Appendix 9). Before we can integrate equation (3.13), we have to reduce the number of variables to two (c and x, or V and x, or c and V). In order to reduce the number of variables, we have to know the mathematical relationship between either c and x, or V and x, or c and V. Hodgkin and Katz reduced the number of variables by assuming that the voltage profile across the membrane was linear. This assumption was first proposed by Goldman and it implies that

$$dV/dx = \text{constant} = -(V_{(0)} - V_{(\delta)})/\delta = -V/\delta$$

Fig.4.1

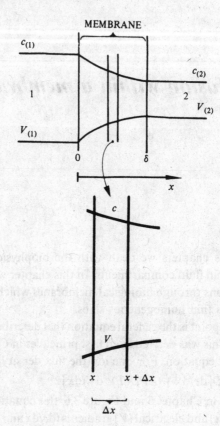

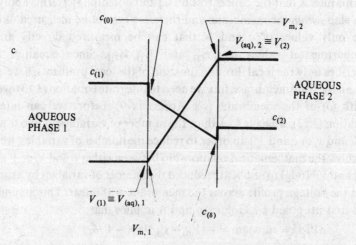

The constant-field assumption

It should be noted here that in Chapter 3 we defined V' as

$$V' = V_{(\delta)} - V_{(0)}$$

which is equivalent to $-V$.

Equation (3.13) can now be rewritten as

$$\bar{J} = -D[dc/dx - (ZF/RT)cV/\delta] \tag{4.1}$$

where $V/\delta = -dV/dx$. If we rearrange equation (4.1) we obtain

$$dc/dx = -\bar{J}/D + (ZF/RT)cV/\delta \tag{4.2}$$

$$dc/dx - (ZFV/RT\delta)c = -\bar{J}/D \tag{4.3}$$

In the steady state, that is, when $\bar{J}$, the flux density, is constant with time and distance, both the concentration and the potential profile must also be constant with time. If $\bar{J}$ is not constant with distance there will be accumulation or depletion of ions and c (and thus V) will change with time. Because there is a net flux ($\bar{J}$) across the membrane and c and V are constant, it is a steady-state situation. This situation is not to be confused with an equilibrium situation where there is no net flux. Since D is constant, as are the terms Z, F, V, R, T, $\bar{J}$ and δ, equation (4.3) can be rewritten as

$$dc/dx - ac = -b \tag{4.4}$$

where

$$a = (ZFV)/(RT\delta) \tag{4.5}$$

and

$$b = \bar{J}/D \tag{4.6}$$

Integration of the Nernst–Planck equation

This equation can be solved by the integrating factor method (see Appendix 10), where $P(x) = -a$ and $Q(x) = -b$, so

$$\int P(x)\, dx = -ax \tag{4.7}$$

and the solution is

$$c = \exp(ax)\left[\int \exp(-ax)(-b)\, dx + B\right] \tag{4.8}$$

where B is a constant of integration.

Integration gives

$$c = (b/a) + B\exp(ax) \tag{4.9}$$

$$c = (\bar{J}/D)/(ZFV/RT\delta) + B\exp(ZFVx/RT\delta) \tag{4.10}$$

When $x = 0$, the concentration is $c_{(0)}$ in the left-hand side of the membrane and is given by

$$c_{(0)} = (RT\delta\bar{J})/(ZFVD) + B \tag{4.11}$$

So, the integration constant (B) is

$$B = c_{(0)} - (RT\delta\bar{J})/(ZFVD) \tag{4.12}$$

Substituting (4.12) into (4.10) we obtain

$$c = (RT\delta\bar{J}/ZFVD) + [c_{(0)} - (RT\delta\bar{J}/ZFVD)] \exp(ZFVx/RT\delta)$$

when $x = \delta$, c is the concentration $c_{(\delta)}$ in the right-hand side of the membrane (see Figure 4.1c).

So, we can write

$$\begin{aligned}
c_{(\delta)} &= (RT\delta\bar{J}/ZFVD) + [c_{(0)} - (RT\delta\bar{J}/ZFVD)] \exp(ZFV/RT) \\
&= (RT\delta\bar{J}/ZFVD)[1 - \exp(ZFV/RT)] + c_{(0)} \exp(ZFV/RT)
\end{aligned} \tag{4.13}$$

If we rearrange equation (4.13) we obtain

$$\bar{J} = (D/\delta)(ZFV/RT)(c_{(0)} \exp(ZFV/RT) - c_{(\delta)})/(\exp(ZFV/RT) - 1) \tag{4.14}$$

where D/δ has the dimensions ($cm \cdot s^{-1}$) of a permeability (P) as defined in Chapter 3.

The partition coefficient at the membrane–solution interphase

This equation only allows us to compute the flux density $\bar{J}$ if we know the concentrations ($c_{(0)}$, $c_{(\delta)}$) and the potential on both *inside* faces of the membrane. But it might be that the concentration and the electrical potential in the solution adjacent to the membrane are different. Hodgkin and Katz made a second assumption that the bulk concentrations of the solutions ($c_{(1)}$, $c_{(2)}$) are at equilibrium with the adjacent membrane concentrations so that the ratios $c_{(0)}/c_{(1)}$ and $c_{(\delta)}/c_{(2)}$ are constant and equal. This means that

$$(c_{(0)}/c_{(1)}) = (c_{(\delta)}/c_{(2)}) = \beta \tag{4.15}$$

β is called the partition coefficient. The partition coefficient is formally defined as the ratio of the concentrations of a substance in two phases at equilibrium.

If we rearrange (4.15) we obtain

$$c_{(0)} = \beta c_{(1)} \quad \text{and} \quad c_{(\delta)} = \beta c_{(2)} \tag{4.16}$$

Substituting (4.16) into (4.14) we obtain

$$\bar{J} = (D\beta/\delta)(ZFV/RT)(c_{(1)} \exp(ZFV/RT) - c_{(2)})/(\exp(ZFV/RT)^{-1}) \tag{4.17}$$

Hodgkin and Katz made a third assumption that the electrical potential is the same on both sides of each membrane–solution interface, that is

$$V_{(1)} - V_{(2)} = V_{(0)} - V_{(\delta)} \tag{4.18}$$

With this final assumption equation (4.17) enables us to define both mathematically and experimentally the 'membrane permeability'.

The membrane permeability

In the case of equation (4.17), the product $D\beta/\delta$ is now the 'membrane permeability' (P_m) and is a measure of the ease with which ions cross the membrane. The membrane permeability (P_m) is given by

$$P_m = \beta D/\delta \quad (\text{cm}\cdot\text{s}^{-1}) \tag{4.19}$$

β is a dimensionless quantity since it is the ratio between two concentrations.

If we substitute (4.19) into (4.17) we obtain

$$\bar{J} = P_m(ZFV/RT)(c_{(1)}\exp(ZFV/RT) - c_{(2)})/(\exp(ZFV/RT) - 1) \tag{4.20}$$

The Goldman–Hodgkin–Katz (constant-field) equation for the membrane current density

The current density ($\bar{I}$) corresponding to the flux ($\bar{J}$) given by equation (4.20) is (see Chapter 3)

$$\bar{I} = ZF\bar{J} = P_m((ZF)^2V/RT)(c_{(1)}\exp(ZFV/RT) - c_{(2)})/(\exp(ZFV/RT) - 1) \tag{4.20a}$$

Equation (4.20a) is sometimes known as the Goldman–Hodgkin–Katz (G–H–K) equation for the membrane current density.

This equation relates the current that flows through a unit area of membrane to an applied field. It is probably the equation that is most often used by electrophysiologists to describe quantitatively the flow of current through a membrane, so we will examine in some detail the assumptions that were made during its derivation.

Assumptions made in the derivation of the constant-field equation

First assumption

We are dealing with a steady-state situation ($\bar{J}$ is constant with distance). This assumption is valid because biological membranes are extremely thin (5–10 nm) and so diffusion is very fast (see Chapter 3), and a steady-state situation is established very quickly (less than 10^{-6} s).

Second assumption

Our second assumption is that dV/dx is a constant. This is valid because, as will be shown in Chapter 5, ions are practically insoluble in the lipid phase of the lipid bilayer. This means that the number of ions present in the lipid phase is negligible, so that the charge density (amount of charge per unit volume of membrane lipid) is also negligible. From Poisson's equation (see Appendix 22)

$$(d/dx)^2(V) \approx 0 \tag{4.21}$$

or

$$(d/dx)(V) = \text{constant} \tag{4.22}$$

since differentiating a constant gives zero.

Third assumption

The third assumption allows us to relate the concentrations just inside the membrane $(c_{(0)}, c_{(\delta)})$ to the solutions on either side of the membrane $(c_{(1)}, c_{(2)})$. Thus the ratios $c_{(1)}/c_{(0)}$ and $c_{(2)}/c_{(\delta)}$ are *assumed* to be equal and constant. The ratios are represented by β which can be thought of as a proportionality constant. That is $c_{(1)} \propto c_{(0)}$ and $c_{(2)} \propto c_{(\delta)}$ which implies

$$c_{(1)} = \beta c_{(0)} \quad \text{and} \quad c_{(2)} = \beta c_{(\delta)} \tag{4.23}$$

Since β is *assumed* to be constant, so the equations in (4.23) imply that $c_{(1)}$ and $c_{(2)}$ are at equilibrium with $c_{(0)}$ and $c_{(\delta)}$. This means that β can be derived from the definition of the electrochemical potential of an ion (i) either in solution (aq) or in the membrane phase (m). So, from equation (2.33)

$$\left. \begin{array}{l} \mu_{i(aq)} = \mu_{i(aq)}^0 + RT \ln(c_{i(aq)}) + ZFV_{(aq)} \\ \mu_{i(m)} = \mu_{i(m)}^0 + RT \ln(c_{i(m)}) + ZFV_m \end{array} \right\} \tag{4.24}$$

At equilibrium

$$\mu_{i(aq)} = \mu_{i(m)} \tag{4.25}$$

If we substitute equations (4.24) into equation (4.25) we obtain

$$\mu_{i(aq)}^0 + RT \ln(c_{i(aq)}) + ZFV_{(aq)} = \mu_{i(m)}^0 + RT \ln(c_{i(m)}) + ZFV_m$$

and rearranging

$$RT \ln(c_{i(aq)}/c_{i(m)}) = \mu_{i(m)}^0 - \mu_{i(aq)}^0 + ZF(V_m - V_{(aq)})$$

or

$$\tag{4.26}$$

$$(c_{i(aq)}/c_{i(m)}) = \beta = \exp((\mu_{i(m)}^0 - \mu_{i(aq)}^0 + ZF(V_m - V_{(aq)}))/RT)$$

As pointed out above, since the membrane is very thin, the concentrations inside the membrane will rapidly attain constant values. So, in practice, $c_{i(aq)}$ will always be in equilibrium with $c_{i(m)}$.

From equation (4.26) we see that β depends upon the difference between the two standard electrochemical potentials $(\mu_{i(aq)}^0)$ and $(\mu_{i(m)}^0)$, and also the difference between the electrical potential of the bulk solution and the lipid phase of the membrane. The standard chemical potentials are assumed to be independent of the concentrations in the corresponding phases, or otherwise activities (see Chapter 2) should be used instead of concentrations. Finally, since it is assumed that the electrical potential is constant at the aqueous lipid interphase, then

$$V_{(aq),1} = V_{m,1}$$
$$V_{(aq),2} = V_{m,2}$$

(4.27)

Because of equation (4.27) (see Figure 4.1)

$$V_m - V_{(aq)} = 0$$

so, equation (4.26) reduces to

$$(c_{i(aq)}/c_{i(m)}) = \beta = \exp(\mu_{i(m)}^0 - \mu_{i(aq)}^0)/RT = \text{constant}$$

(4.28)

The voltage and concentration profiles corresponding to equations (4.20) and (4.28) (see Figure 4.1c) are probably an over-simplification of the profiles that usually occur (see Finkelstein & Mauro).

The constant-field current-voltage curve

To gain further insight into the Goldman–Hodgkin–Katz equation (G–H–K) we plot current density $(\bar{I})$ as a function of voltage (V) (Figure 4.2b) for the case of a positive ion at a higher concentration in compartment (1) than in compartment (2). In this figure, as in equation (4.20), positive currents are due to positive ions moving from left to right (i.e. (1) to (2)). In the sign convention used by electrophysiologists side (1) is the inside of the cell and side (2) is the extracellular medium. Positive current is a current of positive charges that flows from the inside to the outside. Plots of the type in Figure 4.2 are generally known as current/voltage (I/V) curves. If an I/V curve is non-linear it is said to show rectification. An I/V curve which is a straight line is known as a linear I/V curve. Ohm's Law is a classic example of a linear I/V curve, where the conductance is the slope of the line. Under these conditions electrophysiologists refer to the conductance as an ohmic or linear conductance, when the conductance (or the resistance) changes as a function of voltage or current the I/V curve is no longer linear.

Constant-field rectification

The rectification shown in Figure 4.2a(1) is known as constant-field rectification. This rectification occurs when the I/V curve can be fitted with a constant-field I/V curve. Figure 4.2a(2) shows an I/V curve that bends away from the y axis (when $c_{(1)} > c_{(2)}$).

Anomalous rectification

This type of rectification, which can be revealed under certain conditions in skeletal muscle, is different from the constant-field rectification and is thus known as *anomalous rectification*.

Characteristics of constant-field rectification

Rectification occurs when an I/V curve is non-linear. It must be due to changes in conductance (or resistance) with voltage (or current). In order to quantify these changes we can take ratios of conductances at different voltages (or currents). In the case of the G–H–K equation, we can compute the largest value of this ratio by obtaining the value of the conductance for a very large positive and a very large negative V.

At a very large and positive V and when $Z > 0$ the exponential terms of equation (4.20a) containing V are very large, so

$$c_{(1)} \exp(ZFV/RT) \gg c_{(2)}$$

and

$$\exp(ZFV/RT) \gg 1$$

Fig.4.2

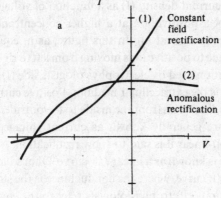

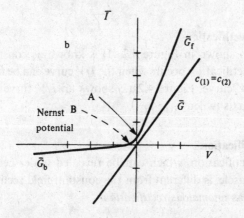

Equation (4.20a) reduces to

$$\bar{I} = P_m((ZF)^2V/RT)c_{(1)}\exp(ZFV/RT)/\exp(ZFV/RT)$$
$$= P_m(ZF)^2c_{(1)}V/RT \tag{4.29}$$
$$= \bar{G}_f V \quad \text{(see Figure 4.2b)}$$

where

$$\bar{G}_f = P_m(ZF)^2c_{(1)}/RT \quad (\text{s} \cdot \text{cm}^{-2}) \tag{4.30}$$

Equation (4.30) shows that when a high current flows from compartment (1) to (2) the conductance becomes a function of only one of the compartment concentrations $(c_{(1)})$.

At a very large and negative V and for $Z > 0$ the exponential terms of equation (4.20a) are very small, so

$$c_{(1)}\exp(ZFV/RT) \ll c_{(2)} \quad \text{and} \quad \exp(ZFV/RT) \ll 1.$$

So equation (4.20a) becomes

$$\bar{I} = P_m(ZF)^2c_{(2)}V/RT$$
$$= \bar{G}_b V \quad \text{(see Figure 4.2b)} \tag{4.31}$$

Equation (4.31) shows that when high currents flow from (2) to (1) the conductance also becomes a function of only one of the compartment concentrations $(c_{(2)})$, where

$$\bar{G}_b = P_m(ZF)^2c_{(2)}/RT \tag{4.32}$$

The maximum value of a constant-field rectification

The ratio between the two limiting conductances given by equations (4.30) and (4.32) is

$$\bar{G}_f/\bar{G}_b = (P_m(ZF)^2c_{(1)}/RT)/(P_m(ZF)^2c_{(2)}/RT) = c_{(1)}/c_{(2)}$$

Since the slope of the curve defined by the G–H–K equation is always positive, $\bar{G}_f/\bar{G}_b$ is the maximum ratio that can be obtained. If we obtain a rectification in a biological membrane that is greater than $c_{(1)}/c_{(2)}$ (that is, $\bar{G}_f/\bar{G}_b$ as defined by equations (4.30) and (4.32)) then the rectification is not constant-field rectification.

When the constant-field equation becomes linear

Equations (4.31) and (4.33) are plotted on Figure 4.2b. They are straight lines which pass through the origin. This means that for large positive or negative voltages a constant-field process approximates to an ohmic one.

Another linear case of the G–H–K equation is when the concentration is the same on both sides of the membrane $(c_{(1)} = c_{(2)} = c)$. Equation (4.20a) now becomes

$$\bar{I} = P_m((ZF)^2 V/RT)(c\,\exp(ZFV/RT)-c)/(\exp(ZFV/RT)-1)$$
$$= P_m((ZF)^2 V/RT)c(\exp(ZFV/RT)-1)/(\exp(ZFV/RT)-1)$$
$$= P_m(ZF)^2 Vc/RT$$
$$= \bar{G}V \tag{4.33}$$

where

$$\bar{G} = P_m(ZF)^2 c/RT \tag{4.34}$$

Since all the terms in equation (4.34) are constant, including c, then $\bar{G}$ is constant, and so the I/V curve is linear. Equation (4.34) is similar to equations (4.32) and (4.30). Since $\bar{G}$ is constant (independent of voltage), equation (4.33) is a statement of Ohm's Law. (See Appendix 15 and Chapter 2.) Equation (4.33) is plotted in Figure 4.2b.

The constant-field equation at zero transmembrane potential

When $(V_{(1)} - V_{(2)})$ is very small (point A in Figure 4.2b), the term
$$(ZFV/RT)/(\exp(ZFV/RT)-1)$$
in equation (4.20a) becomes unity and $\exp((ZFV)/(RT)) \to 1$.

The term $((ZFV)/(RT))/(\exp(ZFV/RT)-1)$ is of the form
$$x/(\exp(x)-1)$$
where
$$x = ZFV/RT$$
and for small x, that is, for small V,
$$\exp(x) = 1 + x/1! + x^2/2! + \cdots + x^n/n!$$
so
$$x/(1+x-1) = x/x = 1$$
so
$$\bar{I} = P_m ZF(c_{(1)} - c_{(2)})$$
If we divide this equation by ZF we obtain
$$\bar{J} = P_m(c_{(1)} - c_{(2)}) = P_m\,\Delta c \tag{4.35}$$
which is a statement of Fick's First Law of diffusion for steady-state diffusion (see Chapter 3).

The constant-field equation at zero current

When the current $\bar{I}$ is zero (point B in Figure 4.2b) we are, by definition, at equilibrium. From the G–H–K equation (4.20a) the only condition when the current $\bar{I}$ is zero is when the terms inside the brackets
$$(c_{(1)}\exp(ZFV/RT) - c_{(2)})$$
sum to zero, that is
$$c_{(1)}\exp(ZFV/RT) - c_{(2)} = 0$$

or

$$\exp(ZFV/RT) = c_{(2)}/c_{(1)}$$

If we take natural logarithms of both sides and rearrange we obtain

$$V = (RT/ZF) \ln(c_{(2)}/c_{(1)})$$

V, that is $(V_{(1)} - V_{(2)})$, is now the equilibrium (Nernst) potential.

The constant-field equation for more than one ion current: the independence principle

So far we have been considering the movement of one ion across a membrane under the influence of an electrical potential and a concentration gradient. In living cells, membranes are permeable to more than one ion species and so the total ionic membrane current density is the sum of the individual ionic current densities. We can write the Nernst–Planck equation for each of the ions (sodium, potassium and chloride ions are the most important) as follows:

$$\bar{J}_{Na}F = \bar{I}_{Na} = -FD_{Na}[d(c_{Na})/dx + (F/RT)c_{Na}\,d(V)/dx]$$
$$\bar{J}_{K}F = \bar{I}_{K} = -FD_{K}[d(c_{K})/dx + (F/RT)c_{K}\,d(V)/dx] \tag{4.36}$$
$$-\bar{J}_{Cl}F = \bar{I}_{Cl} = FD_{Cl}[d(c_{Cl})/dx - (F/RT)c_{Cl}\,d(V)/dx]$$

The equations are derived from equation (3.13) by multiplying both sides by ZF and substituting 1 for Z in the first two and -1 for Z in the third since these values are the respective valencies.

Equations (4.36) can each be integrated with the assumptions used by Hodgkin and Katz to obtain equations (4.37) where U is defined as

$$U = FV/RT$$
$$\bar{I}_{Na} = FP_{Na}(U/(\exp(U)-1))(c_{Na,1}\exp(U) - c_{Na,2})$$
$$\bar{I}_{K} = FP_{K}(U/(\exp(U)-1))(c_{K,1}\exp(U) - c_{K,2}) \tag{4.37}$$
$$\bar{I}_{Cl} = FP_{Cl}(U/(\exp(U)-1))(c_{Cl,2}\exp(U) - c_{Cl,1})$$

Since the total ionic membrane current density is the sum of the individual ionic current densities, we can write

$$\bar{I}_{i} = \bar{I}_{Na} + \bar{I}_{K} + \bar{I}_{Cl}$$
$$= F(U/(\exp(U)-1))(X\exp(U) - Y) \tag{4.38}$$

where

$$X = P_{Na}c_{Na,1} + P_{K}c_{K,1} + P_{Cl}c_{Cl,2}$$

and

$$Y = P_{Na}c_{Na,2} + P_{K}c_{K,2} + P_{Cl}c_{Cl,1}$$

Equation (4.38) implies that the total ionic current $\bar{I}_{i}$ is the sum of three independent ionic currents ($\bar{I}_{Na}, \bar{I}_{K}, \bar{I}_{Cl}$). From equation (4.37) we can see that the same V occurs in all three currents. Thus the currents are effectively coupled through the membrane potential V. However, if V is independently controlled by means of an external circuit, and the ions cross the membrane through separate pathways, the currents become independent of one another. This is the basis of the experimental approach used by electro-physiologists in the analysis of membrane currents.

Although the G–H–K equation was derived assuming a steady-state (that is, the flux density was assumed to be the same at any point inside the membrane), it is frequently used under non-steady-state conditions, that is, when the membrane voltage or the membrane current is changing. For example, although the membrane voltage is constant under voltage-clamp conditions (see Chapter 5), the current density is changing all the time. Although this is a transient condition we assume a steady-state because there is never any sizeable accumulation or depletion of ions within the membrane. This is because the number of ions within the membrane is always very small and hence the charge density is negligible.

The resting membrane potential

When the total ionic membrane current density is zero, the membrane of an excitable cell is said to be in a 'resting state'. Individual ionic currents ($\bar{I}_{Na}$, $\bar{I}_{K}$, $\bar{I}_{Cl}$) may be flowing but the net membrane current ($\bar{I}_{i}$) is zero. Under these conditions equation (4.38) becomes

$$0 = (U/(\exp(U)-1))(X \exp(U) - Y) \tag{4.39}$$

Since numerically $U/(\exp(U)-1)$ can never be zero, then

$$X \exp(U) - Y = 0$$

or

$$X \exp(U) = Y \tag{4.40}$$

The Goldman–Hodgkin–Katz equation for the potential

If we rearrange equation (4.40) and take logarithms we obtain

$$U = \ln(Y/X)$$

or

$$V = (RT/F) \ln[(P_{Na}c_{Na,1} + P_{K}c_{K,1} + P_{Cl}c_{Cl,2})/$$
$$(P_{Na}c_{Na,2} + P_{K}c_{K,2} + P_{Cl}c_{Cl,1})] \tag{4.41}$$

Equation (4.41) is frequently rearranged as

$$V = (RT/F) \ln[(c_{Na,1} + \alpha_1 c_{K,1} + \alpha_2 c_{Cl,2})/(c_{Na,2} + \alpha_1 c_{K,2} + \alpha_2 c_{Cl,1})] \tag{4.42}$$

Where α_1 and α_2 are defined as the permeability ratios

$$\alpha_1 = P_{K}/P_{Na} \quad \text{and} \quad \alpha_2 = P_{Cl}/P_{Na} \tag{4.43}$$

Equations (4.41) and (4.42) give the resting membrane potential as a function of the concentrations of the ions on both sides of the membrane and of the ion permeabilities. The values of α_1 and α_2 for the resting squid axon are around 20 and 0.45 respectively.

The slope conductance

If we now return to Figure 4.2b we see, as pointed out above, that the I/V curve is not linear. Since we are not dealing with an ohmic conductance we need to say what is meant by conductance in the case of a non-linear I/V curve. One way of defining conductance is to consider the conductance at every point along the I/V curve. If we differentiate the I/V curve we obtain the local slope of this curve and this is known as the *slope conductance* (see Figure 4.3a). We can see from this figure that the curve of the slope conductance is always positive and has both a minimum and a maximum value.

To obtain the expression for the constant-field slope conductance we first start with equation (4.20a)

$$\bar{I} = ZFP_m((ZFV/RT)/\exp(ZFV/RT) - 1)(c_{(1)}\exp(ZFV/RT) - c_{(2)})$$

$$(4.20a)$$

If we make the substitution

$$U = ZFV/RT \qquad (4.44)$$

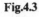

Fig.4.3

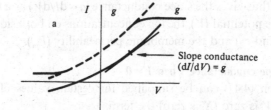

Slope conductance
$(\mathrm{d}I/\mathrm{d}V) = g$

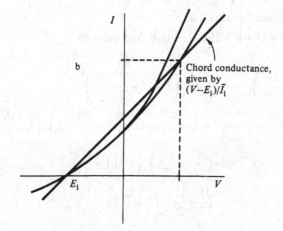

Chord conductance,
given by
$(V - E_i)/\bar{I}_i$

then equation (4.20a) becomes

$$\bar{I} = ZFP_m(U/(\exp(U)-1))(c_{(1)}\exp(U)-c_{(2)}) \tag{4.20b}$$

Differentiating this equation, we obtain from the chain-rule (see Appendix 2)

$$d\bar{I}/dV = (d\bar{I}/dU)(dU/dV) \tag{4.45}$$

Then

$$dU/dV = (d/dV)(ZFV/RT) = ZF/RT \tag{4.46}$$

and

$$d\bar{I}/dU = ZFP_m(d/dx)[(U/(\exp(U)-1))(c_{(1)}\exp(U)-c_{(2)})]$$
$$= ZFP_m[(c_{(1)}\exp(U)-c_{(2)})(d/dx)(U/(\exp(U)-1))$$
$$+ (U/(\exp(U)-1))(d/dx)(c_{(1)}\exp(U)-c_{(2)})]$$
$$= ZFP_m[(\exp(U)(1-U)-1)(c_{(1)}\exp(U)-c_{(2)})/(\exp(U)-1)^2$$
$$+ (U/(\exp(U)-1))c_{(1)}\exp(U)] \tag{4.47}$$

The full formula for the slope conductance

If we now substitute equations (4.46) and (4.47) in equation (4.45) we obtain

$$d\bar{I}/dV = \text{slope conductance} = ((ZF)^2 P_m/RT)$$
$$\times [(\exp(U)(1-U)-1)(c_{(1)}\exp(U)-c_{(2)})/$$
$$(\exp(U)-1)^2 + (U/(\exp(U)-1))c_{(1)}\exp(U)]$$

Equation (4.47) thus gives the slope conductance ($g = d\bar{I}/dV$) as a function of the membrane potential (V), the ion concentrations on both sides of the membrane (c_1 and c_2) and the membrane permeability (P_m).

The slope conductance when $V=0$

Equation (4.47) can be simplified for certain values of V. For example, when V is zero (X is zero) the term

$$(\exp(U)(1-U)-1)/(\exp(U)-1)^2$$

can be simplified, since for small X

$$\exp(U) = 1 + U + U^2/2! + \cdots \quad \text{(see Appendix 2)}$$

so for small U

$$\left(\left(1+U+\frac{U^2}{2!}\right)(1-U)-1\right)\bigg/\left(1+U+\frac{U^2}{2}-1\right)^2$$
$$= \left(1+U+\frac{U^2}{2!}-U-U^2-\frac{U^3}{2}-1\right)\bigg/\left(U+\frac{U^2}{2}\right)^2$$
$$= -\left(\frac{U^2}{2}+\frac{U^3}{2}\right)\bigg/\left(U^2\left(1+\frac{U}{2}\right)^2\right)$$
$$= -\left(\frac{1}{2}+\frac{U}{2}\right)\bigg/\left(1+\frac{U}{2}\right)^2$$

When X is zero this term is equal to $-\frac{1}{2}$ and the terms $U/(\exp(U)-1)$ and $\exp(U)=1$ when $U=0$. So equation (4.47), when $V=0$, becomes

$$d\bar{I}/dV_{(V=0)} \approx ((ZF)^2 P_m/RT)(-(1/2)(c_{(1)}-c_{(2)})+c_{(1)})$$

$$\approx [(ZF)^2 P_m/RT][(c_{(1)}+c_{(2)})/2] \tag{4.48}$$

Equation (4.48) shows that when the membrane potential (V) is zero the slope conductance depends equally on the concentrations of both compartments.

The slope conductance for V positive and very large

Another case is when X is very large and positive. Then e^x is much larger than 1 and so $c_1 e^x$ is much larger than c_2, thus equation (4.47) becomes

$$d\bar{I}/dV_{(V \gg 1)} = ((ZF)^2 P_m/RT)$$

$$\times [\exp(U)(1-U)c_{(1)} \exp(U)/\exp(2U)+Uc_{(1)}]$$

$$= ((ZF)^2 P_m/RT)(c_{(1)}-Uc_{(1)}+Uc_{(1)}) \tag{4.49}$$

$$= ((ZF)^2 P_m/RT)c_{(1)}$$

We note that equation (4.49) is the same as equation (4.30).

The slope conductance for V negative and very large

Finally, for a very large and negative V, $\exp(U)(1-U)$ and $\exp(U)$ become much smaller than 1 and so, $c_{(1)} \exp(U)$ becomes much smaller than $c_{(2)}$, then

$$d\bar{I}/dV = ((ZF)^2 P_m/RT)\left(\frac{-1}{(-1)^2}\right)(-c_{(2)}) = ((ZF)^2 P_m c_{(2)})/RT \tag{4.50}$$

we should also note that equation (4.50) is the same as equation (4.32).

As shown above for very large values of the membrane potential (negative or positive), the G–H–K equation for the current becomes a straight line. Equations (4.49), (4.50) and (4.32) are special conditions where the I/V curves are linear and so the slopes of the curves are constants.

Equations (4.47), (4.49) and (4.50) allow us to examine the relationship between conductance and permeability. For instance, if we take equation (4.49) and imagine a situation where there are two ions at different concentrations in compartment (1); we will let the membrane be more permeable to ion B than to ion A. If the concentration of A is much larger than B and if this means that the product $P_A c_{A,1}$ is larger than $P_B c_{B,1}$, it follows that the fraction of the membrane conductance due to A is larger than that due to B even though the membrane is more permeable to ion B.

The chord conductance

Another way of defining membrane conductances, which are used extensively in electrophysiology, is the membrane *chord conductance*.

This term is a special case of the general expression for chord conductance $\Delta V/\Delta I$ where the ΔV term is replaced by $V - E_i$ so that

$$\left(\begin{array}{l}\text{membrane}\\\text{chord}\\\text{conductance}\end{array}\right) G = (V - E_i)/\bar{I}_i$$

here V is the membrane potential, E_i is the equilibrium potential for ion i (Nernst potential) and $\bar{I}_i$ is the membrane current density of ion i (see Figure 4.3b).

If the I/V curve is linear, the conductance is independent of voltage (or current) and the chord conductance and slope conductance are equal.

Current flow at two different concentrations: scaling of the constant-field equation

Once we know the current at a given concentration the constant-field equation allows us to calculate the current density for an ion at different external concentrations. The way this is done is to take the ratio of equation (4.20) at two different concentrations ($c'_{(2)}$ and $c_{(2)}$) at the same membrane potential and internal concentration ($c_{(1)}$).

This is equivalent to measuring the current that flows through a membrane at two different concentrations in side 2. If $(ZFV/RT) = U$, then

$$\frac{\bar{I}'_i}{\bar{I}_i} = \frac{ZFUP_m(c_{(1)}\exp(U) - c'_{(2)})/(\exp(U) - 1)}{ZFUP_m(c_{(1)}\exp(U) - c_{(2)})/(\exp(U) - 1)} \tag{4.51}$$

provided that the membrane permeability P_m is independent of the current flow or of $c_{(2)}$. Equation (4.51) simplifies to

$$\frac{\bar{I}'_i}{\bar{I}_i} = \frac{c_{(1)}\exp(U) - c'_{(2)}}{c_{(1)}\exp(U) - c_{(2)}}$$

If we divide top and bottom by $c_{(2)}$ we obtain

$$\frac{\bar{I}'_i}{\bar{I}_i} = \frac{(c_{(1)}/c_{(2)})\exp(U) - c'_{(2)}/c_{(2)}}{(c_{(1)}/c_{(2)})\exp(U) - 1} \tag{4.52}$$

But when $\bar{I}_i$ is zero

$$c_{(1)}\exp(U) - c_{(2)} = 0$$

or

$$(c_{(1)}/c_{(2)}) = \exp(-U)$$
$$= \exp(-ZFV/RT) \tag{4.53}$$

and since V is now the Nernst potential (E_i), if we substitute (4.53) into (4.52) we obtain

$$\frac{I_i'}{I_i} = \frac{\exp((ZF/RT)(V-E_i)) - c_{(2)}'/c_{(1)}}{\exp((ZF/RT)(V-E_i)) - 1} \qquad (4.54)$$

or

$$I_i' = I_i \frac{\exp((ZF/RT)(V-E_i)) - c_{(2)}'/c_{(1)}}{\exp((ZF/RT)(V-E_i)) - 1} \qquad (4.55)$$

The independence principle

Equation (4.55) can also be derived by using the independence principle. The independence principle assumes that the net flux (J) of an ion through a membrane is the difference between two independent fluxes (an inward flux, $J_{(1)}$ and an outward flux, $J_{(-1)}$) and this implies that individual ions migrate independently through the membrane. This independence principle can be exemplified using the G–H–K equation. If the flux of an ion obeys the G–H–K equation and if the ions migrate independently through the membrane (that is, $J = J_{(1)} - J_{(-1)}$) then from equation (4.20) with $ZFV/RT = U$ we can write the net flux as

$$\bar{J} = \underbrace{P_m U c_{(1)} \exp(U)/(\exp(U)-1)}_{\bar{J}_{(1)}} - \underbrace{P_m U c_{(2)}/(\exp(U)-1)}_{\bar{J}_{(-1)}}$$

$$(4.56)$$

where $\bar{J}$ is now expressed as the difference between two fluxes in opposite directions $(\bar{J}_{(1)} - \bar{J}_{(-1)})$. This must be the case because $\bar{J}$ is a flux and as we are subtracting two terms, dimensionally, they must also be fluxes. So

$$\bar{J} = \bar{J}_{(1)} - \bar{J}_{(-1)} \qquad (4.56a)$$

where

$$\bar{J}_{(1)} = P_m U c_{(1)} \exp(U)/(\exp(U)-1)$$

and $$(4.56b)$$

$$\bar{J}_{(-1)} = P_m U c_{(2)}/(\exp(U)-1)$$

For a given membrane potential V, equations (4.56) can be written as

$$\bar{J}_{(1)} = k_{(1)} c_{(1)} \quad \text{and} \quad \bar{J}_{(-1)} = k_{(-1)} c_{(2)} \qquad (4.57)$$

These equations were originally used by Hodgkin and Huxley in their derivation of equation (4.55) or (4.65a). If we use the G–H–K equation, $k_{(1)}$ and $k_{(-1)}$ are given by the expressions from (4.56)

$$k_1 = P_m U \exp(U)/(\exp(U)-1) \quad \text{and} \quad k_{(-1)} = P_m U/(\exp(U)-1)$$

so

$$\frac{k_{(1)}}{k_{(-1)}} = \frac{P_m U \exp(U)/(\exp(U)-1)}{P_m U/(\exp(U)-1)} = \exp(U) = \exp(ZFV/RT) \quad (4.58)$$

If $c_{(2)}$ is the concentration at which there is no net flux ($c_{(2)} = c_{eq}$ and $\bar{J} = 0$)

then from (4.56b)

$$(c_{eq}/c_{(1)}) = \exp(U) = \exp(ZFV/RT) \tag{4.59}$$

Also the membrane potential (E_i) at which there is no net flux (Nernst equilibrium potential) is given by

$$(c_{(1)}/c_{(2)}) = \exp(-ZFE_i/RT) \tag{4.60}$$

From equation (4.56) the ratio between two fluxes (J' and J) measured at two different concentrations ($c'_{(2)}, c_{(2)}$) in compartment (2) is

$$\frac{J'}{J} = \frac{J_{(1)} - J'_{(-1)}}{J_{(1)} - J_{(-1)}} \tag{4.61}$$

If we divide top and bottom of the right-hand side of equation (4.61) by $J_{(-1)}$ we obtain

$$(J'/J) = [(J_{(1)}/J_{(-1)}) - (J'_{(-1)}/J_{(-1)})]/[(J_{(1)}/J_{(-1)}) - 1] \tag{4.62}$$

But from equation (4.57)

$$(J_{(1)}/J_{(-1)}) = (k_{(1)}c_{(1)})/(k_{(-1)}c_{(2)}) \tag{4.63}$$

If we substitute (4.58) and (4.60) into (4.63) we obtain

$$(J_{(1)}/J_{(-1)}) = \exp(ZFV/RT)\exp(-ZFE_i/RT)$$
$$= \exp((ZF/RT)(V - E_i)) \tag{4.64}$$

Also by analogy with equation (4.63)

$$J'_{(-1)}/J_{(-1)} = (k_{(-1)}c'_{(2)})/(k_{(-1)}c_{(2)}) = (c'_{(2)}/c_{(2)}) \tag{4.65}$$

If we now substitute (4.64) and (4.65) into (4.62) we obtain

$$J'/J = (\exp(U_i) - (c'_{(2)}/c_{(2)}))/(\exp(U_i) - 1)$$
$$= (ZFJ')/(ZFJ) = \bar{I}'_i/\bar{I}_i \tag{4.65a}$$

where

$$U_i = ZF(V - E_i)/RT$$

which is the same equation as (4.55).

Computation of the membrane permeability

The G–H–K equation can also be used to compute the membrane permeability (P_m) for an ion species.

Rearranging equation (4.20a) and defining $U = ZFV/RT$, then

$$P_m = \bar{I}_i/ZFU((c_{(1)}\exp(U) - c_{(2)})/(\exp(U) - 1)) \tag{4.66}$$

In Chapter 3 we showed that the dimensions of permeability are $cm \cdot s^{-1}$. This is apparent from equation (4.19) and also from the dimensional analysis of equation (4.66). In this equation the exponential term is dimensionless (see Appendix 1). In dimensional terms equation (4.66) reduces to

$$P_m(\text{dimensions}) = \frac{\text{current density}}{\text{charge per mole} \cdot \text{concentration}}$$
$$= \text{coul} \cdot \text{cm}^{-2} \cdot \text{s}^{-1} / \text{coul} \cdot \text{mol} \cdot \text{mol}^{-1} \cdot \text{cm}^{-3}$$
$$= \text{cm} \cdot \text{s}^{-1}$$

In Chapter 8 we shall discuss in more detail electrophysiological applications of the constant-field equation.

5

Membranes, channels, carriers and pumps

Regulation of composition and volume of biological compartments

Living organisms consist of a large number of interdependent fluid compartments (see Chapter 2) and these compartments are bounded by membranes which perform at least two major functions. The first of these is to act as a physical barrier so as to impede the free movement of particles between adjacent compartments. These particles consist of intracellular organelles (for example, mitochondria), macromolecules that exist both intra- and extracellularly (for example, proteins) and small polar molecules (such as water) and ions. The second is that membranes, since they are not passive and impermeable, are able to regulate the volume and composition of the intracellular environment. This regulation means that the composition and volume of the intracellular and extracellular compartments are maintained at constant values despite fluctuations in the external environment.

Membranes regulate the composition of compartments by being selectively permeable. They are also able to utilize free energy (that is stored either in ATP high-energy bonds or in concentration gradients) to transport ions and molecules against electrochemical or chemical potential gradients (see Chapter 3 for discussion of these gradients. For a discussion of free energy see Appendix 25).

Coupling mechanisms in membrane transport

This so-called 'uphill' transport against gradients is possible because membranes contain specialized molecular complexes which are able to couple chemical reactions (for example, $ATP \rightleftharpoons ADP + Pi + free$ energy) to ion fluxes. These complexes are also able to couple ion movements down an electrochemical gradient ('downhill' movements) with the uphill flux of ions or small molecules. For example, the Na/Ca exchange in some excitable cells and Na–glucose co-transport that exists in intestinal cells. It follows then that a study of the molecular structure of membranes is important for our understanding of the way in which membranes function.

Chemical composition of biological membranes

The main molecular constituents of biological membranes are lipids and proteins. The lipids are either amphiphilic molecules or cholesterol (or the derivatives of cholesterol). Amphiphilic molecules contain polar heads (which are able to interact strongly with water) and one or more, usually two, aliphatic chains that are strongly hydrophobic. The two main types of amphiphilic molecules are phospholipids and plasma-logens and both molecules contain phosphate. The head group of the amphiphilic molecules bears the phosphate radicals and is either ionic or neutral polar. While ions bear a net positive (cations) or negative (anions) charge, neutral polar molecules are neutral. But they have an asymmetrical distribution of charge and so become oriented in electrical or magnetic fields.

An example of a polar molecule is water. Because $O - H$ bonds are not in opposition, and because the electronegativity of oxygen is higher than that of hydrogen, the oxygen part of the molecule is partially electronegative. In order to conserve charge the hydrogens of the molecule become partially electropositive

$$
\begin{array}{cc}
\text{H} & \text{H} \\
{}^{+\delta/2}\diagdown & \diagup {}^{+\delta/2} \\
& \text{O}-\delta
\end{array}
$$

Interaction between phospholipids and water

Because the phosphate-containing head groups are polar, these head groups interact electrostatically with water molecules, which are themselves polar molecules (see Figure 5.1a). The tails of the amphiphilic molecules are hydrophobic, so any induced electrostatic interaction that might occur with the water molecules is less than the electrostatic interaction that exists between the water molecules (Figure 5.1b). Because of these electrostatic forces when these phosphate-containing molecules are placed in contact with water their tails become excluded from the water phase. At least three types of molecular arrangements are thus possible when amphiphilic molecules, such as phospholipids, are mixed with aqueous media.

Forms of aggregation of phospholipids in water: monolayers

When the amount of phospholipid in the mixture is very small, the phospholipid molecules form a single layer (monolayer) at the aqueous–air interface (Figure 5.1c). Here the polar heads interact with the water molecules while the fatty-acid chains are in contact with air. These monolayers will spread to fill any available area because of the electrostatic repulsion that occurs between the polar heads. As the number of phospholipid molecules per unit area increases, the aliphatic chains become

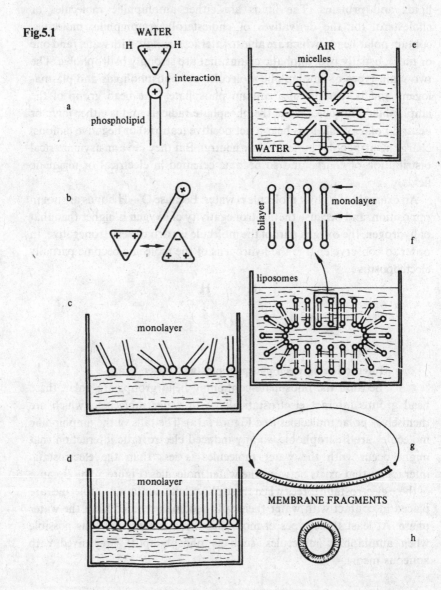

Fig.5.1

less able to move and they become more and more perpendicularly oriented to the water surface until they are so close that they attract each other by van der Waals' forces (Figure 5.1d; see also below).

Micelles

When the phospholipid content of the mixture is much higher a different type of arrangement takes place. Now 'micelles' are formed with the aliphatic chains pointing inwards to the interior of the micelle while the polar heads are in contact with the water phase.

Bilayers – liposomes and microsomes

A third arrangement occurs at even higher concentrations of phospholipids and lipid bilayers are formed (Figure 5.1e). In a bilayer the polar heads are in contact with the water phase while the aliphatic chains are packed parallel to one another (see Figure 5.1e, f). Because the lipid 'core' is hydrophobic it is excluded from the water phase and so lipid bilayers spontaneously round up and form stable vesicles (Figure 5.1g, h).

Gorter and Grundel's experiment

In a classical experiment, Gorter and Grundel produced phospholipid monolayers from red blood cell membranes and showed that the monolayer area was roughly twice the total membrane area from which the lipids were extracted. This experiment shows that cell membranes are composed of lipid bilayers. Because bilayers round up, fragments of biological membranes are always found in vesicular form (these vesicles are known as microsomes).

A study of the aggregation process that takes place when the number of molecules per unit area increases above a certain level allows us to infer some of the physical properties of the lipid core of lipid bilayers. Since biological membranes are lipid bilayers, this implies that with this type of study we can make some statements about the nature of biological membranes.

Phase transitions: surface pressure

The aggregation process is best examined in a Langmuir trough (Figure 5.2a, b). Here a monolayer can be produced by depositing a small amount of phospholipid on the surface of water (or an aqueous solution). If the number of molecules of phospholipid per unit area is sufficiently low (one molecule per 5000 Å^2) the monolayer, because it is a sheet of constant thickness, behaves as if it were a gas in two dimensions, x and y. This means that the monolayers will exert a pressure on the boundaries and, since the

Fig.5.2

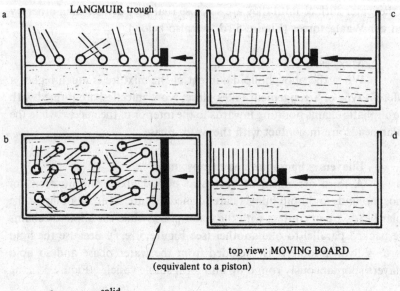

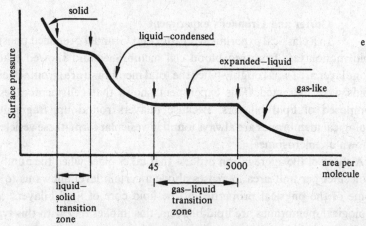

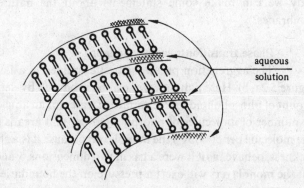

pressure is only in two dimensions, it is called a surface pressure. Since we are dealing with a perimeter the units of pressure will be force per unit length. This force can be measured if one of the sides of the trough is allowed to move (Figure 5.2b). In Figure 5.2b a known force is applied to the moving board and Figure 5.2a, c, d show diagrammatically the effect of compressing the monolayer. The surface pressure will rise as the molecular density of the monolayer rises (that is, the number of molecules per unit area or area available per phospholipid molecule). The behaviour of a monolayer undergoing compression is shown in Figure 5.2e. As the surface pressure is increased the gaseous-type monolayer changes into a liquid type and finally into a solid type. There are specific pressures (see Figure 5.2e) at which these transitions occur. Biological membranes have a phospholipid density of around one molecule per 60 Å^2, which implies that they are in the liquid-like state in the transition zone. It should be emphasized that in the transition zone the monolayer is neither a gas nor a liquid.

Temperature-dependence of phase transitions

The transition zone is a function of temperature because the curve shifts along the pressure axis (Figure 5.2e) and changes shape with temperature. This temperature effect is also seen in biological membranes and is reflected in changes in membrane conductance that occur with temperature. Electrophysiologists call the temperature at which these conductance changes take place the *transition temperature.*

Lipid bilayers as experimental models of biological membranes: liposomes and black lipid membranes

Experimentally lipid bilayers may be produced either from synthetic lipids or from lipids extracted from membranes. When the amount of phospholipids added to an aqueous solution exceeds a certain value, bilayers are formed (see above). These bilayers might form either closed tubes or concentric spheroids called *liposomes* (Figure 5.2f). Sonication of liposomes produces smaller vesicles, whose walls are single bilayers.

Another way to obtain artificial bilayers is to dissolve phospholipids in an organic solvent. This solution is then painted over a small hole (1 mm) in a sheet of a strongly hydrophobic material (such as Teflon) that is under water and separates two aqueous compartments. The organic solvent partitions into the water and evaporates from the water surface. This process continues until a lipid bilayer covers the hole. Membranes formed in this way do not reflect light (because their thickness (5–7 nm) is less than the wavelength of visible light (300–700 nm) and are known as *black lipid membranes* (BLM).

Both liposomes and BLMs have been used extensively in the study of membrane phenomena. Although liposomes are easy to produce and have been used to study permeability, they have a serious experimental drawback in that their inside compartment is inaccessible. But with a BLM both compartments are accessible and so their physical properties can readily be measured. One of the interesting properties of BLMs is that the electrical capacity is found to be similar to the electrical capacity of biological membranes (around $1 \, \mu F \cdot cm^{-2}$).

Permeability of lipid bilayers: fluidity

It is also found that the permeability of the BLMs depends upon their composition. For example, when they are made of unsaturated phospholipids they are more permeable to lipid-soluble substances. In unsaturated phospholipids the aliphatic chains have one or more double bonds. For example, the aliphatic chain oleic acid has one double bond while that of the linoleic acid has two double bonds. Since double bonds prevent the aliphatic chains from stretching out, this means that the chains cannot be packed tightly and so chain interaction is less and the membrane is more fluid. This, then, could explain why unsaturated lipid bilayers are more permeable to lipid-soluble substances, since lipid substances will diffuse more readily through more fluid membrane.

The fluidity of biological membranes was demonstrated clearly by Frey and Edidin when they fused human and mouse cells. Some time after fusion, human and mouse antigens were seen to intermingle completely (the antigens were revealed by reacting them with labelled fluorescent antibodies) (see Figure 5.3).

Fig.5.3

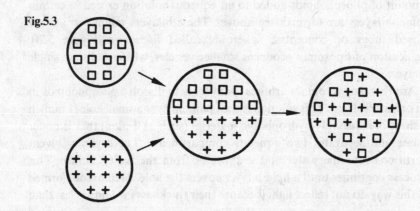

Cholesterol in lipid bilayers

This fluidity of biological membranes is also related to the amount of cholesterol that is within the membrane. Structurally the ring of the cholesterol molecules sits near the polar heads and causes the aliphatic chains to extend in this area (see Figure 5.4). Since the cholesterol steroid ring is rigid it restricts the natural movements of the neighbouring aliphatic chains. This means that the outer part of the lipid becomes less flexible so an increase in the cholesterol concentration of a membrane will result in a decrease in its fluidity. This effect of cholesterol may play a role in nature. Channel-forming antibiotics such as Nystatin only work in cholesterol-containing membranes, and it is possible that the membrane rigidity induced by cholesterol may allow greater stability for the pores.

Flip-flopping of phospholipids in lipid bilayers

The above experiment of Frey and Edidin also shows that cholesterol-containing membranes (such as the plasma membrane of red blood cells) still allows lateral diffusion. However, the phospholipids of lipid bilayers cannot easily jump from one side of the membrane to the other (so-called flip-flopping). This is because polar heads cannot easily pass through the lipid core. As the transport of substances through the membrane is thus unlikely to be due to flip-flopping, we have to postulate other mechanisms. Overton, at the turn of this century, and later on Collander, showed that lipid-soluble substances readily penetrate biological membranes, which suggests that one transmembrane pathway is via the lipid layer.

Fig.5.4

CHOLESTEROL

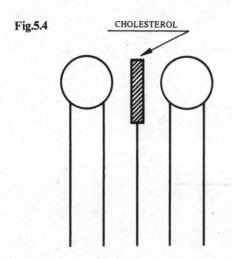

The mechanism of permeation in lipid bilayers: the partition–diffusion model

The simplest model for the translation of a molecule across a membrane via a lipid pathway would involve three steps. The first would be partition of the molecule from a water compartment into the lipid phase. The second step would be diffusion across this lipid layer, and the third would be partition into the water phase of the other compartment (Figure 5.5). Mathematically these three steps can be described as shown below.

First step

In step one the molecule jumps from the solution (1) into the adjacent membrane face or jumps out of this face back into solution (1). The simplest model is to assume that the flux of a molecule into the membrane is proportional to its concentration in the bathing fluid that

$$J \propto c \quad \text{or} \quad J = kc$$

where k is the proportionality or rate constant. This is an example of a first-order reaction. But since, at the same time, there is a back flux of molecules out of the membrane, to obtain the net flux we have to write a similar expression for the back flux. The overall reaction is thus equivalent to a first-order reaction with a forward rate constant (k_{sm}) and a backward rate constant (k_{ms}). The net flow per unit area of membrane from compartment

Fig.5.5

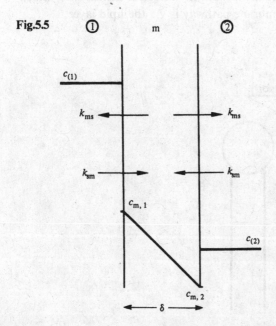

(1) into the membrane ($\bar{J}_{(1)}$) is then given by

$$\bar{J}_{(1)} = k_{sm}c_{(1)} - k_{ms}c_{m,1} \tag{5.1}$$

where k_{sm} is the forward rate constant and k_{ms} is the backward rate constant. Equation (5.1) describes the net flow ($\bar{J}_{(1)}$) from compartment (1) into the membrane and $c_{(1)}$ and $c_{m,1}$ are respectively the concentrations of molecules in compartment (1) and in the membrane near the membrane solution interphase on side (1).

Second step

Membranes are so thin that we can consider step two as being in a steady-state (see Chapter 4 for a discussion of this). Thus the concentration profile (dc_m/dx) is constant with time and, for an homogeneous membrane, we can write from Fick's Law (see Chapter 3) that

$$\bar{J}_{(2)} = (D_m/\delta)(c_{m,1} - c_{m,2}) \tag{5.2}$$

where $c_{m,1}$ and $c_{m,2}$ are the concentrations of the substance in the membrane at both interphases. D_m is the diffusion coefficient in the membrane and δ is the membrane thickness.

Third step

The equation for step three is similar to equation (5.1), that is,

$$\bar{J}_{(3)} = k_{ms}c_{m,2} - k_{sm}c_{(2)} \tag{5.3}$$

$c_{(1)}$ and $c_{(2)}$ in equations (5.2) and (5.3) are the concentrations in compartments (1) and (2) respectively.

At steady-state

$$\bar{J}_{(1)} = \bar{J}_{(2)} = \bar{J}_{(3)} = \bar{J} \tag{5.4}$$

We are able to relate the flux per unit area, $\bar{J}$, to the measurable concentrations $c_{(1)}$ and $c_{(2)}$ because the values of $c_{m,1}$ and $c_{m,2}$ can be obtained from equations (5.1), (5.3) and (5.4).

$$c_{m,1} = (k_{sm}/k_{ms})c_{(1)} - \bar{J}/k_{ms} \quad \text{and} \quad c_{m,2} = (k_{sm}/k_{ms})c_{(2)} + \bar{J}/k_{ms}$$

But the ratio k_{sm}/k_{ms} is the equilibrium constant (K) of reactions (5.1) and (5.3). If we rewrite equation (5.1),

$$\bar{J}_{(1)} - k_{sm}c_{(1)} + k_{ms}c_{m,1} = 0$$

As the unidirectional fluxes are much greater than $\bar{J}_{(1)}$ (the net flux per unit area of membrane)

$$-k_{sm}c_{(1)} + k_{ms}c_{m,1} \approx 0$$

This is the case when step two is rate-limiting (that is, much slower than the unidirectional fluxes in steps one and three). At equilibrium, there is no net flux $(\bar{J}=0)$ so

$$(c_{m,1}/c_{(1)})=(k_{sm}/k_{ms})=K$$

where K is the equilibrium constant also known as the *partition coefficient*. So

$$c_{m,1}=Kc_{(1)}-\bar{J}/k_{ms} \quad \text{and} \quad c_{m,2}=Kc_{(2)}+\bar{J}/k_{ms} \tag{5.5}$$

If we substitute equations (5.4) and (5.5) into equation (5.2) we obtain

$$\bar{J}=(D_m/\delta)(Kc_{(1)}-\bar{J}/k_{ms}-Kc_{(2)}-\bar{J}/k_{ms})$$

$$=(D_mK/\delta)(c_{(1)}-c_{(2)})-(2D_m/\delta)(\bar{J}/k_{ms})$$

$$\bar{J}(1+2D_m/\delta k_{ms})=(D_mK/\delta)(c_{(1)}-c_{(2)})$$

$$\bar{J}=(D_mK/\delta)(c_{(1)}-c_{(2)})/(1+2D_m/\delta k_{ms}) \tag{5.6}$$

The limiting case when diffusion within the membrane is rate-limiting

This equation may be simplified if we assume that

$$2D_m \ll k_{ms} \tag{5.7}$$

so that

$$\bar{J}=(D_mK/\delta)(c_{(1)}-c_{(2)}) \tag{5.8}$$

Permeability of lipid bilayers

The term D_mK/δ has the dimensions $(\text{cm}\cdot\text{s}^{-1})$ of a permeability as described in Chapter 3 and was used in the derivation of the G–H–K equation (Chapter 4). So

$$P_m=D_mK/\delta \tag{5.9}$$

It is possible to measure P_m experimentally with radioisotopes (see Appendix 30) and δ can be inferred from measurements of membrane capacity (see Appendix 24). However, D_m, the diffusion coefficient in the membrane, and K, the partition coefficient between an aqueous compartment and the membrane lipid core cannot be measured directly. The values of D_m and K can be obtained as reasonable approximations from experiments carried out with hydrocarbons. In these measurements the hydrocarbon phase is assumed to represent the membrane lipid core. P_m calculated from equation (5.9) using these values agrees with the experimental measurements of P_m. This means that the assumption made in equation (5.7) is a reasonable one.

Ion permeabilities of lipid bilayers

The partition of small ions into lipids is so small that it is virtually unmeasurable. This is because an enormous energy is needed to transfer an ion from water which has a high dielectric constant $(\varepsilon=80)$ into a lipid which has a low dielectric constant ($\varepsilon \approx 2$–5). The permeability of lipid bilayers to small ions is thus very small (equation (5.9)) because K is very small. This means that at any instant in time the membrane ion concentration is extremely low; this also means that the voltage profile is almost linear (see Chapter 4 and Appendix 22), and that the membrane current can be described by the constant-field equation. It was shown in Chapter 4 that if the constant-field equation applies and if the ion concentration c_i is the same on both sides of the membrane, the membrane conductance is given by

$$\bar{G} = (ZF)^2 P_m c_i / RT \tag{5.10}$$

The value of $\bar{G}$ for lipid bilayers bathed on both sides by 0.1 M NaCl (or KCl solutions) is 10^{-9} to 10^{-8} S·cm^{-2}. $\bar{G}$ is measured by applying a voltage across the BLM and measuring the current flowing through it. For voltages between -100 and $+100$ mV this relationship is approximately linear, so

$$\bar{I} = \bar{G}V$$

in agreement with the constant-field equation for equal concentrations on both sides. From equation (5.10) and for $Z = \pm 1$

$$P_m = \bar{G}RT/(F^2 c_i) = (10^{-9} \times 8.3 \times 298)/(96\,500^2 \times 10^{-4})$$
$$= 2.7 \times 10^{-12} \text{ cm·s}^{-1}$$

Ionophores

From equation (5.9) one can see that membranes can be made more permeable to ions by increasing K or D. K may be increased by incorporating in the membranes hydrophobic molecules which have hydrophilic centres. When an ion combines with one of these molecules it surrounds itself with a hydrophobic atmosphere and so becomes soluble in the lipid core of the membrane. This increase in lipid mobility can be demonstrated in partition experiments between bulk lipid and aqueous phases. An example of such molecule is the antibiotic Valinomycin (see Figure 5.6) which makes lipid bilayers and natural membranes more

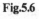
Fig.5.6

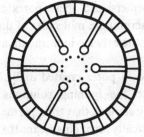

permeable to potassium. As a result of this increase in permeability, the potassium conductance increases by orders of magnitude in proportion to both the antibiotic and to the potassium concentrations.

The relationship between permeability and conductance channels

We should point out that an increase in permeability to an ion does not necessarily mean that there is a concomitant increase in conductance. A conductance (G or g) is always obtained from an I/V curve. If the permeability of a membrane is measured from flux experiments, it is given by

$$R_K = \bar{J}_K / c_K$$

But the experimentally measured flux per unit area, $\bar{J}_K$, is the total unidirectional flux which may be the sum of more than one component. For example, it may consist of a diffusional flux to which the constant-field equation applies and another flux. This other flux might, for example, be an electrically neutral exchange of K^+ by H^+ that is performed by an antibiotic incorporated in the membrane. If the membrane is bathed on both sides by the same solution and if one of the compartments (compartment (1), for example) is labelled with radioactive potassium, the potassium permeability (P_K) is given by

$$P_K = \bar{J}_K^* / c_K^*   \text{(see Appendix 30)}$$

where $\bar{J}_K^*$ is the flux of radioactive potassium into compartment (2) (for example) and c_K^* is the concentration of radioactive potassium in compartment (1). We can also measure the conductance G_K from an I/V curve obtained across the membrane (see Chapter 5). With this conductance we are able to compute a diffusional permeability P_K^D by equation (4.10) (see Chapter 4, where this equation is derived for the special case of diffusion assuming a constant field across the membrane).

The permeability P_K is different from the calculated permeability P_K^D and can be expressed as

$$P_K^D = P_K^D + P_K^E$$

where P_K^E could be due to the antibiotic neutral exchange

If a hole is made in the membrane (pore) this is equivalent to increasing both K and D_m. K is increased because the pore creates a transmembrane water environment (the inside of the pore). Diffusion then occurs from one aqueous environment (compartment (1)) through the pore into the other aqueous compartment (compartment (2)). D_m then must also be different because the diffusion takes place not through the lipid phase but through an aqueous phase.

A number of antibiotics are pore formers and these pores can be examined by studying their ability to discriminate molecules of different diameters (*sieve effect*) or by studying their behaviour in an applied electrical field.

The sieve effect has often been studied in pores created in BLMs by adding Nystatin or Amphotericin B to the bathing solutions. Flux measurements in BLMs doped in this way showed that their permeability to molecules above a certain size was practically zero. This means that there are probably holes in the membrane with specific internal diameters which exclude molecules that have diameters larger than those of the holes.

The kinetics of pore formation

Experimentally, it was found that the antibiotic-dependent permeability to water or other small molecules was linearly related to the antibiotic-dependent conductance. A simple interpretation of these experiments is to assume that both water and ions cross the membrane through the same channels. Furthermore, experimentally the conductance of the doped BLM was proportional to the nth power of the antibiotic concentration (A in $mol \cdot cm^{-3}$) in the bathing solution. That is

$$\bar{G} \propto (A)^n \tag{5.11}$$

where $\bar{G}$ is the membrane conductance (per unit area). If we assume that the antibiotic partitions into the membrane, its concentration in the lipid core is related by the partition coefficient K'

$$K' = [A_m]/[A] \tag{5.12}$$

where $[A_m]$ is moles of antibiotic per unit area. K' can be converted into the dimensionless conventional partition coefficient (K) by dividing it by the membrane thickness δ in cm. The dimensions of A_m are $mol/cm^2 = (mol/cm^3) \cdot cm$, so $K' = ((mol/cm^3) \cdot cm)/(mol/cm^3) = cm$ and $K = (mol/cm^3)/(mol/cm^3) = $ dimensionless.

Furthermore, if we assume that a pore is formed when n molecules of A_m combine, then we can write

$$A + A + \cdots + A \rightleftharpoons (A)_n \quad \text{gives a pore} \tag{5.13}$$

where $(A)_n$ is the complex that results from the combination of n molecules of A. We can also write

$$\bar{G} \propto [A_m]^n$$

or

$$\bar{G} = G_p[A_m]^n \tag{5.14}$$

where G_p is the conductance per pore and $[A_m]^n$ is the nth power of the concentration of pores per cm^2. Dimensionally equation (5.14) can be written as $\bar{G}(= Siemens \cdot cm^{-2}) = G \cdot$ number of pores $\cdot cm^{-2}$ so G_p the proportional constant must be equal to

$$G_p = \frac{Siemens \cdot cm^{-2}}{number\ of\ pores \cdot cm^{-2}} = Siemens/pore$$

If we rearrange equation (5.12) we obtain

$$[A_m] = K'[A] \tag{5.15}$$

If we now substitute (5.15) into (5.14) we arrive at

$$\bar{G} = G_p K'^n[A]^n$$

which is equivalent to (5.11). The implication of the experimental finding that the conductance $\bar{G}$ is proportional to $[A]^n$ is that pores are formed as a result of the association of n antibiotic molecules (for Figure 5.7, $n = 12$). For any given antibiotic concentration the induced conductance is ohmic and this implies that the pore-formation process (equation (5.13)) is independent of the electrical field across the membrane.

Fig.5.7   Pore formation

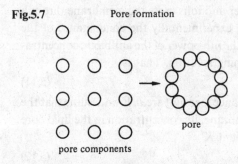

pore components

Pore selectivity

The ion selectivity of the channels may depend upon whether the antibiotic is added to one or both sides of the membrane. If Nystatin is added to one side of the membrane the pore that it forms is cation selective. If the drug is added to both sides of a BLM the membrane becomes permeable to anions (such as chloride). This is an interesting observation because we see the same molecules forming two different selective channels, probably as a result of different intramembrane aggregation.

Fluctuations in membrane conductance

When BLMs are doped with Gramicidin A (another antibiotic) the conductance also increases as a power function of the drug concentration. The pore is probably formed from the combination of two molecules (dimer) as $n = 2$. The molecules are short polypeptides. An interesting feature of this drug is that at very low concentrations very small fluctuations of membrane conductance can be observed in a voltage-clamped BLM (see Figure 5.8). These fluctuations consist of square current pulses, and each pulse is of the same amplitude and duration. For Gramicidin the current pulses are due to elemental conductance changes of about 5×10^{-12} S. Multiple combinations of these 'unit conductances' occur when the drug concentration is increased.

Membrane noise

This implies that for any one instant in time more than one channel is present and conducting. For a given concentration of the antibiotic we either obtain single or multiple combinations of the unit conductances, and because of this we have to talk about the average conductance of a Gramicidin-doped BLM. The instantaneous value of membrane conductance will then fluctuate around this mean value. These fluctuations of an electrical parameter (voltage, current or conductance) around its mean value are known as *noise* and the fluctuations observed with Gramicidin-doped BLM (see Figure 5.8) are a type of membrane noise.

Voltage-dependent conductances

Another class of antibiotics show elemental conductance changes that depend not only on the concentration of the drug but also on the voltage applied across the doped BLM. It can be shown experimentally that the average conductance of a BLM doped with a fixed amount of Alamethicin or Monazomycin increases exponentially with the applied transmembrane voltage and also with nth power of the antibiotic concentration ($n = 6$ for Alamethicin and 5 for Monazomycin). We can thus write

$$\bar{G} \propto [\text{A}]^n e^{BV}$$

where B is a constant (dimensions V^{-1}). The voltage dependence of $\bar{G}$ could be due to the electrical field across the membrane increasing the rate of formation of channels, or it may increase the length of time that a channel is on, or the field may do both.

Voltage-dependent channels in excitable membranes

In Chapters 7 and 8 we will analyse in detail the voltage dependence of channels in excitable cells. These naturally occurring

Fig.5.8

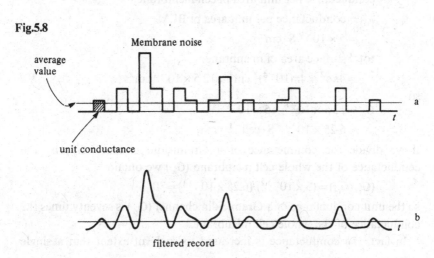

Membrane noise

average value

unit conductance

a

filtered record

b

channels resemble the synthetically formed antibiotic channels in BLMs and many of the inferences that have been made about naturally-occurring channels have come from the experiments of the type described here. This does not mean, however, that the channels in doped BLMs are identical with those found in excitable cells although, interestingly enough, the unit conductances of these artificial channels are similar to those in naturally-occurring membranes.

The conductance of an undoped lipid bilayer bathed by 0.1 M salt is around 10^{-9}–10^{-8} S·cm^{-2}. With the aid of a simple calculation we can show that a single pore in the whole membrane of a cell dramatically increases the conductance of whole membrane.

We can assume that the conductance of a BLM is similar to the conductance of the lipid pathway of a natural membrane. With this assumption we are able to calculate the number of channels (per unit area of membrane) which is roughly equivalent to a conductance of around 5×10^{-9} S·cm^{-2}. As referred to above, the conductance of a Gramicidin channel is around 5×10^{-12} S·channel^{-1}. Thus for a conductance of 5×10^{-9} S,

$$\text{number of channels of membrane per cm}^2$$
$$= (5 \times 10^{-9} \text{ S·cm}^{-2})/(5 \times 10^{-12} \text{ S·channel}^{-1})$$
$$= 10^3 \text{ channel·cm}^{-2}$$

If we take a spherical cell of 10 μm radius and 12.5×10^{-6} cm^2 surface area the conductance G_m will be given by

G_m = conductance per unit area ($\bar{G}$) times total surface area of membrane

conductance per unit area of cell membrane

= conductance per unit area of BLM

$$= 5 \times 10^{-9} \text{ S·cm}^{-2}$$

total surface area of membrane

$$= 4\pi a^2 = 4\pi(10^{-4})^2 \text{ cm}^2 \approx 12.5 \times 10^{-6} \text{ cm}^2$$

so

$$G_m = 12.5 \times 10^{-6} \times 5 \times 10^{-9}$$
$$= 6.25 \times 10^{-14} \text{ S·cell}^{-1}$$

If we divide the conductance of a Gramicidin channel (G_{gr}) by the conductance of the whole cell membrane (G_m) we obtain

$$(G_{gr}/G_m) = (5 \times 10^{-12})/(6.25 \times 10^{-14}) = 70$$

so the unit conductance of a Gramicidin channel (G_{gr}) is seventy times the conductance of the whole cell membrane.

In fact, the conductance is increased to such an extent that a single channel conductance represents almost the total membrane conductance of the cell.

Carriers and pores in natural membranes

Since cell membranes usually have higher permeabilities to ions and polar molecules when compared with undoped BLMs, cells must have specialized mechanisms that increase membrane permeability. These mechanisms may be either carriers or pores and, in practice, it is often difficult to differentiate one from another. The ideal way would be to isolate the molecules or molecular complexes that give rise to these phenomena and to study them in the way that was described above for antibiotics and BLMs. Since there are usually so few channels per unit area of membrane, it is very difficult to isolate them and the distinction between pores and carriers must then be attempted by other means. For instance, calculations of the type described in Chapter 7 show that the number of ions that cross a given conducting site in the membrane is very large. This is a good indication of a pore rather than a carrier because it is difficult to conceive that a single carrier could shuttle forwards and backwards across the membrane almost a million times per second. Another good indicator of the presence of the pore is that the cell membranes have unit-conductance events of the type seen in BLMs doped with Gramicidin. The way in which these unit-conductance events can be studied in cell membranes is discussed in Chapter 7. However, if unit-conductance events cannot be demonstrated, this does not necessarily mean that pores are not present, since their unit conductances or their lifetime may be too small to measure.

Uphill transport

Both carriers and pores are able to increase by orders of magnitude the membrane permeability to ions or polar molecules, but in general they cannot generate concentration gradients across membranes. This is because to generate a gradient an input of free energy (see Appendix 25) is required and the carriers and pores are simply passive elements that sit within the membrane.

In nature, however, every membrane separates compartments of different compositions. Many of the components of these solutions have chemical (for non-charged molecules) or electrochemical (for charged molecules) steady-state gradients. In order to generate and maintain these steady-state gradients there are specialized mechanisms which are able to move solutes against their chemical or electrochemical gradients. The source of free energy for such uphill-transport mechanisms is either the breakdown of ATP or the electrochemical gradient of another ion or polar molecule.

Pumps

When the uphill transport of an ion is directly coupled to the breakdown of ATP, the transport system is known as a '*pump*'. There are several well-known pump systems in biology and probably the best known is the Na/K pump that is found in most animal cells. In the red blood cell this pump exchanges three sodiums for two potassiums per ATP molecule split.

Flux-coupling mechanisms

When the *uphill* transport of molecules is driven by an electrochemical gradient of an ion, there is a specialized mechanism which couples the flux *downhill* of the ion to the uphill flux of the molecule. This process is known as *flux coupling*. A number of flux-coupling mechanisms exist in animal cells. An example is the sodium-driven glucose uptake of the small intestine.

Although kinetics of some of these flux-coupling transporters are known, the underlying molecular events still remain elusive. An *in vitro* example of a flux-coupling transport can be elegantly demonstrated by showing that the movement of water through a Gramicidin channel in a BLM caused by the chemical potential gradient of water can generate an electrical potential across the membrane.

Conventionally when there is a chemical potential gradient for water one says that there is an osmotic gradient. A chemical potential gradient for water between two solutions exists when they contain different amounts of solute. The more concentrated solution is said to exert a higher osmotic pressure (across a semi-permeable membrane) than the more dilute solution. The more concentrated solution has the lower chemical potential.

The key to this experiment is that initially a permeant ion exists at the same concentration on either side of the BLM. An osmotic gradient is then created by adding an impermeant solute to one of the compartments. Water flows down its chemical potential and at the same time an electrical potential develops across the membrane. This potential is due to the drag of the permeant ion by the water flow through the pore. In this case the chemical potential gradient of water is the driving force and the pore couples the flux of water and the flux of the ion.

These flux-coupling mechanisms are able to generate chemical or electrochemical potential gradients. However, the driving forces for the generation of those gradients are gradients that already exist as a result of previous pump activity.

The operation of an ion pump

In order to understand the role of a pump, let us consider a membrane that has a concentration gradient across it. In Figure 5.9a, KCl is at different concentrations in compartments (1) (left) and (2) (right) which are separated by an impermeable membrane. If the membrane is suddenly made permeable to only potassium ions, these ions will flow down their concentration gradients (from compartment (1) to (2)). Before the membrane was made permeable both solutions were electroneutral and so there was no potential across the membrane. As soon as potassium ions begin to flow there is a net loss of positive charge in compartment (1) and a net gain of positive charge in compartment (2) (see Figure 5.7b, d). As time goes on there is a net build-up of positive charge in compartment (2) with a corresponding build-up of negative charge in compartment (1). There is a simultaneous increase in transmembrane potential as shown in Figure 5.7d. The potential is shown as an increasingly positive potential in side (2) because it is measured with reference to side (1). The potential plateaus when it is sufficiently large so as to balance the chemical gradient. This potential is known as the Nernst equilibrium potential (see Chapter 3).

The amount of potassium shifted before equilibrium is reached is very small so that the bulk concentrations are unchanged and the solutions in compartments (1) and (2) are effectively electroneutral (see Chapter 3). If the membrane is now made permeable to chloride ions (see Figure 5.10), but if this membrane permeability (P_{Cl}) is less than the membrane permeability to potassium (P_K), chloride ions will flow down their concentration gradient. One effect of this flow is that the negative chloride ions cancel the net positive charge in compartment (1), thus reducing the membrane potential (see Figure 5.10d). A second effect is that potassium and chloride ions are now moving from compartment (1) to compartment (2). This net flux of KCl will continue until the concentrations on both sides of the membrane are equal and there is now no longer a membrane potential. Increasing P_{Cl} will speed up the process. Since most membranes in biology are permeable to potassium and chloride in order to prevent this run down of concentration gradients, a KCl-pump would be required to remove potassium and chloride from compartment (2) and return them to compartment (1).

In nature the situation is further complicated by the presence of another cation – sodium. All cells are slightly permeable to sodium and during electrical activity excitable cells have an enormously increased sodium permeability. Also during activity, they have a greatly increased potassium permeability (see Chapter 8 for a full discussion of these events). Because the membranes of most animal cells are permeable to sodium, potassium and chloride and because sodium and potassium ions are found not to be in

Fig.5.9

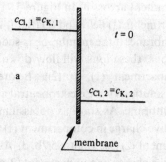

$c_{Cl, 1} = c_{K, 1}$

$t = 0$

a

$c_{Cl, 2} = c_{K, 2}$

membrane

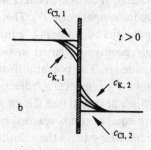

$c_{Cl, 1}$

$t > 0$

$c_{K, 1}$

$c_{K, 2}$

b

$c_{Cl, 2}$

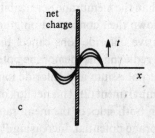

net charge

t

x

c

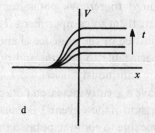

V

t

x

d

Fig.5.10

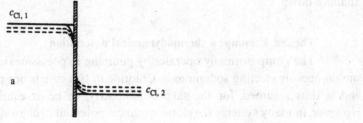

$c_{Cl, 1}$

a

$c_{Cl, 2}$

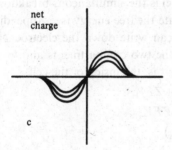

$c_{K, 1}$

b

$c_{K, 2}$

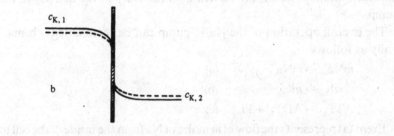

net
charge

c

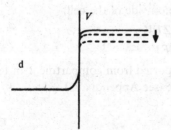

V

d

electrochemical equilibrium across the cell membrane, a Na/K pump is necessary to maintain the ionic gradients and so prevent the system from running down.

The Na/K pump: a thermodynamical description

The pump normally operates by pumping in potassium ions and simultaneously ejecting sodium ions. Chloride in this case is not pumped and is thus assumed, for the sake of simplicity, to be at equilibrium. However, in many systems the electrochemical potential of chloride inside the cells is above equilibrium. This suggests that there is an uphill transport of Cl (inwards). Our aim now is to show how the distribution of ions and the transmembrane potential are related quantitatively to the activity of the pump.

The overall operation of the Na/K pump can be represented schematically as follows:

$$m\mathrm{Na_{In}} \rightarrow m\mathrm{Na_o} \qquad \text{(a)}$$

$$n\mathrm{K_o} \rightarrow n\mathrm{K_{In}} \qquad \text{(b)}$$

$$\mathrm{ATP_{In}} \rightarrow \mathrm{ADP_{In}} + \mathrm{Pi_{In}} \quad \text{(c)}$$

Event (a) represents the flow of m moles of Na from the inside of the cell to the extracellular compartment. Event (b) is the flow of n moles of potassium ions in the opposite direction while (c) is the simultaneous breakdown of one mole of ATP. In order to compute the free energy (see Appendix 25) changes in the overall reaction, we can write down the electrochemical potential (free energy per mole) for the two compartments and for each component. For compartment In, that is, the inside of the cell,

$$\mu_{\mathrm{Na.In}} = \mu^0_{\mathrm{Na.In}} + RT \ln(c_{\mathrm{Na.In}}) + ZFV_{\mathrm{In}}$$

$$\mu_{\mathrm{K.In}} = \mu^0_{\mathrm{K.In}} + RT \ln(c_{\mathrm{K.In}}) + ZFV_{\mathrm{In}}$$

$$\mu_{\mathrm{ATP.In}} = \mu^0_{\mathrm{ATP.In}} + RT \ln(c_{\mathrm{ATP.In}})$$

$$\mu_{\mathrm{ADP.In}} = \mu^0_{\mathrm{ADP.In}} + RT \ln(c_{\mathrm{ADP.In}})$$

$$\mu_{\mathrm{Pi.In}} = \mu^0_{\mathrm{Pi.In}} + RT \ln(c_{\mathrm{Pi.In}})$$

and for compartment o (that is, the outside of the cell)

$$\mu_{\mathrm{Na.o}} = \mu^0_{\mathrm{Na.o}} + RT \ln(c_{\mathrm{Na.o}}) + ZFV_{\mathrm{o}}$$

$$\mu_{\mathrm{K.o}} = \mu^0_{\mathrm{K.o}} + RT \ln(c_{\mathrm{K.o}}) + ZFV_{\mathrm{o}}$$

When m moles of sodium are transported from compartment In to o the change in free energy (ΔG_{Na}) will be (see Appendix 25)

$$\Delta G_{\mathrm{Na}} = m\mu_{\mathrm{Na.o}} - m\mu_{\mathrm{Na.In}}$$

Similarly for n moles of potassium

$$\Delta G_{\mathrm{K}} = n\mu_{\mathrm{K.In}} - n\mu_{\mathrm{K.o}}$$

since potassium moves in the opposite direction. We do not include a term for chloride (ΔG_{Cl}) because this ion is assumed to be at equilibrium across the membrane ($\Delta G_{Cl} = 0$). The flux of chloride across the membrane is given by

$$J_{Cl} = P_{Cl}U[c_{Cl,o}\exp(U) - c_{Cl,In}]/(\exp(U) - 1)$$

where $U = VF/RT$.

Since chloride is not pumped, J_{Cl} is the only flux across the membrane and at steady-state the net flux is zero. That is, $J_{Cl} = 0$. But $(P_{Cl}U/(\exp(U) - 1))$ cannot be zero, so

$$c_{Cl,o}\exp(U) - c_{Cl,In} = 0 \quad \text{or} \quad c_{Cl,o}\exp(U) = c_{Cl,In}$$

then

$$\exp(U) = (c_{Cl,In}/c_{Cl,o}) \quad \text{or} \quad V = (F/RT)\ln(c_{Cl,In}/c_{Cl,o})$$

The change in free energy due to the breakdown of a mole of ATP is

$$\Delta G_{ATP} = \mu_{ADP} + \mu_{Pi} - \mu_{ATP}$$

The total change in free energy (ΔG_T) is then given by

$$\Delta G_T = \Delta G_{Na} + \Delta G_K + \Delta G_{ATP}$$

Because the standard chemical potentials for sodium and potassium are assumed to be the same in both compartments

$$\mu_{Na,o}^0 - \mu_{Na,In}^0 = 0 \quad \text{and} \quad \mu_{K,In}^0 - \mu_{K,o}^0 = 0$$

so

$$\Delta G_{Na} = m(RT\ln(c_{Na,o}) + ZFV_o - RT\ln(c_{Na,In}) - ZFV_{In})$$
$$= m(RT\ln(c_{Na,o}/c_{Na,In}) - ZFV)$$

where $V = V_{In} - V_o$.

Similarly we can write for potassium

$$\Delta G_K = n[RT\ln(c_{K,In}/c_{K,o}) + ZFV]$$

while for ATP

$$\Delta G_{ATP} = \mu_{ADP}^0 + \mu_{Pi}^0 - \mu_{ATP}^0 + RT\ln(c_{ADP}C_{Pi}/c_{ATP})$$
$$= \Delta G_{ATP}^0 + RT\ln(c_{ADP}c_{Pi}/c_{ATP})$$

The overall change in free energy is thus

$$\Delta G_T = mRT\ln(c_{Na,o}/c_{Na,In}) + nRT\ln(c_{K,In}/c_{K,o})$$
$$+ (n - m)FV + \Delta G_{ATP}^0 + RT\ln(c_{ADP}c_{Pi}/c_{ATP}) \quad \text{or}$$
$$\Delta G_T = RT\ln[(c_{Na,o}/c_{Na,In})^n(c_{K,In}/c_{K,o})^n] + (n - m)FV$$
$$+ \Delta G_{ATP}^0 + RT\ln(c_{ADP}c_{Pi}/c_{ATP})$$

since the system cannot cause an increase in free energy ($\Delta G_T \leqslant 0$) (see Appendix 25), then

$$RT\ln[(c_{Na,o}/c_{Na,In})^m(c_{K,In}/c_{K,o})^n] + (n - m)FV + \Delta G_{ATP} \leqslant 0$$

The maximum electrochemical gradient that can be generated by the Na/K pump

The maximum possible gradient that can be obtained is when all the free energy supplied by ATP (ΔG_{ATP}) is completely used up in pumping sodium and potassium uphill, so

$$-\Delta G_{ATP} = RT \ln[(c_{Na,o}/c_{Na,In})^m (c_{K,In}/c_{K,o})^n] + (n-m)FV \qquad (5.16)$$

If we rearrange equation (5.16), we obtain

$$RT \ln[(c_{Na,o}/c_{Na,In})^m (c_{K,In}/c_{K,o})^n] = -\Delta G_{ATP} + (m-n)FV$$

or

$$(c_{Na,o}/c_{Na,In})^m (c_{K,In}/c_{K,o})^n = \exp(-\Delta G_P) \qquad (5.16a)$$

where

$$\Delta G_P = (\Delta G_{ATP} - (m-n)FV)/RT$$

The membrane potential

In this equation ΔG_{ATP} can be found from tables provided we know the concentrations of ATP, ADP and Pi. The membrane potential (V) of the system might be given by the constant-field equation (see Chapter 4).

$$V = (RT/F) \ln(X/Y)$$

where

$$X = P_{Na} c_{Na,o} + P_K c_{K,o} + P_{Cl} c_{Cl,In}$$
$$Y = P_{Na} c_{Na,In} + P_K c_{K,In} + P_{Cl} c_{Cl,o}$$

if the pump does not generate any voltage (neutral pump). In this case m moles of sodium are exchanged for m moles of potassium (that is, $n = m$) and equation (5.16a) simplifies to

$$(c_{Na,o}/c_{Na,In})(c_{K,In}/c_{K,o}) = \exp(-\Delta G_{ATP}/mRT) \qquad (5.17)$$

because $m - n = 0$.

Since in this case only sodium and potassium are pumped, chloride is at equilibrium across the membrane (so it does not contribute to the membrane potential). There are concentration gradients for all three ions but the concentration gradient of the chloride ion is exactly balanced by the membrane potential. Chloride is thus *passively distributed*. As chloride does not contribute to the membrane potential, the constant-field equation reduces to

$$V = (RT/F) \ln[(P_{Na} c_{Na,o} + P_K c_{K,o})/(P_{Na} c_{Na,In} + P_K c_{K,In})]$$

The right-hand side of equation (5.17) enables us to calculate the product of the maximum concentration ratios of sodium and potassium that the pump would be able to generate. To obtain the individual ratios for sodium and potassium we need to take into account the flow of these ions down their concentration gradients. In the case of diffusional flows these can be calculated by equation (4.20) so that, defining U as

$$U = ZFV/RT$$

then

$$\left. \begin{array}{l} \bar{J}_{DNa} = P_{Na}U(C_{Na,In}\exp(U) - C_{Na,o})/(\exp(U) - 1) \\ \bar{J}_{DK} = P_{K}U(C_{K,In}\exp(U) - C_{K,o})/(\exp(U) - 1) \end{array} \right\} \qquad (5.18)$$

where $\bar{J}_{DNa}$ and $\bar{J}_{DK}$ are the diffusional fluxes down their concentration gradients. If the rate of pumping (of sodium and potassium) is $\bar{J}_p$ (positive inwards) in the steady-state

$$\bar{J}_{DNa} = \bar{J}_{PNa}$$

$$-\bar{J}_{DK} = +\bar{J}_{PK} \qquad (5.19)$$

If we substitute equation (5.19) into (5.18) we obtain

$$\bar{J}_{PNa} = P_{Na}U[c_{Na,In}\exp(U) - c_{Na,o}]/(\exp(U) - 1) \qquad (5.20a)$$

$$-\bar{J}_{PK} = P_{K}U[c_{K,In}\exp(U) - c_{K,o}]/(\exp(U) - 1) \qquad (5.20b)$$

We can obtain expressions for the steady-state ratios of sodium and potassium by rearranging equations (5.20a and b).

If we divide equation (5.20a) by

$$P_{Na}Uc_{Na,o}/(\exp(U) - 1)$$

we obtain

$$[\bar{J}_{PNa}/[P_{Na}Uc_{Na,o}/(\exp(U) - 1)]] = (c_{Na,In}\exp(U)/c_{Na,o}) - 1 \qquad (5.21a)$$

Similarly for equation (5.20b)

$$[-\bar{J}_{PK}/(P_{K}Uc_{K,o}/(\exp(U) - 1))] = (c_{K,In}\exp(U)/c_{K,o}) - 1 \qquad (5.21b)$$

Let us define $\mathcal{J}_{Na}$ and $\mathcal{J}_{K}$ as

$$\mathcal{J}_{Na} = P_{Na}Uc_{Na,o}/(\exp(U) - 1) \quad \text{and} \quad \mathcal{J}_{K} = P_{K}Uc_{K,o}/(\exp(U) - 1)$$

Then

$$(c_{Na,In}\exp(U)/c_{Na,o}) = \bar{J}_{PNa}/\mathcal{J}_{Na} + 1$$

$$= (\bar{J}_{PNa} + \mathcal{J}_{Na})/\mathcal{J}_{Na} \qquad (5.22a)$$

and

$$(c_{K,In}\exp(U)/c_{K,o}) = (-\bar{J}_{PK} + \mathcal{J}_{K})/\mathcal{J}_{K} \qquad (5.22b)$$

The relationship between pumping and the membrane potential

If we divide equation (5.22a) by equation (5.22b), we obtain

$$F(V) = (c_{Na,In}/c_{Na,o})(c_{K,o}/c_{K,In})$$

$$= [(\bar{J}_{PNa} + \mathcal{J}_{Na})/\mathcal{J}_{Na}]/[(-\bar{J}_{PK} + \mathcal{J}_{K})/\mathcal{J}_{K}] \qquad (5.23)$$

or

$$F(V) = [1 + \bar{J}_{PNa}/\mathcal{J}_{Na}]/[1 - \bar{J}_{PK}/\mathcal{J}_{K}] \qquad (5.23a)$$

The right-hand side of equation (5.23a) includes the rate of pumping ($\bar{J}_{P\,ion}$), the membrane permeabilities to sodium and potassium (P_{Na} and P_K) contained J_{Na} and J_K and the membrane potential. It is thus a function of the membrane potential ($F(V)$).

If we recall equations (5.17) and (5.23) we can write

$$F(V) = \exp(+\Delta G_{ATP}/mRT) \tag{5.24}$$

Equation (5.24) is the end point of our analysis on the role of a neutral Na/K pump in maintaining the ion gradients. This equation, together with equation (5.23), shows that the membrane potential is determined by a number of factors which are listed below:

> the change in free energy due to the breakdown of ATP (ΔG_{ATP})
>
> the number of sodium (or potassium) ions pumped per ATP split (pump stoichiometry m)
>
> the membrane permeabilities for sodium and potassium ions (P_{Na}, P_K)
>
> the external concentrations of sodium and potassium ions (Na_o, K_o)
>
> the rate of pumping ($\bar{J}_{PNa}$ and $\bar{J}_{PK}$).

The contribution of the rate of pumping to the membrane potential

Although the membrane potential can be computed from the constant-field equation, it is clear from (5.24) that it is due to the operation of the pump. If the pump is blocked, that is, $\bar{J}_{PNa}$ and $\bar{J}_{PK}$ are zero, it can be seen from equations (5.22a, b) that the right-hand sides of equation (5.23) will be one at steady-state and the membrane potential is the Nernst equilibrium potential. This means that

$$(c_{Na,In} \exp(U)/c_{Na,o}) = (c_{K,In} \exp(U)/c_{K,o}) \tag{5.25}$$

where

$$U = FV/RT$$

But as there is only one membrane potential the exponential term has the same value on both sides of equation (5.25). So

$$(c_{Na,In}/c_{Na,o}) = (c_{K,In}/c_{K,o}) \tag{5.25a}$$

Immediately after blocking the pump

$$Na_{In} < Na_o \quad \text{and} \quad K_{In} > K_o$$

and the ions will flow down their concentration gradients until the gradients are dissipated. The concentration ratios will become one – that is, become equal on both sides of the membrane – because initially $c_{Na,In}/c_{Na,o}$ was less than one and $c_{K,In}/c_{K,o}$ was greater than one.

In equation (5.24) we analysed the situation when the pump was neutral. However, this is often not the case and so equation (5.24) no longer applies. The constant-field equation for calculating the voltage now has to include an extra term to take into account the current generated by a non-neutral pump, the so-called *electrogenic pump*.

In order to compute the membrane potential under these conditions, we assume that the chloride flux is zero and we start with the expression for the fluxes of sodium and potassium (5.18) and add a flux term due to pump $\bar{J}_{\text{p ion}}$

$$\left.\begin{aligned}\bar{J}_{\text{Na}} &= \bar{J}_{\text{DNa}} + \bar{J}_{\text{PNa}} \\ \bar{J}_{\text{K}} &= \bar{J}_{\text{DK}} - \bar{J}_{\text{PK}}\end{aligned}\right\} \tag{5.26}$$

where $\bar{J}_{\text{DNa}}$ and $\bar{J}_{\text{DK}}$ are the diffusional (out) fluxes of sodium and potassium ions which can be computed from the G–H–K equation and $\bar{J}_{\text{PNa}}$ is the flux of sodium (outwards) due to the pump and $\bar{J}_{\text{PK}}$ is the flux of potassium (inwards) due to the pump. At steady-state both $\bar{J}_{\text{Na}}$ and $\bar{J}_{\text{K}}$ are zero. So

$$-\bar{J}_{\text{PNa}} = \bar{J}_{\text{DNa}} \tag{5.27}$$

$$\bar{J}_{\text{PK}} = \bar{J}_{\text{DK}} \tag{5.28}$$

Stoichiometry of the pump and the membrane potential

If we divide equation (5.27) by equation (5.28) we obtain the ratio (r) between the sodium and the potassium fluxes through the pump. This ratio is the number of sodium ions exchanged per K ion. Thus

$$-r = -\bar{J}_{\text{PNa}}/\bar{J}_{\text{PK}} = \bar{J}_{\text{DNa}}/\bar{J}_{\text{DK}}$$
$$= [P_{\text{Na}}(c_{\text{Na,In}} \exp(U) - c_{\text{Na,o}})]/[P_{\text{K}}(c_{\text{K,In}} \exp(U) - c_{\text{K,o}})] \tag{5.29}$$

where r is the stoichiometry of the pump and $U = FV/RT$. If we rearrange equation (5.29) we obtain

$$-rP_{\text{K}}(c_{\text{K,In}} \exp(U) - c_{\text{K,o}}) = P_{\text{Na}}(c_{\text{Na,In}} \exp(U) - c_{\text{Na,o}})$$

or

$$\exp(VF/RT)(P_{\text{Na}}c_{\text{Na,In}} + rP_{\text{K}}c_{\text{K,In}}) = P_{\text{Na}}c_{\text{Na,o}} + rP_{\text{K}}c_{\text{K,o}} \tag{5.30}$$

If we divide both sides of equation (5.30) by $P_{\text{Na}}c_{\text{Na,In}} + rP_{\text{K}}c_{\text{K,In}}$ and take natural logarithms, we obtain

$$VF/RT = \ln[(P_{\text{Na}}c_{\text{Na,o}} + rP_{\text{K}}c_{\text{K,o}})/(P_{\text{Na}}c_{\text{Na,In}} + rP_{\text{K}}c_{\text{K,In}})]$$

or

$$V = (RT/F)\ln[(P_{\text{Na}}c_{\text{Na,o}} + rP_{\text{K}}c_{\text{K,o}})/(P_{\text{Na}}c_{\text{Na,In}} + rP_{\text{K}}c_{\text{K,In}})] \tag{5.31}$$

Equation (5.31) was originally derived by Mullins and Noda (1963) and shows that the membrane potential (V) is also a function of the pump stoichiometry. When the pump is neutral ($r = 1$), equation (5.31) reverts to the constant-field equation. Equation (5.31) is thus a more general case of the constant-field equation.

Electrogenicity of the pump

The pump can thus contribute to the membrane potential by setting up the ion gradients and by being electrogenic. Experimentally the electrogenicity of the pump can be tested by the use of a specific pump inhibitor such as ouabain. Before inhibition the membrane potential is given by equation (5.31), while after inhibition ($r = 1$) it is described by the constant-field equation. If the two measurements are different, r is different from 1 and the pump is assumed to be electrogenic. From equation (5.31) if

$$r P_K c_{K,o} \gg P_{Na} c_{Na,o} \quad \text{and if} \quad r P_K c_{K,In} \gg P_{Na} c_{Na,In}$$

then

$$V \approx (RT/F) \ln(c_{K,o}/c_{K,In}) \tag{5.32}$$

Equation (5.32) is the Nernst equation which applies to a membrane which is permeable to only one ion. Equation (5.32) does not include the pump stoichiometry term r. However, the pump is required to set up the concentration difference which is responsible for the membrane potential V.

To conclude, in this chapter we have shown that biological membranes are lipid bilayers that are well modelled by artificially-produced BLMs. Biological membranes are almost impermeable to ions, which means that only a few pumps (per unit area of membrane) are required to set up and maintain long-lasting electrochemical gradients. These gradients, along with the membrane pores, are responsible for the transmembrane potentials. Since membranes are almost impermeable to ions, and as pores are highly permeable structures, only a few pores (per unit area of membrane) are required to set up and control the membrane potential.

6

Membrane equivalent circuits

In the last chapter we examined mechanisms whereby concentration gradients are maintained at steady-state across biological membranes. In this chapter we will analyse the relevance of these gradients to electro-physiology. In Chapter 4 we showed that when there is a concentration gradient for an ion across a membrane and, provided that the membrane is permeable to that ion, an electrical potential difference across the membrane is to be expected.

The equilibrium potentials for K, Na and Cl

If the membrane is permeable to only one ion species the membrane potential is equal to the Nernst potential for that ion species. Thus

$$V = E_i = (RT/ZF)\ln(c_o/c_{In}) \tag{6.1}$$

where R, T, Z and F have their usual meaning, E_i is the Nernst potential for ion i and c_{In} and c_o are the concentrations of the ion inside (In) and outside (o) respectively.

For squid axon

$$E_K = -74\,\text{mV}, \quad E_{Na} = 53\,\text{mV} \quad \text{and} \quad E_{Cl} = -51\,\text{mV}$$

Usually 'In' refers to the intracellular compartment and 'o' to extra-cellular compartment. Although concentrations are most frequently expressed as molar concentrations, in transport biophysics it is often more convenient to use moles per cm^3. If the membrane potential is given by the G–H–K equation (Chapter 4 (4.41)), then,

defining X as

$$X = P_{Na}c_{Na,In} + P_K c_{K,In} + P_{Cl}c_{Cl,o}$$
and Y as

$$Y = P_{Na}c_{Na,o} + P_{K,o} + P_{Cl}c_{Cl,In}$$ \tag{6.2}

$$V = -(RT/F)\ln(X/Y)$$

where P_{Na}, P_K and P_{Cl} are the membrane permeabilities to Na^+, K^+ and Cl^- (in $cm \cdot s^{-1}$) and c_{In}, i and c_o are the concentrations of ion (i) on either side of the membrane.

Equation (6.2) describes a steady-state situation and in the steady-state the concentrations on both sides of the membrane, the membrane potential and the membrane currents are constant. Equation (6.2) can be rewritten as

$$V = -(RT/F) \ln[(c_{Na,In} + \alpha_1 c_{K,In} + \alpha_2 c_{Cl,o})/(c_{Na,o} + \alpha_1 c_{K,o} + \alpha_2 c_{Cl,In})]$$

where $\alpha_1 = P_K/P_{Na}$ and $\alpha_2 = P_{Cl}/P_{Na}$. In the resting axon (see Chapter 7) $\alpha_1 = 25$ and $\alpha_2 = 2.2$.

In equation (6.2) we neglected the contribution of the sodium pump to the membrane potential. The reasons for this were discussed in Chapter 4. An alternative way of expressing the membrane potential as a function of ion concentrations and permeabilities is to represent the membrane by an equivalent circuit.

The equivalent circuit of a membrane

In order to draw the membrane equivalent circuit we first assume that the ions move independently of one another *within* the membrane (independence principle – see Chapter 4). With this assumption we can imagine that the equivalent circuit is composed of the parallel combination of the equivalent circuit for each ion species. In Chapter 3 we derived equivalent circuits for a slab of solution. Although the circuits derived there can be directly applied to the case where we have a slab of membrane instead of a slab of solution, we shall derive them again for the sake of continuity, starting with the Nernst–Planck equation.

The equivalent circuit for one ion can be obtained by first assuming that the membrane is a homogeneous slab of thickness δ through which the ion moves by diffusion (see Figure 6.1). If we now imagine that the membrane is split up into a number of planes parallel to the two membrane faces, then for one plane the relationship between the local current of ion i and the local

Fig.6.1

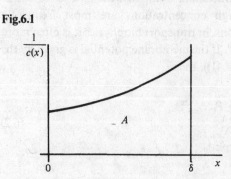

concentration and electrical potential gradient is given by the Nernst–Planck equation (see Chapter 2)

$$\bar{I}_i = -ZFu_ic_i(x)(d/dx)(RT \ln(c_i(x)) + ZFV(x)) \tag{6.3}$$

where u_i is the mobility of the ion in the membrane and $c_i(x)$ and $V(x)$ are the local concentration of the ion and the local electrical potential, respectively. If we divide both sides of equation (6.3) by $-(ZF)^2u_ic_i(x)$ we obtain

$$-\bar{I}_i/((ZF)^2u_ic_i(x)) = (d/dx)((RT/ZF) \ln(c_i(x))) + dV/dx \tag{6.4}$$

In order to understand the physical meaning of equation (6.4) we first divide the membrane up into n slabs of thickness δ, where n is sufficiently large for δ/n to be very small (Δx) (see Figure 6.2c, d).

The first term on the right-hand side of equation (6.4) can be approximated by

$$(d/dx)(RT/Z_iF) \ln(c_i(x)) \approx (RT/ZF)(\ln(c_i(x+\Delta x)) - \ln(c_i(x)))/\Delta x$$
$$= (RT/ZF) \ln(c_i(x+\Delta x)/c_i(x))/\Delta x \tag{6.5}$$

But $(RT/ZF) \ln(c_i(x)/(c_i(x)+\Delta x))$ is the Nernst potential across the slab (ΔE_i). Thus

$$(d/dx)(RT/ZF) \ln(c_i(x)) \approx -\Delta E_i/\Delta x \tag{6.6}$$

The second term on the right-hand side of equation (6.4) can also be approximated by

$$dV/dx \approx (V(x+\Delta x) - V(x))/\Delta x \tag{6.7}$$

But $(V(x+\Delta x) - V(x))$ is the electrical potential difference across the slab (ΔV). If we substitute (6.6) and (6.7) into (6.4) we obtain

$$-\bar{I}/((ZF)^2u_ic_i(x)) \approx (-\Delta E_i + \Delta V)/\Delta x \tag{6.8}$$

Multiplying throughout by Δx we obtain

$$+\bar{I}(\Delta x/(ZF)^2u_ic_i(x)) \approx \Delta E_i - \Delta V \tag{6.9}$$

Since the two terms on the right-hand side of equation (6.9) are electrical potential differences (volts), and $\bar{I}$ is the current that flows through the slab (amp·cm^{-2}), the term

$$\Delta x/((ZF)^2u_ic_i(x)) \tag{6.10}$$

must be a resistance (ΔR, ohm·cm^2).

If we rearrange equation (6.9) we obtain

$$1/((ZF)^2u_ic_i(x)) = ((\Delta E_i - \Delta V)/\Delta x)(1/\bar{I})$$

The right-hand side of this equation is, by definition, a resistivity since it is the ratio between the electric field (($\Delta E_i - \Delta V)/\Delta x$) and the current density

Fig.6.2

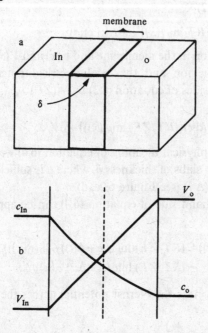

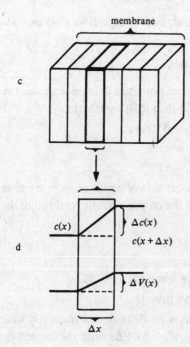

$(\bar{I})$

$$\text{resistivity} = \frac{\text{electric field}}{\text{current density}} = \frac{\text{volt} \cdot \text{cm}^2}{\text{cm} \cdot \text{amp}} = \text{volt} \cdot \text{cm} \cdot \text{amp}^{-1}$$

Ohm's Law is a special case of this relationship where the resistivity is constant (that is, independent of V or I). A membrane obeying Ohm's Law is said to have an ohmic conductance.

Similarly, a conductivity is defined as

$$\text{conductivity} = \frac{\text{current density}}{\text{electrical field}} = \text{amp} \cdot \text{cm}^{-2}/\text{volt} \cdot \text{cm}^{-1}$$

$$= \text{amp} \cdot \text{volt}^{-1} \cdot \text{cm}^{-1}$$

$$\text{Siemens} = \frac{\text{cm}^2}{\text{cm ohm}} = \text{A} \cdot \text{V}^{-1}$$

We can thus rewrite (6.9) as

$$\bar{I} \Delta \bar{R}_i \approx \Delta E_i - \Delta V \tag{6.11}$$

or if we define

$$\Delta \bar{G}_i = 1/\Delta \bar{R}_i \tag{6.12}$$

$$\bar{I} \approx \Delta \bar{G}_i(j)(\Delta E_i(j) - \Delta V(j)) \tag{6.13}$$

Equation (6.11) can be directly translated into a simple equivalent circuit of the type shown in Figure 6.3a. Furthermore, the whole membrane can be represented as a series combination of n equivalent circuits (Figure 6.3b). Figure 6.3b can be further simplified (6.3c). To do this we use Kirchhoff's Laws, for the addition of voltages (see Appendix 15).

$$I_i = \sum_{j=1}^{j=n} \Delta E_i(j) \tag{6.14}$$

and

$$V = \sum_{j=1}^{j=n} \Delta V(j) \tag{6.15}$$

Membrane resistance and conductance

If the current density $(\bar{I})$ through the membrane is constant with time, the left-hand side of equation (6.11) becomes, for the whole membrane

$$\sum_{j=1}^{j=n} \bar{I} \Delta \bar{R}(j) = \bar{I} \bar{R}_i$$

where $\bar{R}_i$, the membrane resistance to the flow of ion i, is given by

$$\bar{R}_i = \sum_{j=1}^{j=n} (\Delta x/(ZF)^2 u_i c_i(x))$$

For small Δx ($\Delta x \rightarrow 0$), since $\delta = n \Delta x$ where δ, the membrane thickness, is

constant, then $n \to \infty$ and

$$\sum_{\substack{j=1 \\ n \to \infty \\ \Delta x \to 0}}^{j=n} (\Delta x/(ZF)^2 u_i c_i(x)) \to \int_0^\delta \mathrm{d}x/((ZF)^2 u_i c_i(x)) \qquad (6.16)$$

so

$$\bar{R}_i = \int_0^\delta \mathrm{d}x/((ZF)^2 u_i c_i(x))$$

$$= (1/(ZF)^2 u_i) \int_0^\delta \mathrm{d}x/c_i(x) \qquad (6.16a)$$

Fig.6.3

a

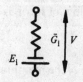

b

c

and

$$\bar{G}_i = 1/\bar{R} = 1 \Big/ \int_0^\delta dx/((ZF)^2 u_i c_i(x)) \qquad (6.16b)$$

where $\bar{G}_i$ is the membrane conductance to ion i per cm^2.

The membrane equilibrium potential for an ion

Equation (6.14) can be expanded, as

$$E_i = \sum_{j=1}^{j=n} E_i(j) = E_i(1) + E_i(2) + \cdots + E_i(j)$$

where

$$E_i(n) = (RT/ZF)\ln(c_i(n)/c_i(n+1))$$

But

$$c_i(1) = c_{i,\text{In}}$$

and

$$c_i(n) = c_{i,o}$$

thus

$$E_i = (RT/ZF)[\ln(c_{i,\text{In}}/c_i(2)) + \ln(c_i(2)/c_i(3)) + \cdots$$
$$+ \ln(c_i(n-1)/c_{i,o})]$$

$$= (RT/ZF)\ln[(c_{i,\text{In}}/c_i(2))(c_i(2)/c_i(3)) \cdots$$
$$(c_i(n-1)/c_{i,o})]$$

this equation reduces to

$$E_i = (RT/ZF)\ln(c_{i,\text{In}}/c_{i,o}) \qquad (6.17)$$

Equation (6.15) can also be expanded as

$$V' = (V(1) - V(0)) + (V(2) - V(1)) + (\quad) + \cdots + (V(n) - V(n-1))$$
$$= V(n) - V(0)$$

where $V(0), V(1), \ldots, V(n)$ are the electrical potentials when

$$x = 0, \Delta x, 2\Delta x, \ldots, n\Delta x$$

Since

$$\delta = n\Delta x$$

then

$$V' = V(\delta) - V(0)$$

so

$$\bar{I}\bar{R}_i = E_i - V'$$

or if we define V as

$$V = -V' = V(0) - V(\delta)$$
$$\bar{I}_i \bar{R}_i = E_i + V \qquad (6.18)$$

and

$$\bar{I}_i = \bar{G}_i(E_i + V) \qquad (6.18a)$$

The meaning of the integral on the right-hand side of equation (6.16a) is shown in Figure 6.1. If, as a result of a change in membrane potential, the concentration profile ($c(x)$) within the membrane changes (and this usually happens) we would expect that the area under the curve shown in Figure 6.1 will change, which means that the $\bar{R}_i$ of equation (6.18) and $\bar{G}_i$ of equation (6.18a) will also change.

The relationship between chord and slope conductance

If the I/V relationship across the membrane is of the constant-field type (see Chapter 4), then the changes of $\bar{G}_i$ with voltage can be expressed in two different ways. One way is by a slope conductance (which was discussed in Chapter 4), and the other by a chord conductance (also discussed in Chapter 4). The $\bar{G}_i$ in equation (6.18) is, by definition, a chord conductance, since

$$\bar{G}_i = \bar{I}_i/(E_i + V) \quad \text{(see Figure 6.4)}$$

Fig.6.4

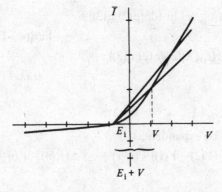

The relationship between *chord* and *slope* conductance in equation (6.18a) is obtained by differentiating the equation with respect to voltage

$$\bar{I}_i = \bar{G}_i(E_i + V) \tag{6.18a}$$

$$\text{slope conductance} = d\bar{I}_i/dV = (d/dV)(\bar{G}_i(E_i + V))$$
$$= (E_i + V)\,d\bar{G}_i/dV + \bar{G}_i\,d(E_i + V)/dV$$
$$= (E_i + V)\,d\bar{G}_i/dV + \bar{G}_i(dE_i/dV + dV/dV)$$
$$\qquad\qquad\qquad\qquad\quad \underset{0}{\parallel} \qquad \underset{1}{\parallel}$$
$$= (E_i + V)\,d\bar{G}_i/dV + \bar{G}_i \tag{6.19}$$

When the I/V relationship is linear then the slope conductance and the chord conductance are the same since $d\bar{G}_i/dV = 0$.

From the independence principle we are now able to represent the membrane as a parallel combination of equivalent circuits of the type shown in Figure 6.3c (Figure 6.5).

The full equivalent circuit of a membrane

The total current flowing across the circuit shown in Figure 6.5 is, from Kirchhoff's Laws, the sum of the currents flowing through each branch or

$$\bar{I}_t = \bar{I}_{Na} + \bar{I}_K + \bar{I}_{Cl} \tag{6.20}$$

From equation (6.18), $\bar{I}_i$ can be expanded as follows

$$\bar{I}_i = \bar{G}_{Na}(E_{Na} + V) + \bar{G}_K(E_K + V) + \bar{G}_{Cl}(E_{Cl} + V) \tag{6.20a}$$

In the steady-state and when $I_t = 0$ this equation can be rearranged as follows

$$0 = \bar{G}_{Na}(E_{Na} + V) + \bar{G}_K(E_K + V) + \bar{G}_{Cl}(E_{Cl} + V)$$
$$= \bar{G}_{Na}E_{Na} + \bar{G}_K E_K + \bar{G}_{Cl}E_{Cl} + V(\bar{G}_{Na} + \bar{G}_K + \bar{G}_{Cl}) \tag{6.21}$$

But

$$\bar{G}_m = \bar{G}_{Na} + \bar{G}_K + \bar{G}_{Cl} \tag{6.22}$$

where $\bar{G}_m$ is the total membrane conductance per cm^2.

Fig.6.5

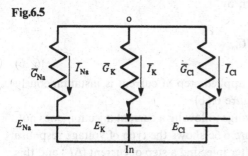

The open-circuit potential

If we substitute (6.22) into (6.21) and rearrange we obtain

$$V = V_{oc}$$
$$= -(E_{Na}(\bar{G}_{Na}/\bar{G}_m) + E_K(\bar{G}_K/\bar{G}_m) + E_{Cl}(\bar{G}_{Cl}/\bar{G}_m)) \tag{6.23}$$

where V is the open-circuit potential (V_{oc}). The open circuit potential is the resting membrane potential, that is, the membrane potential when no net current flows ($\bar{I}_t = 0$). It is known as an open-circuit potential as it is equivalent to the situation in which the connection between the membrane and any external source of current is broken. The external source of current might be an external circuit or another part of the membrane through which current is flowing. This equation gives the membrane potential as a function of the ion concentrations on both sides of the membrane and of the conductance of the membrane to sodium, potassium and chloride. The ratios $\bar{G}_i/\bar{G}_m$ are known as *transport numbers*. Equation (6.23) is comparable with equation (6.2), except that the membrane potential is defined in terms of conductances rather than permeabilities. (The relationship that exists between conductance and permeability is discussed in Chapter 4). It is clear from equations (6.21) and (6.23) that the membrane potential will be changed if the ion composition on either side of the membrane is changed (that changes E_i). An alternative way of changing V is to inject a current (I_t) through the membrane either into or out of the cell. From equation (6.20a) we obtain

$$\bar{I}_t = \bar{G}_m V + (E_{Na}\bar{G}_{Na} + E_K\bar{G}_K + E_{Cl}\bar{G}_{Cl}) \tag{6.24}$$

this equation can be rearranged as follows

$$V = (\bar{I}_t/\bar{G}_m) + (E_{Na}\bar{G}_{Na} + E_K\bar{G}_K + E_{Cl}\bar{G}_{Cl})/\bar{G}_m \tag{6.24a}$$

From equation (6.23)

$$V = (\bar{I}_t/\bar{G}_m) + V_{oc} \tag{6.25}$$

The membrane capacitance

If we instantaneously change the current ($\bar{I}_t$) to $\bar{I}_t + \Delta\bar{I}_t$ then the membrane voltage will be given by

$$V = (\bar{I}_t + \Delta\bar{I}_t)/G_m + V_{oc}$$
$$V = (\bar{I}_t/\bar{G}_m + V_{oc}) + \Delta\bar{I}_t/\bar{G}_m$$
$$= (\bar{I}_t/\bar{G}_m + V_{oc}) + \Delta V \tag{6.26}$$

Equation (6.26) states that an applied step of current is instantaneously followed by a voltage step (Figure 6.6b).

An instantaneous voltage change following a current injection does not, however, occur in nature. Figure 6.6c shows the type of voltage response obtained across a membrane after injecting a step of current ($\Delta\bar{I}_t$) and this type of response is found in electrical circuits of the type represented in Figure 6.6d. It is a circuit which includes a capacitance ($\bar{C}_m$) in parallel with a resistance ($\bar{R}_m$). The explanation of the curve in 6.6c might be that the membrane has a capacitance (see Appendix 15). This would seem to be a reasonable explanation since the membrane is a poor conductor separating two highly conductive media (intra- and extra-cellular fluids). The slow rise of the voltage (Figure 6.6c) is thus due to the time taken to charge up the membrane capacity.

Charge separation across a membrane

Charging involves a net accumulation of positive ions (and a net depletion of negative ions) on the positive side of the membrane and a net

Fig.6.6

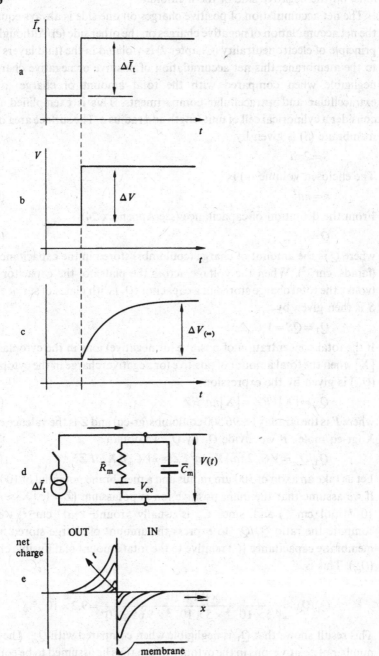

depletion of positive ions (together with a net accumulation of negative ions) on the negative side of the membrane.

The net accumulation of positive charges on one side is always equal to the net accumulation of negative charges on the other side (e). Although the principle of electroneutrality (Chapter 2) is violated in the fluid layers next to the membrane, this net accumulation of positive or negative charge is negligible when compared with the total amount of charge in the extracellular and intracellular compartments. This is exemplified if we consider a cylindrical cell of unit length and radius a. The surface area of the membrane (S) is given by

$$S = 2\pi a \tag{6.27}$$

The enclosed volume (v) is

$$v = \pi a^2 \tag{6.28}$$

From the definition of capacitance (see Appendix 24)

$$Q = V\bar{C}_m \tag{6.29}$$

where Q is the amount of charge (coulombs) stored in the capacitance C_m (farads $\cdot$ cm^{-2}). When the voltage across the plates of the capacitor is V (volts), the total charge stored in a capacitor (Q_T) with plates of surface area S is then given by

$$Q_T = QS = V\bar{C}_m 2\pi a \tag{6.30}$$

If the total concentration of positive (or negative) ions in the cytoplasm is [X] when the total amount of positive (or negative) charge in the cytoplasm (Q_{cy}) is given by the expression

$$Q_{cy} = [X]VFZ = [X]\pi a^2 FZ \tag{6.31}$$

where F is the faraday ($\simeq 96\,500$ coulombs/gr-eq) and Z is the valence of ion X (gr-eq/mole). If we divide Q_T by Q_{cy} we obtain

$$Q_T/Q_{cy} = V\bar{C}_m 2\pi a/[X]\pi a^2 FZ = 2V\bar{C}_m/[X]aFZ \tag{6.32}$$

Let us take an axon of 500 μm radius and a membrane potential of 100 mV. If we assume that the main positive ion is potassium ($Z = 1$; $[X] \approx 4.5 \times 10^{-4}$ mol $\cdot$ cm^{-3}) and, since $\bar{C}_m$ is usually around 1 μF $\cdot$ cm^{-2}, we can compute the ratio Q_T/Q_{cy} to express the amount of charge stored in the membrane capacitance (C) relative to the total amount of diffusible charge (Q_{cy}). This is

$$Q_T/Q_{cy} \approx \frac{2 \times 0.1 \times 10^{-6}}{4.5 \times 10^{-4} \times 5 \times 10^{-2} \times 9.65 \times 10^4} = 9.2 \times 10^{-8}$$

This result shows that Q_T is negligible when compared with Q_{cy}. The total number of positive ions in the cytoplasm can thus be assumed to be equal to the total number of negative ions.

The capacitance current

Since we have concluded that the membrane has a capacitance, whenever there is a transient change in voltage across the membrane two types of current will flow. These are the ionic current ($\bar{I}_i$), due to the flow of ions through the membrane, and the capacitative current ($\bar{I}_c$) due to charge accumulation and depletion on either side of the membrane. The total current $\bar{I}_t$ is then given by

$$\bar{I}_t = \bar{I}_i + \bar{I}_c \tag{6.33}$$

As shown above, $\bar{I}_i$ can be obtained from equation (6.25)

$$\bar{I}_i = (V - V_{oc})\bar{G}_m \tag{6.34}$$

$\bar{I}_t$ in equation (6.24) is equal to $\bar{I}_i$ in equation (6.33) since at steady-state $\bar{I}_c$ is zero.

The capacitative current ($\bar{I}_c$) can be obtained by differentiating equation (6.29) with respect to time. This is because the capacitative current is equal to the rate of accumulation or depletion of charge. Thus

$$Q = V\bar{C}_m \tag{6.35}$$

so

$$\bar{I}_c = dQ/dt = \bar{C}_m(dV/dt) \tag{6.36}$$

Thus, in order to describe quantitatively the voltage response obtained across cell membranes (Figure 6.6c), it is necessary to split the total membrane current ($\bar{I}_t$) into its two components, and express it as a function of voltage.

If we substitute equations (6.36) and (6.34) into equation (6.33) we obtain

$$\bar{I}_t = \underbrace{(V - V_{oc})\bar{G}_m}_{\bar{I}_i} + \underbrace{\bar{C}_m(dV/dt)}_{\bar{I}_c} \tag{6.37}$$

Equation (6.37) is a first-order differential equation, in V, which is easily solved when $\bar{I}_t$ is a constant current.

The membrane voltage in response to a current step

Rearranging equation (6.37) we obtain

$$\bar{C}_m\, dV/dt + \bar{G}_m V = I_t + V_{oc}\bar{G}_m \tag{6.38}$$

and

$$\begin{aligned} dV/dt &= -[(\bar{G}_m/\bar{C}_m)V - (\bar{I}_t + V_{oc}\bar{G}_m)/\bar{C}_m] \\ &= -(\bar{G}_m/\bar{C}_m)[V - (\bar{I}_t + V_{oc}\bar{G}_m)/\bar{G}_m] \end{aligned} \tag{6.39}$$

At steady-state the voltage is not changing with time ($dV/dt = 0$), and the membrane voltage (V) becomes the steady-state voltage (V_∞) so

$$V_\infty - (\bar{I}_t + V_{oc}\bar{G}_m)/\bar{G}_m = 0$$

or

$$V_\infty = \bar{I}_t/\bar{G}_m + V_{oc} \tag{6.40}$$

If we substitute (6.40) into (6.39) we obtain

$$dV/dt = -(\bar{G}_m/\bar{C}_m)(V - V_\infty) \tag{6.41}$$

But since

$$\bar{G}_m = 1/\bar{R}_m$$

then

$$\bar{G}_m/\bar{C}_m = 1/\bar{C}_m\bar{R}_m$$
$$= 1/\tau_m \tag{6.42}$$

The membrane time constant

The product $R_m C_m$ is called the membrane time constant τ_m. Equation (6.41) can now be rewritten as

$$dV/dt = -(1/\tau_m)(V - V_\infty) \tag{6.43}$$

This equation can be solved if we separate the variables (see Appendix 9) and we obtain

$$dV/(V - V_\infty) = -(1/\tau_m)\,dt \tag{6.44}$$

Integrating

$$\ln(V - V_\infty) = -t/\tau_m + B \tag{6.45}$$

where B is the constant of integration.

Immediately before current flows through the circuit ($\bar{I}_t = 0$) the membrane potential (V) is equal to V_0 at $t = 0$. From equation (6.25) we can see that V_0 is the steady-state open-circuit potential (V_{oc}), so

$$t = 0, \quad V = V_0 \quad \text{and} \quad B = \ln(V_0 - V_\infty)$$

If we substitute for B and rearrange, we obtain

$$\ln((V - V_\infty)/(V_0 - V_\infty)) = -t/\tau_m$$

Taking antilogs and rearranging

$$V - V_\infty = (V_0 - V_\infty)\exp(-t/\tau_m)$$

so that

$$V = V_\infty + (V_0 - V_\infty)\exp(-t/\tau_m) \tag{6.46}$$

If we add and subtract V_0 to the right-hand side of equation (6.46) we obtain

$$V = V_0 + (V_\infty - V_0) + (V_0 - V_\infty)\exp(-t/\tau_m)$$

which is

$$V = V_0 + (V_\infty - V_0)(1 - \exp(-t/\tau_m)) \tag{6.47}$$

Equation (6.47) provides a complete quantitative description of the voltage response that follows the injection of a constant current into a spherical cell (Figure 6.6c). For the case where $\bar{I}_t$ is zero before the application of the current step ($\Delta \bar{I}_t$), V_0 will be equal to the open circuit potential V_{oc}. This equation is plotted in Figure 6.7b.

When $t = \tau_m$ equation (6.47) reduces to

$$(V - V_0)/(V_\infty - V_0) = 1 - \exp(-1) = 0.632\dots$$

If the membrane resistance $(\bar{R}_m)$ or conductance $(\bar{G}_m)$ is known, then the membrane capacitance $(\bar{C}_m)$ can be obtained from equation (6.42) as

Fig.6.7

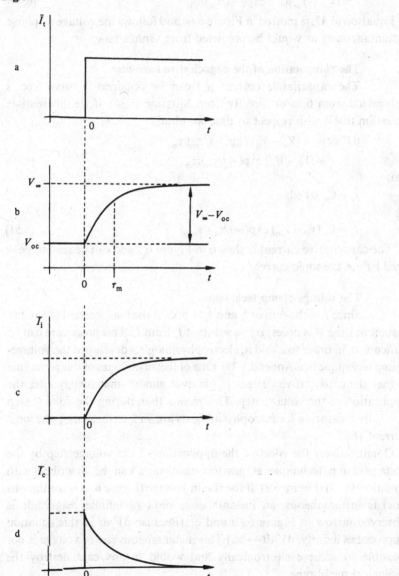

follows:

$$\bar{C}_m = \tau_m/\bar{R}_m = \bar{G}_m\tau_m \tag{6.48}$$

In order to describe the current flow through both branches of Figure 6.6d we can compute $\bar{I}_i$ from equations (6.34), (6.40) and (6.47)

$$\begin{aligned}
\bar{I}_i &= (V - V_{oc})\bar{G}_m \\
&= [V_{oc} + (V_\infty - V_{oc})(1 - \exp(-t/\tau_m)) - V_{oc}]\bar{G}_m \\
&= (V_\infty - V_{oc})(1 - \exp(-t/\tau_m))\bar{G}_m
\end{aligned} \tag{6.49}$$

Equation (6.49) is plotted in Figure 6.6c and follows the voltage response instantaneously as would be predicted from Ohm's Law.

The computation of the capacitative currents

The capacitative current (I_c) can be obtained if curve 6.6c is subtracted from 6.6a or directly from equation (6.36). If we differentiate equation (6.47) with respect to time we obtain

$$\begin{aligned}
dV/dt &= -(V_\infty - V_0)\exp(-t/\tau_m)/\tau_m \\
&= (V_0 - V_\infty)\exp(-t/\tau_m)/\tau_m
\end{aligned} \tag{6.50}$$

But

$$\bar{I}_c = \bar{C}_m \, dV/dt$$

so

$$\bar{I}_c = \bar{C}_m(V_0 - V_\infty)\exp(-t/\tau_m)/\tau_m \tag{6.51}$$

The capacitative current is shown in Figure 6.7 and can be seen to peak well before the ionic current.

The voltage-clamp techniques

Since $\bar{I}_t$ is the sum of $\bar{I}_c$ and $\bar{I}_i$ to obtain the ionic current ($\bar{I}_i$) at any instant in time, it is necessary to subtract $\bar{I}_c$ from $\bar{I}_t$. This procedure can be difficult so, in order to avoid it, electrophysiologists developed the voltage-clamp technique (see Appendix 31). One of the advantages of this technique is that the capacitative current ($\bar{I}_c$) is over almost immediately after the application of the voltage step. This means that, during the voltage step $\bar{I}_t = \bar{I}_i$, by measuring $\bar{I}_t$ electrophysiologists are, in fact, measuring the ionic current ($\bar{I}_i$).

Quantitatively the effect of the application of the voltage step by the voltage-clamp technique across the membrane can be described with equation (6.37) (Figure 6.8). If the rise in voltage (Figure 6.8a – continuous line) is instantaneous, an instantaneous peak of infinite magnitude is observed (arrow in Figure 6.8b and c). (Because dV/dt in this equation approaches infinity, $dV/dt \to \infty$.) This instantaneous rise of voltage is not possible to achieve electronically and would in any case destroy the biological membrane.

In practice, the voltage step is blunted (Figure 6.8a – smooth curved line), but the capacitative current transient is still of very short duration (see Figure 6.8b, c – smooth curved lines), since soon after the application of the voltage step $dV/dt = 0$ and so $\bar{I}_c = 0$. Equation (6.37) then becomes

$$\bar{I}_t = (V - V_{oc})\bar{G}_m = \bar{I}_i \qquad (6.52)$$

Fig.6.8

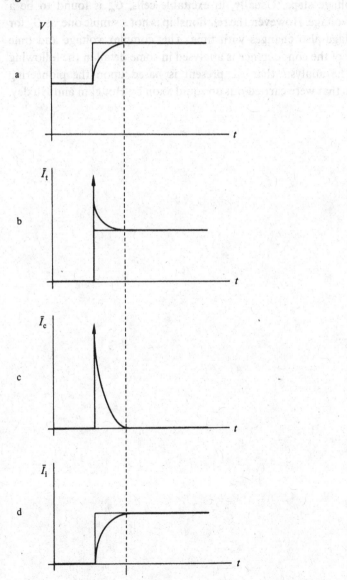

If we rearrange this equation we obtain the membrane conductance

$$\bar{G}_m = \bar{I}_t/(V - V_{oc}) \tag{6.53}$$

$\bar{G}_m$ is easily obtained from this equation because V, the voltage, is clamped and both V_{oc} and $\bar{I}_t$ can be measured. Equation (6.53) is of the same type as equation (6.18) and in both equations $\bar{G}_m$ is not necessarily a function of voltage. The voltage-clamp technique allows the electrophysiologist to test whether or not $\bar{G}_m$ depends on V. To do this, $\bar{I}_t$ is measured for a number of different voltage steps. Usually, in excitable cells, $\bar{G}_m$ is found to be a function of voltage. However, the relationship is not a simple one, as $\bar{G}_m$ for a fixed voltage also changes with time. This complex voltage and time dependence of the conductance is analysed in some detail in the following chapters. The analysis that we present is based upon the pioneering experiments that were carried out on squid axon by Hodgkin and Huxley.

7

Voltage-sensitive channels: the membrane action potential

Introduction

In Chapter 6 we described how electrical potentials may be recorded across membranes. In the absence of any externally applied currents, or spontaneous activity, these potentials take the form of steady-state membrane potentials. In excitable cells, and as a result of transient changes in the membrane properties, we can also record transient changes of the membrane potential. Some of those changes result in reversal of the polarity of the membrane potential. In this chapter we will examine the basis of this electrical activity which is the action potential. The action potential is a transient change in transmembrane electrical potential.

Although action potentials can be generated in different ways (and they may have a variety of different waveforms) the underlying electrical event is always a change in membrane conductances. The purpose of this chapter is to analyse this conductance change, so that we are able to understand action potential generation in any excitable cell.

Propagated and local action potentials

Action potentials can be recorded either as propagating electrical waves, or as electrical events that take place at a specific point in a cell membrane (local action potential). In the inset of Figure 7.1 an action potential propagates from left to right after electrical stimulation. Records obtained from the shaded area of the inset are displayed in the rest of the figure. The closed circles are voltages recorded at the same instant of the time (t_0) by electrodes placed at different positions along the fibre (x_1 to x_5). While Figure 7.1 shows the way in which propagated action potentials may be recorded, Figure 7.2 shows a local action potential obtained at a specific point in an axon (that is, at position x_5, Figure 7.1, for few milliseconds (starting at time t_0)).

If Figures 7.1 and 7.2 are compared, we notice that the waveforms obtained are mirror images of one another. This is because an observer at position x_5 will see the waveform displayed in Figure 7.1 sweep through from left to right. This means that the point in the curve corresponding to x_4 will precede the point corresponding to x_3 and so on. If each point of the waveform in Figure 7.1 is travelling at velocity v we can relate t exactly to x by the equation $x = v(t_0 - t)$.

Fig.7.1

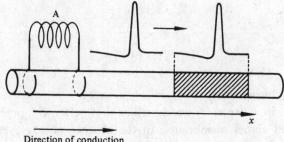

Direction of conduction

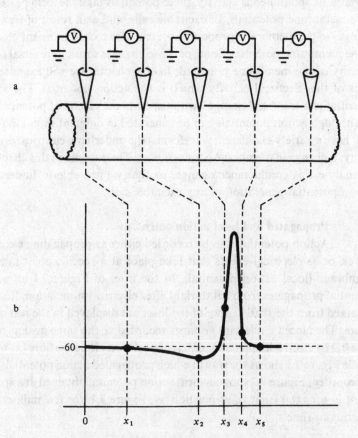

The action potential and the membrane current

The electrical potential transients seen in Figures 7.1 and 7.2 are almost entirely due to the transient flow of ionic currents. (A small fraction of the membrane currents will be 'asymmetrical displacement currents'. These are not ionic currents and are discussed later.) The quantitative relationship that exists between voltage and current will be determined entirely by the physical properties of the membrane. If we are able to define this relationship mathematically we should then be in a position to say something about the physical properties of the membranes. (This approach is used when we derive equivalent electrical circuits for membranes (in Chapter 6).) Thus, one of the aims of an electrophysiologist is to relate membrane voltage mathematically to the membrane current. The simplest way for the electrophysiologist to do this is to make one of them the independent variable.

Voltage and current clamps

Experimentally one fixes or 'clamps' the waveform of either the current or the voltage and this is known as either current or voltage clamping. In Appendix 31 the principles of these clamping techniques are discussed in more detail.

The squid axon as an idealized experimental model

For the sake of simplicity, let us imagine a cylindrical cell whose membrane has the same properties as the membrane of a squid axon. The cell is impaled with one microelectrode (Figure 7.3) and a silver wire is

Fig.7.2

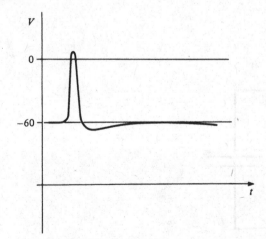

inserted along the axis of the cylinder. The silver wire is connected to a constant-current generator and the tip of the microelectrode is placed inside the cell, near the membrane, and records the transmembrane potential. As discussed in Chapter 6, the simplest electrical representation of a membrane is provided by Figure 7.4.

The lumped electrical equivalent circuit of the membrane

The constant-current generator can be thought of as a voltage source (V_s) in series with a very large resistor R_s (Figure 7.5). In this figure, R_m is the lumped resistance of the whole membrane. We shall ignore the cytoplasmic resistance as it is very small compared with R_m. It is the current flowing across the total area of cell membrane and is given by Ohm's Law:

$$I_t = V_s/(R_s + R_m) = (V_s/R_s)(1 + R_m/R_s) \tag{7.1}$$

If R_s is made much larger than R_m then the ratio R_m/R_s is very much smaller than unity and $I_t = V_s/R_s$. This implies that the injected current from the generator is independent of the membrane resistance.

Fig.7.3

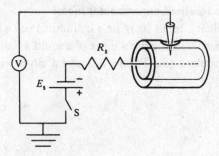

Fig.7.4

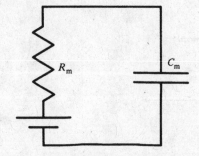

Current sign convention

Electrophysiologists have a sign convention when they describe current flow across a membrane. We have already pointed out that positive currents leave the positive terminal of a battery and flow through the external circuit into the negative terminal. Negative currents (i.e. electron flow) are in the opposite direction. Membrane potentials are measured with respect to the outside (Figure 7.3) and they are usually found to be negative potentials. When a microelectrode impales a cell and a positive current is injected through the membrane, positive ions accumulate in the solution adjacent to the *inside* of the membrane, and ions will flow away from the solution adjacent to the *outside* of the membrane. This is so because (from the Kirchhoff's Law for the currents), the current is the same at all points around a loop and so the membrane potential becomes less negative. Later on we will show that during an action potential sodium ions flow into a cell as a result of the electrochemical potential gradient, and of the change in sodium membrane conductance. Although this is also a positive current flowing into the cell, the effect will be to increase (slightly) the number of positive ions (sodium ions) inside the cell and thus to depolarize the cell. If we recall equation (6.24a)

$$V = \bar{I}_t / \bar{G}_m + (E_{Na} \bar{G}_{Na} + E_K \bar{G}_K + E_{Cl} \bar{G}_{Cl}) / \bar{G}_m \qquad (6.24a)$$

the effect on the membrane potential of injecting a positive current into a cell through a microelectrode is completely described by the first term on the right-hand side. In the course of an action potential $\bar{G}_m$ and $\bar{G}_{Na}$ are also changing, so that the second term on the right-hand side moves towards the value of E_{Na} which is positive, so the membrane is depolarized. The increase in negativity is called 'hyperpolarization' and the decrease is called 'depolarization'. In electrophysiology the present convention is to call the inward flow of positive charge (cations such as Na^+ or K^+) a negative

Fig.7.5

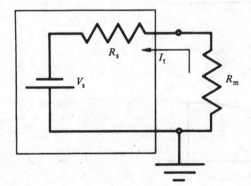

current. (Inward means positive charges move across the cell membrane from outside into the cytoplasm.) Positive current is then the outward flow of positive charges or the inward flow of negative charges (anions such as Cl^-, HCO_3^-).

Membrane potential transients under current clamp

In an experimental set up described in Figure 7.3, closing the switch S causes an outward flow of positive charge. This depolarizes the membrane and a voltage response is observed. If the cell membrane was an undoped lipid bilayer, its electrical behaviour would be, as described earlier, an exponential rise in potential (see Figure 7.6). The numerical value of the time constant (τ_m) of the rise would be given by the product $R_m C_m$ and the ΔV value is $I_t R_m$. In excitable cells, however, membranes behave differently. Figure 7.7 shows the voltage response of a membrane which has the same properties of a squid axon membrane to both depolarizing and hyper-polarizing constant-current pulses ($\bar{I}_t$). It is obvious from Figure 7.7 that the shape of the voltage transient depends on both the amplitude and sign of the constant current step.

Figure 7.8 compares the transient computed using the values of $\bar{R}_m$ and $\bar{C}_m$, before current injection, with the actual response of the system. The curve in Figure 7.8a was computed using values of $\bar{R}_m$ and $\bar{C}_m$ (both quantities expressed per cm^2) for squid axon at $t = 0$. Since the steady-state

Fig.7.6

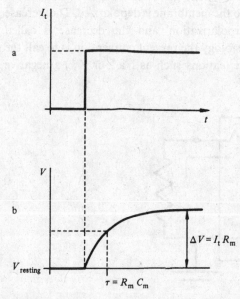

values of potential are different from those predicted, this can only be explained by changes in membrane conductances. This is because the steady-state value of membrane potential is dependent only on the membrane resistance and is independent of the membrane capacitance. As shown in Chapter 6, the equivalent circuit of the resting membrane described in Figure 7.4 can be further expanded into that of Figure 7.9. Although the transient behaviour displayed in Figure 7.7 is partly explained by the membrane capacity, $\bar{C}_m$, we have to assume that there have

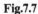

Fig.7.7

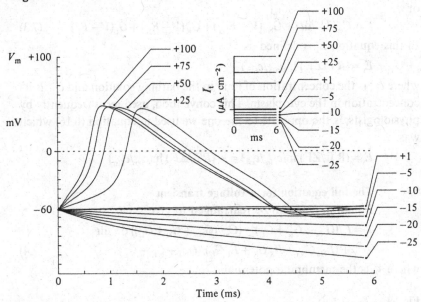

Fig.7.8

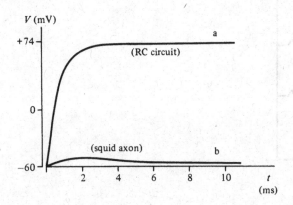

been changes in $\bar{G}_{Na}$, $\bar{G}_K$ or $\bar{G}_L$, or any combination of these conductances. The membrane capacity is involved here because the membrane potential does not follow the current step instantaneously. This is because it takes time to charge or discharge the membrane capacity.

As discussed in Chapter 6, and using the equivalent circuit from Figure 7.9, we can write a quantitative description of the total membrane current that flows during any of the voltage transients shown in Figure 7.7. $\bar{I}_t$ is, of course, the sum of the currents flowing through the four branches of the equivalent circuit shown in Figure 7.9. Thus

$$\bar{I}_t = \bar{I}_c + \bar{I}_{Na} + \bar{I}_K + \bar{I}_L \tag{7.2}$$

or

$$\bar{I}_t = \bar{C}_m (dV/dt) + \bar{G}_{Na}(V - E_{Na}) + \bar{G}_K(V - E_K) + \bar{G}_L(V - E_L) \tag{7.3}$$

In this equation E_i is defined as

$$E_i = (RT/ZF)\ln(c_{i,o}/c_{i,In})$$

where $c_{i,o}$ is the concentration of ion i in the bathing solution and $c_{i,In}$ is its concentration in the cytoplasm. This convention, used most frequently by physiologists, is the opposite to the one we used in equation (6.16) which was

$$E_i = (RT/ZF)\ln(c_{i,In}/c_{i,o}) = -(RT/ZF)\ln(c_{i,o}/c_{i,In})$$

The full equation for a voltage transient

Equation (7.3) can be rearranged to give

$$V = \bar{I}_t/(\bar{G}_{Na} + \bar{G}_K + \bar{G}_L) - (\bar{C}_m/(\bar{G}_{Na} + \bar{G}_K + \bar{G}_L))\,dV/dt$$
$$+ (E_{Na}\bar{G}_{Na} + E_K\bar{G}_K + E_L\bar{G}_L)/(\bar{G}_{Na} + \bar{G}_K + \bar{G}_L) \tag{7.4}$$

where V is the membrane potential.

Fig.7.9

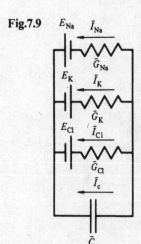

This equation can be more easily understood if we take three cases. In the open-circuit case (i.e. switch S open in Figure 7.3) no current is injected into the cell. This means that the membrane current $\bar{I}_t$ is zero and the membrane potential does not change with time, so $\bar{I}_i = 0$, $d(V)/dt = 0$, and equation (7.4) reduces to

$$V_{oc} = (E_{Na}\bar{G}_{Na} + E_K\bar{G}_K + E_L\bar{G}_L)/(\bar{G}_{Na} + \bar{G}_K + \bar{G}_L) \qquad (7.5)$$

where V_{oc} is defined as the open-circuit potential. In the steady-state case (obtained after closing the switch S in Figure 7.3), $\bar{I}_t$ is not zero but the membrane potential is still not changing with time, so $dV/dt = 0$ and equation (7.4) becomes

$$V = \bar{I}_t/(\bar{G}_{Na} + \bar{G}_K + \bar{G}_L) + V_{oc} \qquad (7.6)$$

which can be rewritten as

$$V = \bar{I}_m \bar{R}_m + V_{oc} \qquad (7.6a)$$

where

$$\bar{R}_m = 1/\bar{G}_m = 1/(\bar{G}_{Na} + \bar{G}_K + \bar{G}_L) \qquad (7.7)$$

Equation (7.6) describes the circuit shown in Figure 7.10 and the relationship between voltage and current at the terminals is shown in Figure 7.11.

For the third case (which occurs during the voltage transient), all three terms in equation (7.4) have to be included. It is of interest that the second term on the right-hand side of equation (7.4), the fraction

$$\bar{C}_m/(\bar{G}_{Na} + \bar{G}_K + \bar{G}_L)$$

is equal to $\bar{C}_m\bar{R}_m$ (equation (7.7)). This is the membrane time constant τ_m which will determine the rate of rise of the membrane potential.

Conductance changes in excitable membranes

With equation (7.4) and because $\bar{I}_t$ is constant, we are now in a position to analyse the voltage curves displayed in Figure 7.7. Changes in

Fig.7.10

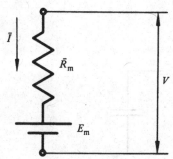

equilibrium potential (E_{Na}, E_K, E_L) in equation (7.4) will depend upon the surface:volume ratio of the cell and the size and duration of the membrane currents. We will assume that the equilibrium potentials in equation (7,4) are constant. (Although not always valid, this is a common assumption made by electrophysiologists.) As pointed out above, the most likely explanation that the excitable cell membrane shown (Figure 7.7) is not like an undoped lipid bilayer, is that transient conductance changes do take place. Figure 7.12 shows the way in which these conductance changes may be incorporated into an equivalent circuit. It is usual to represent ionic conductances as variable conductors.

The independence of the membrane conductances: ion substitutions and the use of inhibitors

Since we have decided that the transient changes in membrane voltage are due to conductance changes, we have to obtain a quantitative description of the dynamic behaviour of the three conductances $\bar{G}_{Na}$, $\bar{G}_K$, and $\bar{G}_L$. The classical way in which electrophysiologists have approached this problem was to first assume that $\bar{G}_{Na}$, $\bar{G}_K$ and $\bar{G}_L$ were independent of one another. They then examined the total membrane conductance ($\bar{G}_m$)

Fig.7.11

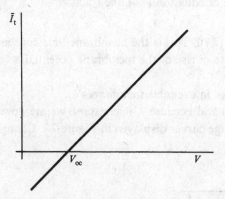

Fig.7.12

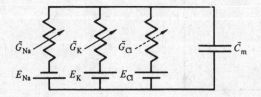

with one or more of the individual membrane conductances turned off. Hodgkin & Huxley did this by removing different ion species from the external solution. This technique is known as *ion substitution* because, in practice, one substitutes an impermeant ion for a permeant one. For example, in the case of sodium, Hodgkin & Huxley replaced it with choline. More recently, electrophysiologists have used pharmacological agents that block (with a high degree of specificity) different ion conductances. For example, tetrodotoxin (TTX) will block $\bar{G}_{Na}$ and tetraethylammonium ions (TEA) will block $\bar{G}_{K}$.

In order to understand the basis of the ion substitution technique, let us consider the case of a single sodium-specific channel through which current flows as a result of an applied electric field (Figure 7.13). In the first figure (7.13a) sodium is on both sides of the membrane and current flows inwards. In 7.13b we have substituted choline for sodium in the outside bathing fluid.

Fig.7.13

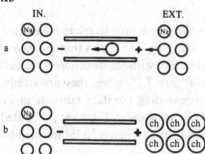

Since choline is unable to carry current inwards, through the channel, the channel becomes non-conducting. In a real system the situation is more complex as, generally, there will be an outward diffusional sodium current through the channel (see Chapter 3). But for these purposes this diffusional current is so small that it is usually ignored.

The mechanism by which pharmacological agents block channels can be pictorially represented by Figure 7.14. We can consider that conceptually ion substitution (Figure 7.13) and a pharmacological block (Figure 7.14) have the same effect because the end result of both techniques is the blocking of ion channel conductances.

Fig.7.14

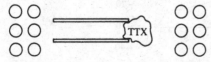

Elimination of sodium conductance

In an ion substitution experiment of the type described in Figure 7.13, but, instead of sodium, chloride is removed from the external bathing fluid, the voltage transients obtained are similar to those shown in Figure 7.7. (In this experiment, chloride ions are substituted with impermeant ions such as sulphate or isothionate.) If we now block the sodium conductance we obtain the responses shown in Figure 7.15, the delayed change in resistance seen with the more positive depolarizing current pulses is generally known as 'delayed rectification' and is due to the delayed changes in the potassium membrane conductance which we describe later. Because of the large number of transients displayed, the comparison between the two sets of curves in Figures 7.7 and 7.15 is difficult, so we shall compare only one curve from each set (Figure 7.16). Thus, Figure 7.16 represents the voltage transient obtained before and after blocking the sodium current. The constant current step was the same for both the transients.

I/V curves

We have seen already in Chapter 6 how to relate membrane I/V curves to membrane conductances. Figure 7.15 shows that the membrane conductance changes with both time and with the direction of the current. The values of the voltages from Figure 7.15, when they are steady, are plotted as a function of the corresponding constant currents in Figure 7.17a. In addition, in Figure 7.17 we show I/V curves computed for membranes containing only ohmic channels (Figure 7.17b) and membranes

Fig.7.15

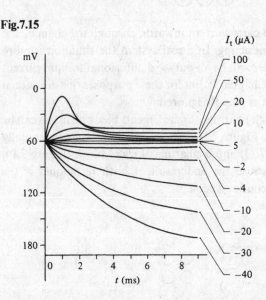

containing only channels which obey the Goldman–Hodgkin–Katz equation (Figure 7.17c) (see Chapter 4). The G–H–K I/V curve was calculated, with a $\bar{G}_K$ obtained at the resting membrane potential of Figure 7.15. The same value of $\bar{G}_K$ was used to compute the ohmic I/V curve.

Fig.7.16

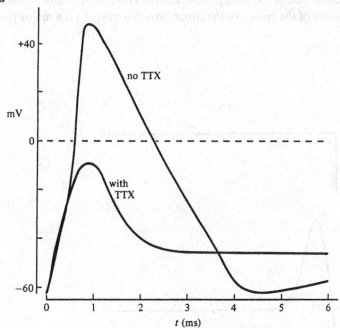

Fig.7.17

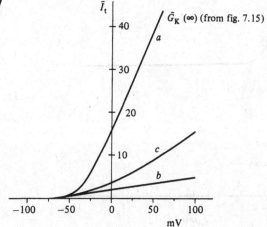

The capacitative current

In the experiment described in Figure 7.14 the main carrier of the membrane current is potassium. However, the voltage transient shown in Figure 7.15 does not entirely reflect the dynamic behaviour of the potassium conductance. This is because in the transient part of the response a large part of the membrane current is capacitative. This is more clearly shown in Figures 7.18 and 7.19 where the separate components of $\bar{I}_t$ have been plotted for one of the voltage transients (V) taken from Figure 7.15. In the early phase of the response the capacitative current ($\bar{I}_c$) is a major part of $\bar{I}_t$.

Fig.7.18

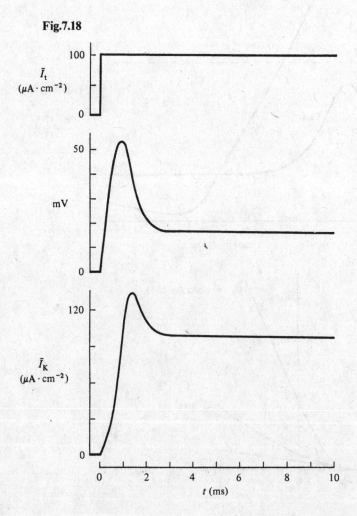

Removal of capacitative current by voltage clamp

Whenever rapid changes in transmembrane voltage take place, large membrane capacitative currents $(\bar{I}_c)$ occur. This is because $\bar{I}_c = \bar{C}_m \, dV/dt$. One way of controlling $\bar{I}_c$ is to choose a constant waveform for V, controlling its time course by a voltage-clamp technique. Figure 7.20 shows a very simplified diagram of a voltage-clamp arrangement. The ground reference electrode G, the voltage (V) and the current (I) electrodes are designed so that the membrane voltage and current are the same at every point along the membrane. By the action of amplifier A the

Fig.7.19

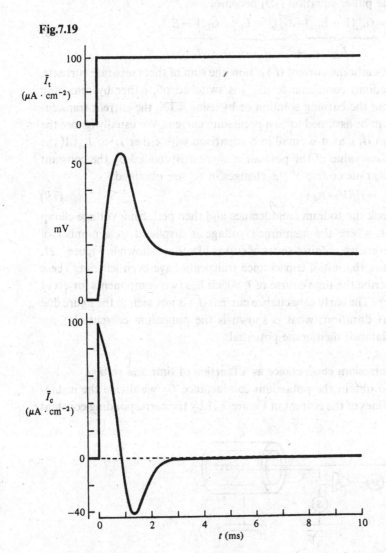

membrane voltage follows the output of the source voltage S, and the current waveform is displayed in D.

The usual waveform is a quickly rising step so that the membrane capacity is very rapidly either charged or discharged. When the membrane is either fully charged or discharged, $\bar{I}_c$ is zero because dV/dt is zero ($\bar{I}_c = \bar{C}_m(dV/dt)$).

If we recall equation (7.3)

$$\bar{I}_t = \bar{C}_m(dV/dt) + \bar{G}_{Na}(V - E_{Na}) + \bar{G}_K(V - E_K) + \bar{G}_L(V - E_L) \qquad (7.3)$$

Under voltage-clamp conditions, except for a very short period during the onset of the pulse, equation (7.3) becomes

$$\bar{I}_t = \underbrace{\bar{G}_{Na}(V - E_{Na})}_{\bar{I}_{Na}} + \underbrace{\bar{G}_K(V - E_K)}_{\bar{I}_K} + \underbrace{\bar{G}_L(V - E_L)}_{\bar{I}_L} \qquad (7.8)$$

The total membrane current ($\bar{I}_t$) is now the sum of three separate currents.

If the sodium conductance ($\bar{G}_{Na}$) is switched off, either by removing sodium from the bathing solution or by using TTX, the current transient recorded can be assumed to be a potassium current. We usually ignore the leak current ($\bar{I}_L$), as it is small in comparison with either $\bar{I}_K$ or $\bar{I}_{Na}$. If the instantaneous value of the potassium current is divided by the constant $(V - E_K)$ the time course of the changes in $\bar{G}_K$ are obtained

$$\bar{G}_K = I_t/(V - E_K) \qquad (7.9)$$

If we block the sodium conductance and then perform a voltage-clamp experiment, where the membrane voltage is displaced to a number of different levels, we obtain a series of curves like those shown in Figure 7.21. In this figure the initial capacitance transients have been left out. These curves describe the time course of $\bar{I}_t$ which has two components for every voltage step. The early capacitance current ($\bar{I}_c$) is not seen in the figure due to its short duration; what is shown is the potassium current ($\bar{I}_K$), for different clamped membrane potentials.

Potassium conductance as a function of time and voltage

To obtain the potassium conductance $\bar{G}_K$ we divide the instantaneous values of the current in Figure 7.21 by the corresponding constant

Fig.7.20

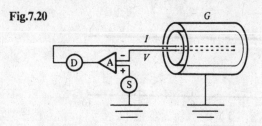

$(V - E_K)$ values and so obtain the family of curves displayed in Figure 7.22. This shows that the potassium conductance depends upon both time and voltage or, mathematically, we can write that

$$\bar{G}_K = f(V, t) \tag{7.10}$$

The potassium conductance $\bar{G}_K$ might be a function of the membrane current but, as we shall see later, this is unlikely. This voltage and time dependence of the potassium conductance can be explained by at least two mechanisms:

Fig.7.21

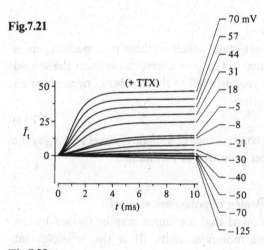

Fig.7.22

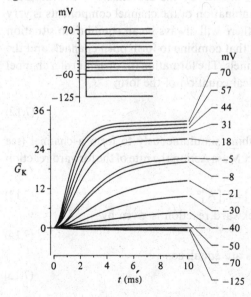

(i) that potassium crosses the membrane through a constant number of ion-specific channels. The permeability of these channels changes with both time and membrane potential; or

(ii) that the potassium channels can only exist in either an opened or closed state. The fraction of the channel population in either state changes with time and is voltage dependent.

Both these explanations are based on the assumption that potassium crosses the membrane through channels. The basis of this assumption was discussed in Chapter 5.

Potassium channels

At present we cannot state which of these two mechanisms is correct, but evidence presented in Chapter 5 seems to support the second case. If $\bar{G}_K$ is assumed to be proportional to the number of open channels per unit area of membrane, then

$$\bar{G}_K = G_{Kch} N_{ch} \qquad (7.11)$$

where G_{Kch} is the potassium conductance of a single channel and N_{ch} is the number of open channels per unit area of membrane.

The formation or opening of potassium channels

In Chapter 5 we showed that a channel may be formed by the aggregation of two or more molecular units. (It is also possible that channels may be opened (or closed) by the movement of two or more blocking particles.) If the combination of the channel components is very fast (almost instantaneous), there will always be an equilibrium situation between the number of units that combine to form open channels and the existing number of open channels. The formation (or opening) of a channel can be described by a chemical equation of the form

$$\underbrace{A + A + \cdots + A}_{a} \rightleftharpoons ch \qquad (7.12)$$

where a particles of A combine simultaneously to form a channel (see Figure 7.23). From the Law of Mass Action the rate of the forward reaction can be written as

$$v_f = k_f[A][A] \cdots [A] = k_f[A]^a \qquad (7.13)$$

Similarly the rate of the backward reaction is given by

$$v_b = k_b[ch] \qquad (7.14)$$

At equilibrium the two rates are equal, so

$$v_f = v_b \qquad (7.15)$$

and
$$k_b[ch] = k_f[A]^a \tag{7.16}$$
then
$$[ch] = K[A]^a \tag{7.17}$$
or more simply
$$N_{ch} = KN^a \tag{7.18}$$
where K is the equilibrium constant and N is the number of particles of A per unit area of membrane. (We can think of N as the number of particles in a cylinder whose height is the thickness of the cell membrane and with a base of unit area, while $[A]$ is the number of particles per unit volume.) The total number of channels per unit area of membrane (M_{chT}) is then given by
$$N_{chT} = KN_T^a \tag{7.19}$$
where N_T is the maximum number of particles per unit area of membrane, N can be related to N_T by
$$N = nN_T \tag{7.20}$$
where n is the fraction of the total number of particles available to form channels. By substituting equations (7.18), (7.19) and (7.20) in equation (7.11) we get
$$\bar{G}_K = (G_{Kch}N_{chT})n^a \tag{7.21}$$

The maximum potassium conductance

The term $(G_{Kch}N_{chT})$ is the maximum possible value that the membrane potassium conductance can reach ($\bar{G}_K$) and equation (7.21) can be rewritten as
$$\bar{G}_K = \bar{G}_K n^a \tag{7.22}$$

Fig.7.23

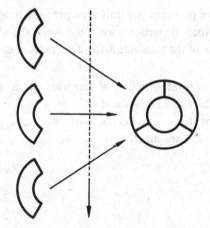

The approach of relating conductance to the opening (formation) of channels was first used by Hodgkin and Huxley in their classical study of the squid axon. They proposed that for any instant of time a certain number of channels are being opened and that, at the same time, a certain number of open channels are being closed. As discussed above, the conversion of closed to open channels can mean either the opening of closed channels or the formation of new channels.

The Hodgkin–Huxley model of channel opening (formation)

In order to describe this conversion process the simplest assumption to make is to assume that in a unit area of membrane there are a fixed number of particles (N_T). N of these N_T particles are in a position or conformation so that a channel can be formed (opened) and $\bar{N}$ of N_T particles are in an inactive form and unable to form (open) channels. At any moment in time, the rate of conversion of an inactive into an active particle is proportional to the number of inactive particles ($\bar{N}$). Also the rate of inactivation of active particles is proportional to the number of available or active particles (N). Thus the net rate of formation of active particles (dN/dt) is given by

$$dN/dt = \underset{\substack{\text{rate of}\\\text{conversion}\\\text{of inactive}\\\text{particles}}}{\alpha_n \bar{N}} \quad - \quad \underset{\substack{\text{rate of}\\\text{conversion}\\\text{of active}\\\text{particles}}}{\beta_n N} \tag{7.23}$$

where α_n and β_n are the rate constants. The rate constant in this case is the fraction of the inactive particles (active particles) that are inactive (active) per unit time and membrane area. The product of rate constant and the number of inactive particles has the dimensions of

$$(1/t)(\bar{N}/\text{area})$$

which is the number of inactive particles per unit area per unit time.

Instead of using actual number of particles we could write the above equation in terms of the fraction of the total numbers of particles in each of the two states where

$n=$the fraction of the total number of particles for a given membrane area which are active, and

$\bar{n}=$the fraction of the total number of particles for a given membrane area which are inactive.

Then

$$n + \bar{n} = 1.0 \tag{7.24 (i)}$$

and

$$N = nN_T \tag{7.24 (ii)}$$

$$\text{and } \bar{N} = \bar{n}N_T \tag{7.24 (iii)}$$

Substituting (7.24)(i), (ii) and (iii) in equation (7.23) we obtain

$$dn/dt = \alpha_n(1-n) - \beta_n n \tag{7.25}$$

It should be remembered that equation (7.25) was derived in order to describe how the potassium conductance shown in Figure 7.22 changes with time and voltage. In physical terms n can be assumed to have a constant value (n_0) before a voltage-clamp pulse is applied. If sufficient time is allowed to elapse after switching on the voltage pulse, n reaches a steady-state and becomes constant (n_∞). Before the application of the pulse ($t=0$)

$$dn/dt = 0 \quad n = n_0 \tag{7.26}$$

and at steady-state ($t \to \infty$)

$$dn/dt = 0 \quad n = n_\infty \tag{7.27}$$

Substituting (7.27) in equation (7.25) we obtain

$$0 = \alpha_n(1-n) - \beta_n n \tag{7.28 (i)}$$

$$n = \alpha_n/(\alpha_n + \beta_n) \tag{7.28 (ii)}$$

Both of the two mechanisms described earlier, to explain the switching on of the potassium conductance, imply that $\bar{G}_K$ is directly related to the number of open channels (N_{ch}) and thus to n (see equations (7.14) to (7.17)). In the steady state, it is clear from Figure 7.22 that $\bar{G}_K$ is a function of voltage only. This means that n_0 and n are also voltage dependent, and it is also implied from equation (7.28) that the rate constants α_n and β_n are voltage dependent. If we now assume that α_n and β_n are functions of voltage, the integration of equation (7.25) becomes relatively simple. Rearranging equation (7.25)

$$dn/dt = -(\alpha_n + \beta_n)[n - \alpha_n/(\alpha_n + \beta_n)]$$

which on substitution for (7.28) becomes

$$dn/dt = -(\alpha_n + \beta_n) \tag{7.29}$$

The equation may be integrated (see Appendix 10) to give

$$n = n_\infty + (n_0 - n_\infty)\exp(-kt) \tag{7.30}$$

where

$$k = \alpha_n + \beta_n$$

If n_0 is added and subtracted to the right-hand side of (7.30) we obtain

$$n = n_0 + (n_\infty - n_0)(1 - \exp(-kt)) \tag{7.31}$$

In order to relate n to $\bar{G}_K$, n is obtained from equation (7.22)

$$(\bar{G}_K/\bar{G}_K)^{1/a}$$

and substituted into equation (7.31) to give

$$(\bar{G}_K/(G_{Kch}N_{chT}))^{1/a} = (\bar{G}_o/(G_{Kch}N_{chT}))^{1/a}$$
$$+ [(\bar{G}_{K_\infty}/(G_{Kch}N_{chT}))^{1/a} - (\bar{G}_{K_0}/(G_{Kch}N_{chT}))^{1/a}]$$
$$\times [1 - \exp(-kt)] \tag{7.32}$$

As can be seen from Figure 7.24, for a fixed value of K, as the value of a is increased from 1 to 4, better fits are obtained of the experimental $\bar{G}_K$ curves shown in Figure 7.22. Although the choice of K used in equation (7.32) to draw Figure 7.24 (y_1) was arbitrary, it can still be noted that Figure 7.24 (y_1) is a smoothly rising exponential while the curves in Figure 7.24 (y_2–y_4) and Figure 7.22 all have points of inflexion.

Fig.7.24

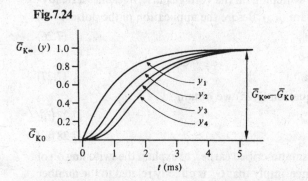

Since a best fit is obtained with a equal to at least four, the conclusion we draw is that a channel is opened when at least four particles are activated by the transmembrane voltage. As $\bar{G}_K$ is dependent on the fraction of activated particles (n), so it must be voltage dependent (as shown in Figure 7.22).

We have obtained an analytical expression (equation (7.32)) which describes the course of $\bar{G}_K$ under voltage-clamp conditions. The way in which we set out to derive this expression is represented schematically in Figure 7.25. In this figure particles in the inactive state ($\bar{n}$) are activated (n) before they form an open channel. The combination of the n particles to form a channel is assumed to be very fast so that the rate-limiting step is the conversion of $\bar{n}$ to n. Equation (7.13) describes the combination of n particles to form a channel, while the much slower process ($\bar{n}$ to n) is described by equation (7.23). (It should be remembered that Figure 7.25 only pictorially describes the formation of an open channel; as to what really happens in nature we are, as yet, unable to say!)

Charge movements inside the membranes of excitable cells: displacement currents

An alternative scheme that might easily be proposed to Figure 7.25 is shown in Figure 7.26. This is a more elaborate scheme where the particles are the gates which move (or deform) under the influence of an electric field. In order to derive equation (7.13) using this model, we still have to assume that the four gates are independent of one another. This movement of gates (or deformation) corresponds to a displacement of charge in the membrane. An interesting recent development is that these displacements of charge have been measured in different types of excitable cells. A movement of charge inside the membrane is detected externally as a very small current (displacement current). The way in which these currents are measured is first to block all the ionic currents using appropriate pharmacological agents. The residual total current records obtained under voltage clamp are then digitized and stored in a computer. With reasonably sophisticated programmes the capacitative current obtained when there are no conductance changes occurring in the membrane is subtracted from the total

Fig.7.25

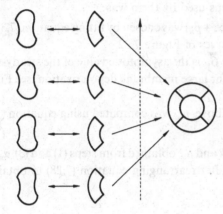

Fig.7.26

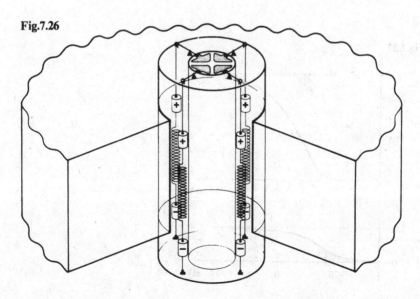

current record to obtain the displacement current. A clear voltage dependence of the displacement current has been observed.

At this point we have obtained a general expression in equation (7.32) which, with an appropriate choice of k, can be made to fit the experimental curves shown in Figure 7.22.

In order to derive a full analytical description of $\bar{G}_K$ as a function of voltage as well as of time, we have to obtain a relationship between k (which is $\alpha_n + \beta_n$) and V. A number of different ways of doing this are available. For example, a computer programme could be run to carry out a repetitive search of the parameter values ($\bar{G}_{K_0}$, $\bar{G}_K$, a and k). The end point of the search is when the experimental curves are well fitted by equation (7.32). We shall limit ourselves here to the numerical strategy used by Hodgkin and Huxley. The sequence of steps used by them was:

(1) A value of k (that is, $\alpha_n + \beta_n$) was chosen by fitting equation (7.32) to the experimental curves of Figure 7.22.

(2) Then $\bar{G}_K$ was found. $\bar{G}_K$ is the asymptotic value of the steady-state conductance ($\bar{G}_{K_\infty}$) for large membrane depolarization (see Figure 7.27).

(3) With $\bar{G}_K$ obtained above, n_∞ was computed using equation (7.22)

$$n_\infty = (\bar{G}_K/\bar{G}_K)^{1/4} \tag{7.33}$$

(4) Using the values of k and n_∞ obtained from steps (1) and (3), α_n and β_n were calculated after rearranging equation (7.28) to obtain

$$\alpha_n = n_\infty k \tag{7.34}$$

$$\beta_n = (1 - n_\infty)k \tag{7.35}$$

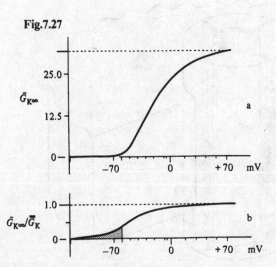

Fig.7.27

The voltage dependence of the rate constants

The results obtained using the above four steps allow α_n and β_n to be plotted as functions of V (Figure 7.28). It should be pointed out that for values of membrane potential near or below the resting potential (shaded in Figures 7.27 and 7.28), $\bar{I}_K$ is small. This means that curve fitting using equation (7.33) is difficult and k cannot be estimated. The way this problem

Fig.7.28

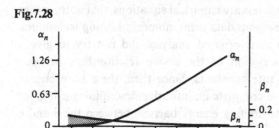

is overcome is to first displace the membrane potential to a level where there is a measurable steady-state $\bar{I}_K$, and then to switch the membrane potential back to levels around and below the resting potential (Figure 7.29). The exponential decline of $\bar{G}_K$, shown in Figure 7.29, depends on the values of α_n and β_n which have been instantaneously set by the hyperpolarizing pulse. By curve fitting the declining $\bar{G}_K$ with the expression (7.34), we are now able to estimate k and hence α_n and β_n.

It should be noted that Figure 7.28 displays the relationship between energy per coulomb (V) and a rate constant. An intuitive interpretation of this relationship is to assume that particles in the $\bar{n}$ or n states have a spectrum of energy levels given by the Boltzmann distribution (see Appendix 21). We further assume that in order for a particle to change from the $\bar{n}$ state into the n state, its energy must be above a certain level ($\vec{E}$). The same thing applies to transitions from n to $\bar{n}$ but the energy required for the transition ($\overleftarrow{E}$) is different. At any given temperature there will be an equilibrium distribution of particles in the n and $\bar{n}$ states when the number of particles changing from $\bar{n}$ to n (that is, having energies above $\vec{E}$) is equal to the number of particles changing from n to $\bar{n}$ (that is, having energies above $\overleftarrow{E}$). If we suddenly change the membrane potential, and thus the particle energies, a new readjustment has to take place since more (or fewer) particles will now have enough energies to make the transition. At each membrane voltage there will be a rate at which particles change from $\bar{n}$ to n

and from n to $\bar{n}$. Thus the rate constants α_n and β_n are themselves functions of voltage. The voltage functions which Hodgkin and Huxley fitted to their voltage-clamp data for the rate constants were

$$\alpha_n = 0.01(V+10)/(\exp(V+10)/10)-1)$$

and

$$\beta_n = 0.125 \exp(V/80)$$

(but see Appendix 32 for equations currently used by electrophysiologists).

These rate-constant equations are empirical equations, that is, they were obtained from the voltage-clamp data using numerical fitting techniques. Hodgkin and Huxley, in their original analysis, did not try to give a complete biophysical description of the above relationships between membrane potential and rate constants. Since then, there have been a number of attempts to give complete quantitative descriptions using, for example, one or multi-rate-limiting energy barriers between the $\bar{n}$ and n states. But, as we consider these models beyond the scope of this book, we shall limit our approach to the above intuitive description of the rate constant-voltage relationship.

Fig.7.29

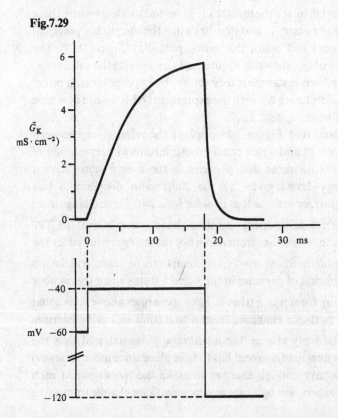

We have so far been able to show that equation (7.27), together with equations (7.22), (7.28) and (7.29), provide an analytical description of $\bar{G}_K$ as function of both time and voltage, and these equations allow all the experimental curves shown in Figure 7.22 to be reconstructed.

Potassium channels are ohmic: instantaneous I/V curves

There is, however, an assumption that was made but not yet analysed. Equation (7.9), when used to calculate $\bar{G}_K$, assumes that potassium channels are ohmic conductors. By definition I/V (current divided by voltage) is a conductance but it is not necessarily an ohmic (i.e. linear) conductance. However, Hodgkin and Huxley assumed that when $\bar{I}_K$ was divided by $(E_K + V)$ the $\bar{G}_K$ obtained was an ohmic conductance. This assumption can be tested experimentally by obtaining I/V curves at a constant $\bar{G}_K$. By constant this means that the number of open potassium channels is fixed. If $\bar{G}_K$ follows Ohm's Law, the I/V curve should be linear. Experimentally a constant $\bar{G}_K$ is obtained with the voltage protocol described in Figure 7.30 and Figure 7.29. Initially the membrane is depolarized with a single voltage step and this step is always of a fixed amplitude and duration and is responsible for setting a constant $\bar{G}_K$. A second pulse is then applied and sets the membrane at different voltage levels. The first pulse is often known as the *conditioning* pulse and the second pulse is often known as the *test* pulse. (Figure 7.30 plots the extrapolated currents against the test pulse voltage.) If the membrane had no capacity the family of curves obtained would be similar to those shown in the insets of Figure 7.30. But, since there always is a membrane capacity,

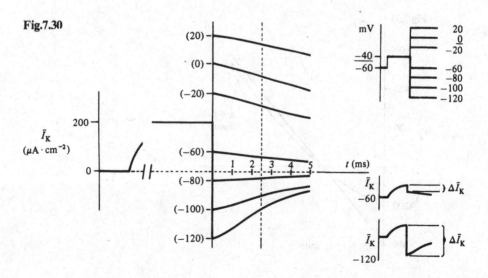

Fig.7.30

to obtain the values of $\bar{I}_K$ the transient curves have to be extrapolated (either graphically or numerically) back to the instant of time at which the membrane was either hyperpolarized or depolarized by the test pulse. Alternatively, with the use of a computer, a scaled capacitative transient may be subtracted from the current response to obtain curves similar to the inserts. The resulting so-called instantaneous I/V curve obtained in squid axon is shown in Figure 7.31a.

The potassium equilibrium potential

Curves a and b are I/V curves obtained at different moments in time (see Figure 7.30) and with a changing $\bar{G}_K$. Curve a, which is linear, can be used to determine the potassium equilibrium potential (E_K, Chapters 2, 3 and 6). From equation (7.9), where $\bar{I}_K$ is zero, $V = E_K$, and this is the value of the membrane potential when $\bar{I}_K$ is zero.

We can thus conclude that during an action potential in the squid axon, potassium current flows through voltage-sensitive channels, and that these channels act as ohmic conductors when they are open. Although, as in the case of the squid axon, the channels behave as ohmic conductors, this is not always so. Thus, for example, in the node of Ranvier of the myelinated nerve fibre of the frog, the voltage-dependent potassium channels are not ohmic and they show constant-field rectification. It is perhaps more accurate to say that the Hodgkin–Huxley model leads to the derivation of quantitative relationships which accurately predict the behaviour of the potassium currents. The voltage-sensitive channels are conceptual components of the model.

Fig.7.31

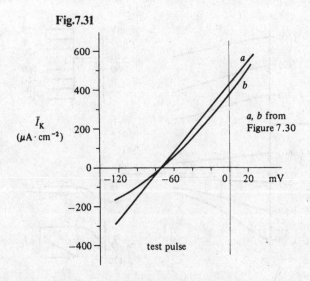

Although we are unable to describe the exact physical nature of either the conductance changes or the way in which membrane voltage controls channel opening, we have been able to describe these relationships quantitatively. Moreover, the set of quantitative relationships that were derived above provides a very accurate description of the time and voltage dependence of the potassium currents.

The sodium current

In order to provide a description of the sodium current we have to characterize $\bar{G}_{Na}$ in a similar manner. For this purpose the relationship

$$\bar{G}_{Na} = \bar{I}_{Na}/(V - E_{Na}) \tag{7.36}$$

is used and this equation may be directly compared with equation (7.9). To obtain the $\bar{I}_{Na}$ term in equation (7.36) we can either follow the approach of Hodgkin and Huxley and subtract the $\bar{I}_K$ from $\bar{I}_t$ (see equation (7.8)), or we can pharmacologically block $\bar{I}_K$. In Figure 7.32, panel a shows a family of $\bar{I}_t$ curves obtained after the membrane potential was voltage clamped at a number of different levels. In panel b we show the corresponding $\bar{I}_K$ curves that have already been described in Figure 7.21. The family of curves in panel c can be recorded directly by blocking $\bar{I}_K$ or computed by subtracting $\bar{I}_K$ curves (panel b) from $\bar{I}_t$ curves (panel a).

The sodium conductance

From any of the curves of panel c in Figure 7.32 we can calculate (with equation (7.36)) the instantaneous value of $\bar{G}_{Na}$. One of these curves is plotted in Figure 7.33 together with the $\bar{G}_K$ curve for the same voltage-clamp pulse. Comparison of the two curves reveals three major differences:

(i) $\bar{G}_{Na}$ is switched on before $\bar{G}_K$,

Fig.7.32

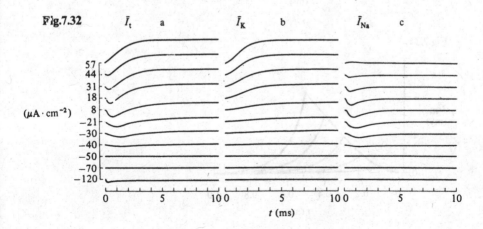

(ii) $\bar{G}_{Na}$ rises more steeply than $\bar{G}_K$, and

(iii) $\bar{G}_{Na}$ rises and then falls while the $\bar{G}_K$ rises and then remains constant.

The time course of the $\bar{G}_{Na}$ curve suggests that $\bar{G}_{Na}$ is independent of membrane potential. However, if the clamp pulse is switched off earlier (Figure 7.34), $\bar{G}_{Na}$, like $\bar{G}_K$, is turned off (compare Figure 7.34 with Figure 7.29) and this shows that $\bar{G}_{Na}$ is also a continuous function of the membrane voltage. Mathematically we can imagine that $\bar{G}_{Na}$ is being controlled by the separate, activating and inactivating voltage-dependent processes. If only the activation process was in operation, $\bar{G}_{Na}$ would follow curve *a* in Figure 7.35. But inactivation occurs, and $\bar{G}_{Na}$ is increasingly turned off (curve *b*, Figure 7.35). Pictorially this could be imagined in Figure 7.36, where depolarization simultaneously sets in motion the opening (activation) of a fast gate (m) and the closing (inactivation) of a slower blocking gate (h). From Figure 7.35 and by direct comparison with $\bar{G}_K$ (Figure 7.22, equation

Fig.7.33

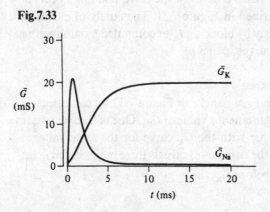

Fig.7.34

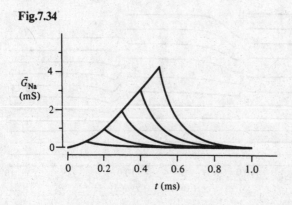

(7.22)) we can write for curve *a* the following function

$$\tilde{G}_{Na} = \overline{G}_{Na} m^a \tag{7.37}$$

where $\overline{G}_{Na}$ is the *maximum* sodium conductance, per unit area of membrane, and *m* is the fraction of the total number of activating particles. Curves like $\tilde{G}_{Na}$ can be obtained experimentally if curves are initially perfused with pronase. This enzyme is thought to remove the inactivation process.

Sodium inactivation

Curve *b* in Figure 7.35 is the sodium conductance ($\overline{G}_{Na}$). If we now define arbitrarily a voltage and time-dependent inactivation function, *h*, as

Fig.7.35

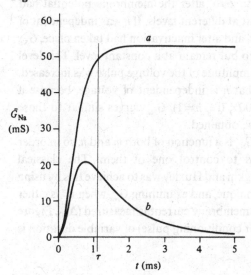

Fig.7.36

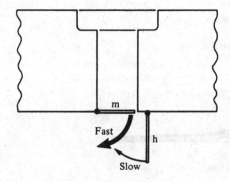

$$h = \bar{G}_{Na}/\tilde{G}_{Na} \tag{7.38}$$

curves *a* and *b* in Figure 7.35 can be related by

$$\bar{G}_{Na} = \tilde{G}_{Na}h = \overline{\overline{G}}_{Na}m^a h \tag{7.39}$$

The inactivation function h varies between zero and one. When $h=0$ (full inactivation) there is no $\bar{G}_{Na}$, when $h=1$ (no activation) $\bar{G}_{Na}$ depends on m.

Figure 7.37 shows $\bar{G}_{Na}$ calculated from Figure 7.32 using equation (7.36) and illustrates that h is a function of time. This is because the conductance decreases with time, which means that channel inactivation also increases with time.

Voltage dependence of inactivation

Figure 7.37 also suggests that h might be a function of voltage because $\bar{G}_{Na}$ always returned to zero, after the membrane potential had been changed and kept constant at different levels. If h was independent of voltage for a given clamp pulse, and after inactivation had taken place, $\bar{G}_{Na}$ values would not return to zero but remain at a constant level. This level would also increase when the amplitude of the voltage pulse was increased. However, it is also possible that h is independent of voltage, because if inactivation always became 100% (i.e. $h=1$), $\bar{G}_{Na}$ curves similar to those shown in Figure 7.37 would be obtained.

Equation (7.39) shows that $\bar{G}_{Na}$ is a function of both m and h, so in order to measure m or h we need to control one of them. The classical experimental approach of Hodgkin and Huxley was to achieve this by using a two-pulse voltage-clamp technique, and examining $\bar{G}_{Na}$ when m^a is either small or constant. Initially the membrane current is measured ($\Delta \bar{I}_0$, Figure 7.38a). Then a pre-test pulse (or conditioning pulse) of variable duration is

Fig.7.37

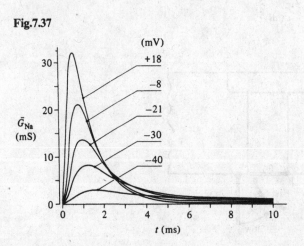

applied before the membrane is returned to the test pulse value (Figure 7.38b). The peak current obtained $(\Delta \bar{I}_t)$, for a conditioning pulse of t ms, is shown in Figure 7.38b, along with the voltage profile. Mathematically, the double-pulse technique may be analysed as follows:

If we rearrange equation (7.36) we obtain

$$\bar{I}_{Na} = \bar{G}_{Na}(V - E_{Na}) \tag{7.36a}$$

Before the test pulse is applied this equation can be rewritten as

$$\bar{I}_{Na_0} = \bar{G}_{Na}(V_0 - E_{Na}) \tag{7.36b}$$

If we apply a test pulse we obtain

$$\bar{I}_{Na_t} = \bar{G}_{Na}(V_t - E_{Na}) \tag{7.36c}$$

By subtracting (7.36b) from (7.36c) we obtain

$$\begin{aligned} \Delta \bar{I}_0 &= \bar{I}_{Na_t} - \bar{I}_{Na_0} \\ &= \bar{G}_{Na}(V_t - V_0) \\ &= \bar{G}_{Na} \, \Delta V \end{aligned}$$

From equation (7.39), and in the absence of the conditioning pulse, $\bar{I}_0$ is given by

$$\Delta \bar{I}_0 = \bar{G}_{Na} m^a h(0) \, \Delta V \tag{7.40}$$

while after a conditioning pulse of duration t

$$\Delta \bar{I}_t = \bar{G}_{Na} m_t^a h(t) \, \Delta V \tag{7.41}$$

so that

$$y(t) = \Delta \bar{I}_t / \Delta \bar{I}_0 = (\bar{G}_{Na} m_{(t)}^a \, \Delta V h(t))/(\bar{G}_{Na} m_0^a \, \Delta h(0)) \tag{7.42}$$

Fig.7.38

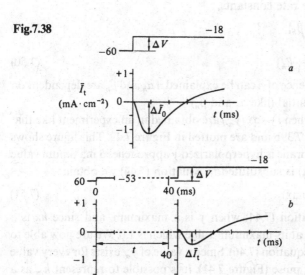

Time dependence of the inactivation

If the conditioning pulse turns on an appreciable $\bar{G}_{Na}$, $m^a_{(t)}$ may be different from m^a_0. For small depolarization, as is usually the case, $\bar{G}_{Na}$ is small and so $m^a_{(t)} \approx m^a_0$. Equation (7.42) becomes

$$y(t) = h(t)/h(0) \tag{7.43}$$

or

$$h(t) = h(0)y(t) \tag{7.44}$$

Figure 7.39a displays the set of records in an experiment where the time dependence of y (i.e. $\Delta\bar{I}_{(t)}/\Delta\bar{I}_0$) is examined. Each of the records provides a value of y at time t and the curve obtained in this experiment can be fitted with the function

$$y(t) = 1 + (y_\infty - 1)(1 - \exp(-t/t_y)) \tag{7.45}$$

where y_∞ is the value of y when t tends to infinity ($t \to \infty$) and t_y is the time constant of y (see Figure 7.40).

If we substitute (7.45) in (7.44) and define h_∞ for $t \to \infty$ by

$$h_\infty = h_0 y_\infty \tag{7.46}$$

we obtain

$$h(t) = h_0 + (h_\infty - h_0)(1 - \exp(-t/t_y)) \tag{7.47}$$

which is an analytical expression for h as a function of t. It should be noted that equation (7.48) is in the same form as equation (7.25), which means that h can be analysed in the same way as n. Thus, equation (7.47) is the solution of the differential equation

$$dh/dt = \alpha_h h - \beta_h(1-h) \tag{7.48}$$

where α_h and β_h are rate constants,

$$\tau_y = 1/(\alpha_h + \beta_h) \tag{7.49}$$

and

$$h_\infty = \alpha_h/(\alpha_h + \beta_h) \tag{7.50}$$

The voltage dependence of h can be explained if α_h and β_h are dependent on the membrane potential (like α_n and β_n).

The values of y when $t \to \infty$ (y_∞) are obtained in an experiment like that described in Figure 7.39b and are plotted in Figure 7.42. This figure shows that when the membrane is hyperpolarized y approaches a maximum value $y_\infty(\text{max})$. If $y_\infty(\text{max})$ is substituted in equation (7.44) we obtain

$$h_0 = 1/y_\infty(\text{max}) \tag{7.51}$$

If we recall equation (7.44) when y is a maximum, and since h_0 is a constant, h must be at its maximum value which is 1.0. We are now able to calculate h_∞ using equation (7.46). Since a value of y_∞ exists for every value of the conditioning pulse (Figure 7.41), it is possible to represent h_∞ as a

Fig.7.39

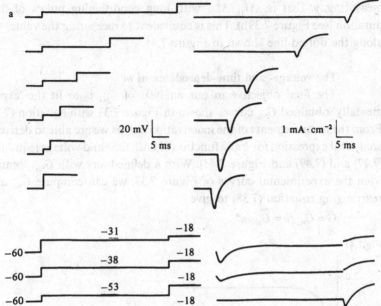

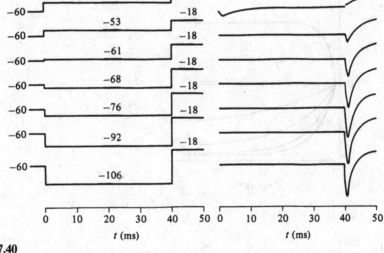

Fig.7.40

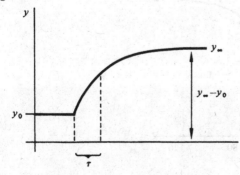

function of voltage (Figure 7.43). Experimental h_∞ curves are obtained by measuring y, that is, $\Delta \bar{I}_{(t)}/\Delta \bar{I}_0$, with long conditioning pulses of fixed duration (see Figure 7.39b). This is equivalent to measuring the values of y along the dotted line shown in Figure 7.41.

The voltage- and time-dependence of m

The final objective in our analysis of $\bar{G}_{Na}$ is to fit the 'experimentally' obtained $\bar{G}_{Na}$ curves shown in Figure 7.37 with equation (7.39). From the measurements of the inactivation curves we are able to derive an analytical expression for h as a function of both time and voltage (equations (7.47) and (7.49) and Figure 7.43). With h defined and with $\bar{G}_{Na}$ obtained from the experimental curves of Figure 7.37, we can compute $\tilde{G}_{Na}$ after rearranging equation (7.38) to give

$$\tilde{G} = \bar{G}_{Na}/h = \overline{\overline{G}}_{Na} m^a \tag{7.52}$$

Fig.7.41

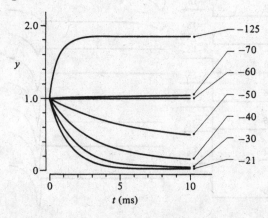

Fig.7.42

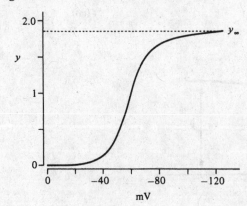

$\tilde{G}_{Na}$ has the same form as $\bar{G}_K$ (compare curves in Figures 7.22 and 7.44) and so can be analysed in an identical way. Thus, we have a first-order differential equation of the type:

$$dm/dt = \alpha_m(1-m) - \beta_m m \tag{7.53}$$

which when solved gives

$$m = m_0 + (m_\infty - m_0)(1 - \exp(-t/\tau_m)) \tag{7.54}$$

where

$$m_\infty = \alpha_m/(\alpha_m + \beta_m) \tag{7.55}$$

and

$$\tau_m = 1/(\alpha_m + \beta_m) \tag{7.56}$$

In equation (7.53), α_m and β_m are the voltage-dependent rate constants. If we use the same procedure to determine m^a as was used to determine n^a, we obtain a set of curves as displayed in Figure 7.45. From this figure, it is clear that m^3 gives the best fit to the 'experimental curve'. If we treat all the

Fig.7.43

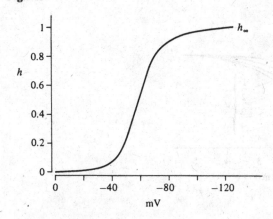

Fig.7.44

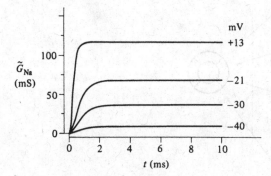

'experimental curves' of Figure 7.44 in the same way, we would obtain a value of 3 for m in each case.

Four-particle models of the sodium channel

We can now write equation (7.39) as

$$\bar{G}_{Na} = \bar{\bar{G}}_{Na} m^3 h \tag{7.57}$$

which pictorially can be represented as in Figures 7.46 and 7.47. In this figure we represent the formation of a sodium channel as being made up of four particles, three of type m in the $\bar{m}$ state and one of type h in the $\bar{h}$ state. The conversion of $\bar{m}$ to m is considered to be a slow step and the conversion of $\bar{h}$ to h is even slower. The assembly of a channel from the four particles is considered to be very fast and so is not the rate-limiting step. As particles in state $\bar{h}$ convert into particles in state h, the channels are disassembled (inactivated) and no longer conduct.

An alternative model (Figure 7.47) could be that, in order for the channel to conduct, the sodium gates have to move away from the channel. While

Fig. 7.45

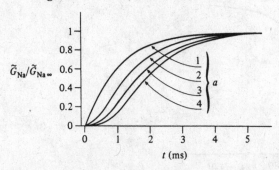

$\tilde{G}_{Na}/\tilde{G}_{Na\infty}$

t (ms)

Fig. 7.46

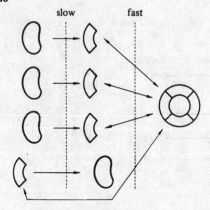

slow   fast

this takes place the inactivating gate moves in at a slower pace towards the opening of the channel so that in the end the channel will be blocked (inactivated) again.

If we substitute the full expressions for m and h in equation (7.57), we obtain

$$\bar{G}_{Na} = \bar{G}_{Na}[m_0 + (m_\infty - m_0)(1 - \exp(-t/\tau_m))]^3$$
$$\times [h_0 + (h_\infty - h_0)(1 - \exp(-t/\tau_h))] \quad (7.58)$$

The full analytical expression for the voltage- and time-dependence of the sodium channel

In order to fit equation (7.58) to the experimental $\bar{G}_{Na}$ curves, Hodgkin and Huxley used a simplified version where

$$\bar{G}_{Na} = \bar{G}_{Na} m^3 h_0 (1 - \exp(-t/\tau_m))^3 \exp(-t/\tau_h) \quad (7.59)$$

This equation applies for depolarizations larger than $30\,mV$ from the resting membrane potential. Under these conditions, h_0 (see Figure 7.43) is much smaller than h_∞ and m_0 is much smaller than m_∞. At the resting potential $\bar{G}_{Na}$ will be very small. Thus, m_0 will be negligible when compared with m_∞ after the membrane is depolarized by some $30\,mV$.

The end result of fitting equation (7.59) (or (7.58)) to the 'experimental curves' displayed in Figure 7.37 is that τ_m and m_∞ can be defined for every membrane voltage. Rearranging equations (7.49) and (7.50), and redefining

Fig.7.47

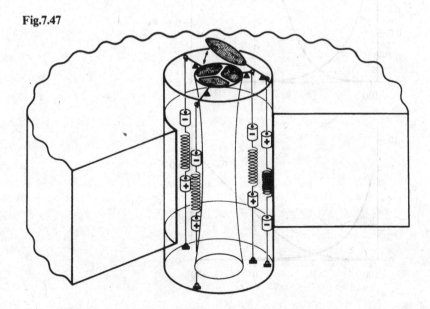

them for m, we obtain

$$\alpha_m = m_\infty/\tau_m \qquad \alpha_h = h_\infty/\tau_h \tag{7.60a}$$

$$\beta_m = (1 - m_\infty)/\tau_m \qquad \beta_h = (1 - h_\infty)/\tau_h \tag{7.60b}$$

The sodium channels are ohmic conductors

Equations (7.60a, b) allow us to plot the rate constants as functions of voltage (Figure 7.48). With this knowledge of the rate constants, we now have a quantitative description of $\bar{G}_{Na}$ as a function of voltage and time. However, the assumption implicit in equation (7.36), which is that $\bar{G}_{Na}$ is an ohmic conductance, has not yet been analysed.

Hodgkin and Huxley used the same double-pulse procedure as outlined in Figure 7.30 for $\bar{G}_K$. They used very short first pulses (short pulses used were between 0.3 and 1.5 ms so that potassium currents would be negligible and could be neglected), and found that the instantaneous I/V relationship was linear (Figure 7.49). This curve can also be used to determine the sodium equilibrium potential E_{Na}.

The end of our analysis of the biophysics of excitability is approaching, for we are now almost in the position to give a complete quantitative

Fig.7.48

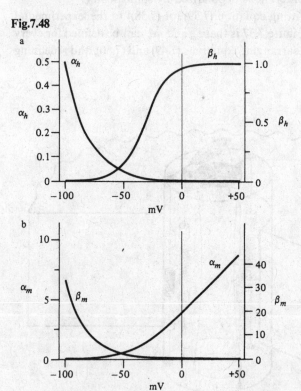

description of the membrane current. But first we have to define the voltage dependence of the rate constants shown in Figures 7.28 and 7.48.

Voltage-dependence of the rate constants

The functional relationship between the rate constants and voltage has not, as yet, been derived from first principles. Electrophysiologists use empirical relationships, derived from those first proposed by Hodgkin and Huxley, for n, m and h and these are given below:

$$\alpha_n = \bar{\alpha}_n(V - \bar{V}_n)/(1 - \exp(-(V - \bar{V}_n)/10))$$
$$\beta_n = \bar{\beta}_n \exp(-(V - \bar{V}_n)/80)$$
$$\alpha_m = \bar{\alpha}_m(V - \bar{V}_m)/(1 - \exp(-(V - \bar{V}_m)/10))$$
$$\beta_m = \bar{\beta}_m \exp(-(V - \bar{V}_m)/18)$$
$$\alpha_h = \bar{\alpha}_h \exp(-(V - \bar{V}_h)/20)$$
$$\beta_h = \bar{\beta}_h/(1 + \exp(-(V - \bar{V}_h)/10))$$

These relationships imply that the rate constants are instantaneous functions of voltage alone. It should be emphasized that these relationships are empirical and that other functions could equally well be used, as long as they describe adequately the experimentally obtained relations between rate constants and membrane potential.

The leak conductance

There is one more current that we have to consider and this is the leak current. We have described the voltage and time dependence of the sodium and potassium conductances, but there is a conductance that is not a function of voltage and time and Hodgkin and Huxley called this the

Fig.7.49

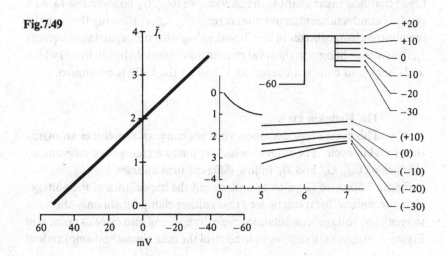

leakage conductance. They assumed that any other ions involved in the action potential currents crossed the membrane through this leakage conductance. These currents would be composed of chloride ions and sodium and potassium ions that did not pass through voltage-sensitive channels.

The leak conductance is a linear conductance that does not change with voltage and time, so we can represent the leak current as

$$\bar{I}_L = \bar{G}_L(V - E_L)$$

where $\bar{G}_L$ is the leak conductance per unit area of membrane. Since the leakage conductance is a constant the maximum leak conductance per unit area $\overline{\bar{G}_L}$ is equivalent to the leak conductance $\bar{G}_L \equiv \overline{\bar{G}_L}$.

Action potential generation

We can now describe quantitatively the mechanism of action potential generation. In Figure 7.50a we reproduce a summary of all the important equations derived in this chapter and show how they interact. From this figure it can be seen that if the membrane potential (V, see box in line 2) is disturbed by one or more of the following:

(a) local injections of current ($\bar{I}_t$)
(b) changes in equilibrium potentials (E_{Na}, E_K, E_L), or
(c) changes in membrane conductance ($\bar{G}_m$),

instantaneous changes in the rate constants will occur (see boxes in line 3). These changes will result in changes in the rate of conversion (dn/dt, dm/dt, dh/dt boxes of line 4) of the particles (n, m, h, boxes of line 5) from the state associated with closed channels to the state associated with open channels. Open channels cause changes in conductance ($\bar{G}_{Na}$, $\bar{G}_K$ boxes in line 6). As a result of conductance changes, the currents ($\bar{I}_K$, $\bar{I}_{Na}$, $\bar{I}_L$) flowing through the membrane change (boxes in line 7) and, along with the capacitative current $\bar{I}_c$, this causes changes in the total membrane current ($\bar{I}_t$, box in line 8) which feeds back and causes a change in V and so the cycle is continued.

The Hodgkin cycle

This cycle of conductance–voltage changes is sometimes known as the Hodgkin cycle. The rates at which m, n and h change are different, so changes of $\bar{G}_{Na}$, $\bar{G}_K$ and $\bar{G}_L$ follow different time courses.

Figure 7.50a also helps us to understand the importance of the voltage-clamp technique, for it can be seen that voltage clamping not only allows us to break the voltage–conductance cycle (by entering into cycle at point A in Figure 7.50a), but also allows us to control the time course and amplitude of

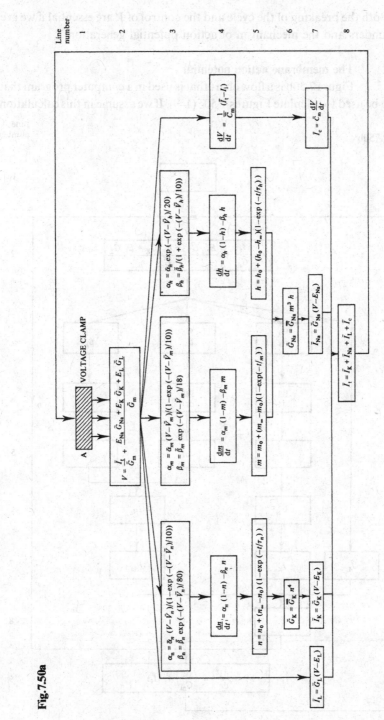

Fig.7.50a

V. Both the breaking of the cycle and the control of *V* are essential if we are to understand the mechanism of action potential generation.

The membrane action potential

Figure 7.50b is a flow chart that is used in a computer program that can be used to calculate Figures 7.50c (1–9). If we assume in this calculation

Fig.750b

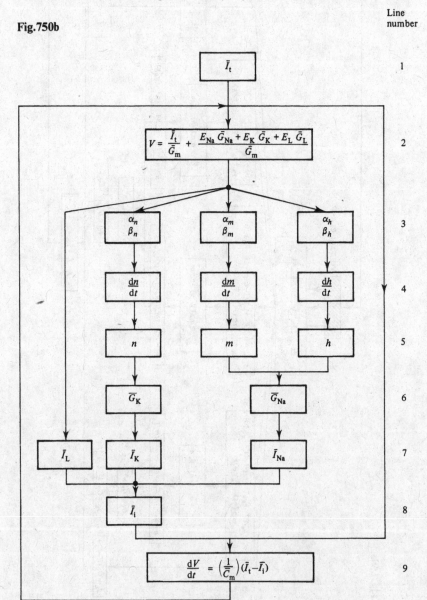

that the potential is the same at any instant of time for any point in the membrane, and so there is no current flow along the inside of the fibre, we are able to calculate a so-called *membrane* action potential. At rest $\bar{I}_t$ is equal to zero (line 2, Figure 7.50b) and except during a stimulus the membrane current is always assumed to be zero in a membrane action potential. Thus from equation (7.2)

$$\bar{I}_t = \bar{I}_c + \bar{I}_{Na} + \bar{I}_K + \bar{I}_L$$

Fig.7.50c

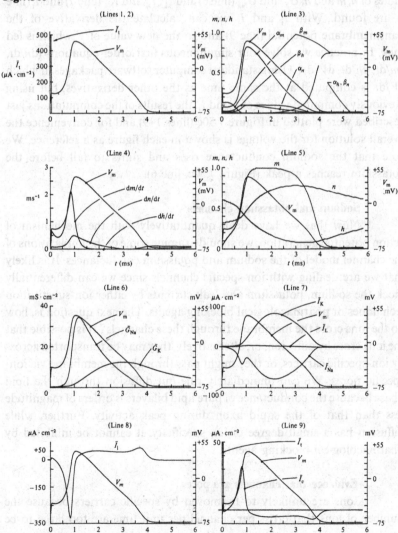

so except for a very brief constant current stimulus we set out to solve equation (7.3) with $\bar{I}_t = 0$, $V = V_{r.p}$ and m, n, h with their resting steady-state values. The brief constant current stimulus ($\bar{I}_t$) causes the membrane potential (V) to change (line 2) and so the voltage-dependent rate constants are changed (line 3). These values are then fed into the three first-order differential equations for n, m and h (line 4). As yet, these equations cannot be solved analytically but there are a number of numerical procedures which allow us to compute the new values of n, m and h once we know their derivatives (for example, the Runge–Kutta methods) (line 5). With the new values of n, m and h, $\bar{G}_K$ and $\bar{G}_{Na}$ (line 6) and $\bar{I}_L$, $\bar{I}_K$ and $\bar{I}_{Na}$ (line 7) and $\bar{I}_i$ (line 8) are found. With $\bar{I}_i$ and $\bar{I}_t$ we can calculate the derivative of the transmembrane potential (line 9) and so the new value of V which is fed back. In practice we solve four simultaneous first-order equations ($\mathrm{d}n/\mathrm{d}t$, $\mathrm{d}m/\mathrm{d}t$, $\mathrm{d}h/\mathrm{d}t$, $\mathrm{d}V/\mathrm{d}t$). Using standard computer software packages in which $\mathrm{d}V/\mathrm{d}t$ is computed at the same time as the other derivatives, but using previously computed values of $\bar{I}_i$ and $\bar{I}_t$, the results of the computations just described were plotted in Figure 7.50c (lines 1–9) and for convenience the overall solution for the voltage is shown in each figure as a reference. We note that the sodium conductance rises and starts to fall before the potassium reaches a peak (Figure 7.50c, line 6).

Sodium and potassium channels

Now that we have dealt quantitatively with the mechanism of action potential generation, we should examine some of the implications of the channel model of the sodium and potassium conductances. It is likely that we are dealing with ion-specific channels since we can differentially block the sodium, potassium and leak currents by either ion-substitution techniques or pharmacological blocking agents. The next question is, how do the ions cross the membrane through these channels? It is possible that the ions cross by diffusion, or, alternatively, they may be transported across by ion-specific carriers, or they might pass through the membrane via ion-specific pores. We can immediately rule out diffusion through the lipid phase because the conductance of pure lipid bilayers is orders of magnitude less than that of the squid axon during peak activity. Further, while diffusion has a small degree of ion specificity, it cannot be inhibited by pharmacological blocking agents.

Evidence that channels are pores

Ions are unlikely to be moved by specific carriers because the number of ions that cross per channel per unit time are too large to be carried across. The number of ions that cross per channel per unit time can be calculated by dividing the maximum ionic current per unit area ($\bar{I}_t$) by the number of channels per unit area (N_T). Channels can be counted by labelling them using radioactive pharmacological blocking agents. A simple calculation of the following type is able to show this. If a milliamp of sodium current flows through a square centimetre of membrane (Figure 7.32c) and if there are 500 sodium channels per micron square then

Number of sodium ions that flow through a single channel per second

$$= \frac{\overbrace{(10^{-3} \ \text{coul} \cdot \text{s}^{-1} \cdot \text{cm}^{-2}}^{\text{sodium current (1 mA)}} \times \overbrace{6 \times 10^{23} \ \text{ions} \cdot \text{mol}^{-1})}^{\text{Avogadro's number}}}{\underbrace{10^8 \ \mu\text{m}^2 \cdot \text{cm}^{-2}}_{\substack{\text{membrane area} \\ (\text{cm}^2) \text{ in } \mu\text{m}^2}} \times \underbrace{500 \ \text{channels} \cdot \mu\text{m}^{-2}}_{\substack{\text{number of channels} \\ \text{per cm}^2}} \times \underbrace{96\,500 \ \text{coul} \cdot \text{mol}^{-1}}_{\text{faraday}}}$$

$$= 1.24 \times 10^5 \cdot \text{ions} \cdot \text{channel}^{-1} \cdot \text{s}^{-1}$$

This number of ions is about three orders of magnitude larger than the rate of sodium pumping that occurs in the squid axon membrane. Similar calculations can be made for the potassium channel and these types of calculations strongly support the proposal that the ionic channels are ion-specific pores.

Patch-clamp technique

Further important evidence for ion-specific pores comes from a new voltage-clamp technique which clamps small membrane areas. This technique is known as a 'patch-clamp'. Patch-clamp is assumed to be able to record faithfully the switching 'on' and 'off' of channels. This assumption is made because the records obtained are similar to those observed when black lipid membranes were doped with channel-forming ionophores. Patch-clamp records show that the conductance rises rapidly, stays constant and then sharply falls away. The most likely explanation for this is that current flows through a pore (or hole) in the membrane that rapidly opens and closes. The associated conductance would thus rise quickly, remain at a constant value (the unit conductance), and then rapidly fall.

Membrane noise

When a number of pores are open at once, records should be obtained which are integral multiples of the unit conductance. This is found experimentally and is drawn schematically in Figure 7.51a–e. This figure shows that when a membrane is subject to depolarizing voltage-clamp steps, the unit conductances sum until eventually a continuous current record is obtained (Figure 7.51e). Figure 7.51e also shows an average direct current (d.c.) level. The membrane currents $(\bar{I}_t, \bar{I}_K, \bar{I}_{Na})$ that we have examined up to now have been these d.c. levels around which the current fluctuates in an apparently random manner (thin line x in e). These random fluctuations of current are known as current noise. If we were current clamping, we would measure a voltage noise.

Basic properties of the unit conductance

Since current noise is the sum of randomly occurring unit conductances, we should be able to analyse this noise mathematically and so obtain the basic properties of the unit conductance which are its amplitude, its duration and average frequency. By average frequency we mean that for any given current noise record we add up the number of unit conductances and divide the sum by the duration of the record. As the number of open channels increases we can calculate the average frequency over a shorter time. In the limit we can talk about an instantaneous number of channels open and this is equivalent to N_{ch} of equation (7.11).

Fig.7.51

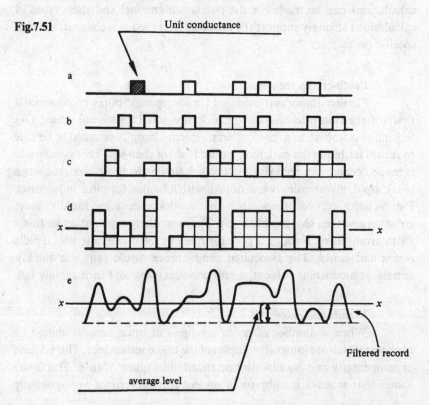

Unit conductance

Filtered record

average level

While the amplitude and duration of the unit conductance are assumed to be fixed, the average frequency is, at least, a function of the membrane voltage. Thus, the further a membrane is depolarized the greater the current noise. This increase in noise is predicted by the previously developed Hodgkin–Huxley model. This mathematical analysis will not, however, be simple. This is because there are other noise sources in the membranes (for example, undoped lipid bilayers also display current noise) and a certain number of untested statistical assumptions have to be made.

Unit conductances

From unit conductance (G_{ch}) values experimentally obtained from either patch-clamping or from noise analysis of squid axon membranes, it is possible to obtain the sodium or potassium channel density (that is, the number of channels per unit area of membrane (N_T)). For sodium and potassium channels unit conductances of about 10 pS have been measured. If we rearrange equation (7.11) and substitute N_T for N_{ch}, we obtain

$$N_T = \bar{G}_{max}/G_{ch} \tag{7.61}$$

where $\bar{G}_{max}$ is the maximum value of the sodium ($\bar{G}_{Na}$) or potassium ($\bar{G}_K$) conductance obtained from Hodgkin–Huxley voltage-clamp experiments. With a $\bar{G}_{Na}$ value of $120\,\text{mS}\cdot\text{cm}^{-2}$ (see Appendix 32) we obtain a sodium channel density of 120 channels and for a $\bar{G}_{K\,max}$ value of $35\,\text{mS}\cdot\text{cm}^{-2}$ (see Appendix 32) we obtain a potassium channel density of 35 channels/μm^2.

Estimates of the number of sodium channels (tetrodotoxin-binding studies) and potassium channels (from the kinetics of TEA inhibition) have given values of channel density within the same order of magnitude. These pharmacological methods show that there is a limited number of permeating sites per unit area of membrane, which suggests that each site must have a high conductance and so be a pore.

Effective pore diameters

We can proceed further with our analysis of the sodium and potassium channels if we assume that they are ion-specific pores of similar conductances of around 10 pS. With this value of conductance we can estimate the cross-sectional area of a cylindrical pore. In this chapter we have shown that both the sodium and potassium channels in squid axon are ohmic conductors. It is possible to derive the conductance of small cylinders of solution and for the case of a cylinder acting as an ohmic conductor the approximate expression for its radius is

$$a_{pore} = [(G_p\,\delta RT)/(\pi D(ZF)^2 \bar{c}]^{1/2} \tag{7.62}$$

and is obtained as follows.

Let us assume that the pore is bathed on both sides by an electrolyte solution (NaCl, for example) of concentration (c), where $c = [\text{Na}^+] + [\text{Cl}^-]$, which also fills its interior. If we treat the pore as a resistor its conductance is given approximately by

$$G_p = kA/\delta$$

where k is the conductivity of the solution that fills the pore, A the cross-sectional area and δ the length of the pore.

From Chapter 2

$$k_i = u_i(ZF)^2 c_i$$

Let us assume an average mobility (u) for the salt, then, for $z = \pm 1$

$$k = uF^2 c$$

But $A = \pi a_{pore}^2$ and $D = uRT$ or $u = D/RT$ where D is the diffusion coefficient of the salt. So

$$k = (D/RT)F^2 c \quad \text{and} \quad G_p = \pi a_{pore}^2 F^2 Dc/(\delta RT)$$

If c is not the same on both sides of the membrane we substitute c by an average value $\bar{c}$. So

$$G_p = \pi a_{pore}^2 F^2 D\bar{c}/\delta RT$$

from which equation (7.62) is derived. If we make a further assumption that the pore allows only sodium (sodium channel) or only potassium (potassium channel), the concentration $\bar{c}$ will refer only to sodium or potassium. This expression can be used to derive the radius of the membrane pore since sodium and potassium pores are ohmic conductors and they can be thought of as cylinders of solution connecting two compartments (Figure 7.52). The concentration of the salt in the cylinder $(\bar{c})$ is the average concentration of ions (sodium or potassium) on either side of the membrane $(c_{(1)}$ and $c_{(2)})$. The diffusion coefficient, D, in equation (7.62) is the value for diffusion in free solution and the dimensions of the cylinder (Figure 7.52) correspond to the inside dimensions of the pore.

Fig.7.52

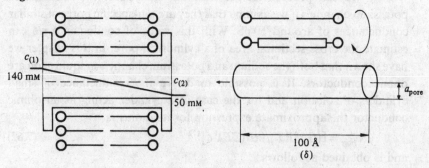

$c_{(1)}$
140 mM
$c_{(2)}$
50 mM
a_{pore}
100 Å
(δ)

Substituting appropriate values (see Figure 7.52) in equation (7.62), we obtain a value of 1.3 Å for the potassium pore radius. This gives a cross-sectional area of 5.32 Å. Independent estimates give similar values for pore size. These estimates were obtained through studying the permeation of different sizes of monovalent cations through potassium and sodium channels. This approach showed that the potassium channel was permeable to ions of unhydrated diameter of less than 3.3 Å (Cs is impermeant and has a diameter of 3.3 Å). Sodium channels will pass potassium ions and they are also permeable to large organic cations that will fit into a slit of maximum height 3 Å and maximum width 5 Å.

Channel selectivity

Although both channels seem to have similar pore sizes, the channels are specifically permeable to different ions. Thus, the sodium channel is twelve times less permeable to potassium than it is to sodium and the potassium channel is a hundred times less permeable to sodium than to potassium. However, the ionic radii of sodium and potassium are respectively 0.95 and 1.33 Å and this shows that, providing the permeating ion has a radius of less than 3 Å, pore size alone cannot determine channel specificity. Some form of channel–ion interaction has yet to be established which describes the permeation process.

Activation energy of ion permeation

The interaction does not, however, seem to involve a high activation energy since the Q_{10} (see Appendix 26, about 1.2–1.3) of the sodium and potassium currents is similar to that of diffusional currents in free solution. Thus, it can be imagined that the sodium and potassium ions move along the pore in a similar way to their movement in a water phase.

8

The propagated action potential

Non-uniform distribution of currents and voltages along the axon

In the last chapter we assumed that the membrane potential of excitable cells was at all times uniform. In nature this is generally not the case and, in an axon for example, the potential (and the membrane current) are different for each instant in time, along its length. If measurements are made with microelectrodes positioned at equal intervals along an axon (Figure 8.1a), and if a constant current is injected into the middle of an axon (at $x = 0$), we find that after a steady-state has been obtained the membrane potential decays with distance (Figure 8.1b). The voltage drop between any two consecutive electrodes is also seen to decay (Figure 8.1c). Since the resistance (per unit length) of axoplasm is constant, this means that the current that flows through any given cross-section of the axoplasm must also decay with distance. If the membrane properties are uniform (with distance) then we can conclude that the current that flows across the membrane must also fall with distance. This is pictorially represented in Figure 8.2 where the spaces between the current lines become wider at greater distances from the current source.

Three-dimensional analysis of current distribution along the axon

A better representation of the current distribution along an axon is given in Figure 8.3, which shows the current pattern described in Figure 8.2 that corresponds to only a small wedge-shaped segment of the axon. To obtain the full instantaneous three-dimensional picture we can imagine that the point P (and the current lines associated with it) are rotated in space around the axon axis. But this three-dimensional picture is difficult to analyse mathematically. So, in order to simplify this analysis, we imagine that the axon is composed of a series of wedge-shaped segments. One of these wedges is shown in Figure 8.4, where P is now represented by the dotted area and there are a series of identical elements $E_{(1,2,\ldots)}$ spaced at equal intervals along the surface of the axon wedge. A constant current is injected inwards at element E_1 of plane P and flows outwards through elements E_1, E_2, E_3, ... of the same plane P. The relative sizes of these

Fig.8.1

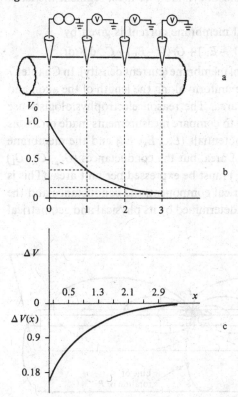

Curve c is the derivative of curve b.

Fig.8.2

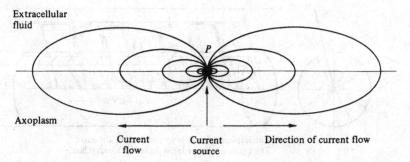

currents are pictorially represented in the figure by the widths of the arrows. But the current is flowing out in a ring around the periphery of the axoplasm, so it is not possible to analyse current distribution by conceptually splitting the axon longitudinally and laying it out as slab. Because current is flowing along the core of the axon, that is, through the whole cross-sectional area of the axoplasm cylinder, we must segment the axon into a series of wedges.

From equation (7.3) the total membrane current is given by

$$\bar{I}_t = \bar{G}_{Na}(V - E_{Na}) + \bar{G}_K(V - E_K) + \bar{G}_L(V - E_L) + \bar{C}_m \, dV/dt$$

where $\bar{I}_t$ is current per unit area of membrane (current density). In Chapter 7 current flow was assumed to be uniform along the length of the axon and expressed as current per unit area. The reason electrophysiologists use current density is to allow them to compare measurements made on axons of different sizes. The Nernst potentials (E_{Na}, E_K, E_L) and the membrane potential (V) are independent of area, but the conductances ($\bar{G}_{Na}, \bar{G}_K, \bar{G}_L$) and membrane capacitance ($\bar{C}_m$) must be expressed per unit area. (This is reasonable since, like any electrical component, the conductance and the capacitance of a membrane are determined by its physical and geometrical properties.)

Fig.8.3

Fig.8.4

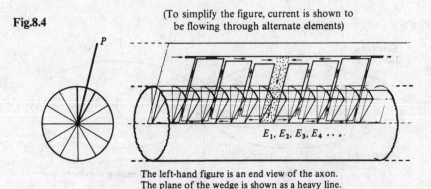

(To simplify the figure, current is shown to be flowing through alternate elements)

$E_1, E_2, E_3, E_4 \ldots$

The left-hand figure is an end view of the axon. The plane of the wedge is shown as a heavy line.

In order to describe Figure 8.4 mathematically, it is more convenient to express the total membrane current as current per *unit length* instead of current per unit area. This is because we want to describe the distribution of the membrane potential and of the flow of current with distance (x). However, we shall first define the conductances and capacitances as per unit area and then go on to express them per unit length.

If we consider the *sector of area* ΔA of Figure 8.5a, and if we drop a perpendicular b to radius a, Figure 8.5b, and let ΔA become very small, then the length of the arc approximately equals b, and the area of Figure 8.5b is given by

$$\Delta A \approx ab/2 \quad \text{(from the area of a triangle)} \tag{8.1}$$

b can be written in terms of a and $\Delta\phi$, since

$$\sin \Delta\phi = b/a = b/\text{radius} \tag{8.2}$$

and so

$$b = a \sin \Delta\phi \tag{8.3}$$

If we define

$$\Delta z = \text{length of the arc/radius} \tag{8.4}$$

Fig.8.5

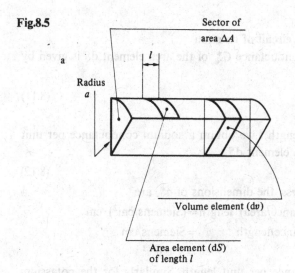

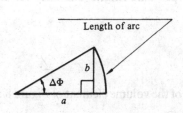

and as for very small $\Delta\phi$, $\Delta\phi \rightarrow d\phi$, so

$$dz \approx b/\text{radius} = \sin d\phi \tag{8.5}$$

where dz is the angle $d\phi$ expressed in radians. (One radian is an arc whose length is equal to the radius; so a circle contains 2π radians. Since a radian is a ratio of two lengths it has no dimensions.) So

$$b = a\,z \tag{8.6}$$

but the length of the arc $\approx a\,dz \tag{8.7}$

so

$$dA = (a^2/2)\,dz \tag{8.8}$$

We can now compute the area of the *area element* represented in Figure 8.5a as

$$dS \approx \text{length of the arc} \times l = la\,dz \tag{8.9}$$

We can also obtain the volume of the volume element dv in Figure 8.5a as

$$dv = \text{area of the area sector } (dA) \times l$$
$$= dAl$$
$$= \frac{a^2}{2} l\,dz \tag{8.10}$$

The equivalent circuit of an axon

The sodium conductance G_{Na}^* of the area element dS is given by

$$G_{Na}^* = \bar{G}_{Na}\,dS$$
$$= \bar{G}_{Na}\,\underset{dS}{\underline{la\,dz}} \tag{8.11}$$

Dividing G_{Na}^* by the length l we obtain a sodium conductance per unit length (g_{Na}^*) of the area element dS

$$g_{Na}^* = \bar{G}_{Na}a\,dz \tag{8.12}$$

Since dz is dimensionless, the dimensions of g_{Na}^* are

$$g_{Na}^* = (\text{conductance/area}) \cdot \text{length} = (\text{Siemens/cm}^2) \cdot \text{cm}$$
$$= \text{conductance/length} \qquad = \text{Siemens/cm}$$
$$= \text{S} \cdot \text{cm}^{-1}$$

g_{Na}^* is thus a conductance per unit length. Similarly for the potassium conductance

$$g_K^* = \bar{G}_K a\,dz \tag{8.13}$$

and the leak conductance

$$g_L^* = \bar{G}_L a\,dz \tag{8.14}$$

The longitudinal resistance of the volume element of Figure 8.5 (R_i^*) is given by (see Appendix 15)

$$R_i^* = \rho_{In} l / dA \tag{8.15}$$

the dimensions of R_i^* are ohm·cm·cm·cm^{-2}=ohm, since ρ_{In} (the resistivity of the axoplasm) has dimensions of ohm·cm.

If we substitute dA we obtain the longitudinal resistance of the volume element in ohms

$$R_i^* = (\rho_{In} l) / ((a^2/2)\, dz) \tag{8.16}$$

If we express the resistance of the axoplasm in terms of resistance per unit length (r_i). Then the resistance of the volume element axoplasm (r_i^*) is given by

$$r_i^* = R_i^* / l \tag{8.17}$$

where r_i^* has the dimension of ohm·cm^{-1}. The capacitance of the area element of Figure 8.5a is given by

$$c_m = \bar{C}_m\, ds \tag{8.18}$$

c_m is in farads because its dimensions are farad·cm^{-2}·cm^2=farads. If we substitute dS from (8.9) into (8.18) we obtain

$$c_m = \bar{C}_m la\, dz \tag{8.19}$$

The dimensions of $\bar{c}_m$ are farads·cm^{-1} or farads per unit length. We are able to rewrite equation (7.3), for the area element dS, where the total membrane current is expressed as per unit length (i_t^*)

$$i_i^* = g_{Na}^*(V - E_{Na}) + g_K^*(V - E_K) + g_L^*(V - E_L) + c_m^*(dV/dt) \tag{8.20}$$

We can also draw the equivalent circuit corresponding to this equation (see Figure 8.6). By reducing $\Delta\phi$ of Figure 8.5b to a small value ($d\phi$) we have

Fig.8.6

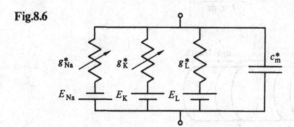

effectively reduced the wedge segment to a plane and the total membrane current now can be imagined to flow along and up this plane (Figure 8.7a). The equivalent circuit of Figure 8.6 can be considered to lie in this plane and the axon will be composed of a series of identical radially oriented planes (Figure 8.7b). Since there are many planes and equation (8.21) applies to only one of them (P), i_t^* should be rewritten

$$i_i^*(P) = g_{Na}^*(P)(V - E_{Na}) + g_K^*(P)(V - E_K) + g_L^*(P)(V - E_L)$$
$$+ c_m^*(P)(dV/dt) \tag{8.21}$$

In a similar way the conductances and capacitances for a single plane (P) should be rewritten using equations (8.13), (8.14), (8.17) and (8.21)

$$g_{Na}^*(P) = \bar{G}_{Na} a \, dz \tag{8.22}$$

$$g_K^*(P) = \bar{G}_K a \, dz \tag{8.23}$$

$$g_L^*(P) = \bar{G}_L a \, dz \tag{8.24}$$

$$r_i^*(P) = 2\rho_{in}/(a^2 \, dz) \tag{8.25}$$

$$c_m^* = \bar{C}_m a \, dz \tag{8.26}$$

Fig.8.7

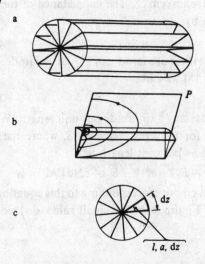

a

b

c

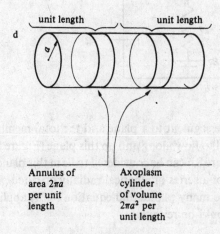

d

unit length   unit length

Annulus of
area $2\pi a$
per unit
length

Axoplasm
cylinder
of volume
$2\pi a^2$ per
unit length

Since we are dealing with a series of n radially oriented planes, the current flowing through the whole surface of the axon membrane and through the whole cross-section of the axoplasm is the sum of all the currents flowing along and up each individual plane. Mathematically we write this as

$$i_t = \sum_{P=1}^{n} i_t^*(P)$$

$$= \sum_{P=1}^{n} [g_{Na}^*(P)(V-E_{Na}) + g_K^*(P)(V-E_K)$$

$$+ g_L^*(P)(V-E_L) + c_m^*(P)\, dV/dt] \quad (8.27)$$

This can be represented as

$$i_t = g_{Na}(V-E_{Na}) + g_K(V-E_K) + g_L(V-E_L) + c_m\, dV/dt \quad (8.28)$$

where

$$g_{Na} = \sum_{P=1}^{n} g_{Na}^*(P) = \bar{G}_{Na} a 2\pi \quad (8.29)$$

$$g_K = \sum_{P=1}^{n} g_K^*(P) = \bar{G}_K a 2\pi \quad (8.30)$$

$$g_L = \sum_{P=1}^{n} g_L^*(P) = \bar{G}_L a 2\pi \quad (8.31)$$

and

$$c_m = \sum_{P=1}^{n} c_m^*(P) = \bar{C}_m a 2\pi \quad (8.32)$$

Since there are n dzs

$$\sum_{P=1}^{n} \bar{G}_{Na} a\, dz = \bar{G}_{Na} a \sum_{P=1}^{n} dz \quad (8.33)$$

and

$$\sum_{P=1}^{n} dz = 2\pi \quad (8.34)$$

$\sum_{P=1}^{n} dz$ is the circumference of the cross-section of the axon membrane measured in radians (Figure 8.7c).

In order to derive an expression for the resistance of the axoplasm per unit length (r_i), we rearrange equation (8.25) so as to obtain the internal conductance for each plane ($g_i^*(P)$).

$$g_i^*(P) = 1/r_i^*(P) = a^2\, dz/2\rho_{In} \quad (S \cdot cm) \quad (8.35)$$

The total internal conductance (g_i) is thus

$$g_i = \sum_{P=1}^{n} g_i^*(P) = \sum_{P=1}^{n} (a^2\, dz)/2\rho_{In}$$

$$(8.36)$$

$$= (a^2/(2\rho_{In})) \sum_{P=1}^{n} dz \quad (S \cdot cm)$$

From equation (8.34)

$$g_i = (2\pi a^2)/2\rho_{In} = \pi a^2/\rho_{In} \tag{8.37}$$

Therefore

$$r_i = \rho_{In}/\pi a^2 \quad (\text{ohm} \cdot \text{cm}^{-1}) \tag{8.38}$$

We can now rewrite equation (8.20) for unit length of axon

$$i_t = g_{Na}(V - E_{Na}) + g_K(V - E_K) + g_L(V - E_L) + c_m \, dV/dt \tag{8.39}$$

It should be emphasized that the conductances (g_{Na}, g_K, g_L) and the capacitance (c_m) are for annuli of unit length (see Figure 8.7d) of axon and so the total membrane current (i_t) is thus per unit length of axon. The equivalent circuit for equation (8.39) is identical to Figure 8.6 except that g_{Na}, g_K, g_L and c_m have to be substituted for g_{Na}^*, g_K^*, g_L^* and c_m^* respectively. The total membrane current (i_t) is for a three-dimensional system, the current flowing along the axoplasm and radially out through all the annuli. Instead of using the above approach where we started with a wedge element, it is possible to derive equations (8.29)–(8.32) and (8.37) by a more direct analysis of the currents that flow through the axoplasm cylinder and out through the annulus (the annulus and the axoplasm cylinder are shown in Figure 8.7d). For example, equation (8.11) can be written as

$$\bar{G}_{Na}^* = \bar{G}_{Na} 2\pi a l$$

where $\bar{G}_{Na}^*$ is the total conductance of an annulus of length l and radius a. So

$$g_{Na} = \bar{G}_{Na}^*/l$$

Also R_i can be written as

$$R_i = \rho_{In} l/\pi a^2$$

so that

$$r_i = R_i/l = \rho_{In}/\pi a^2 \quad (\text{ohm} \cdot \text{cm}^{-1})$$

where R_i is the resistance of a cylinder of length l and radius a, and ρ_{In} is the resistivity of the axoplasm.

From Ohm's Law

$$i(x) = (V(x - \Delta x) - V(x))/r_i \, \Delta x \tag{8.40}$$

where $V(x)$, $V(x + \Delta x)$ and $V(x - \Delta x)$ refer to depolarization (or hyper-polarizations) around the resting membrane potential. Similarly

$$i(x + \Delta x) = (V(x) - V(x + \Delta x))/r_i \, \Delta x \tag{8.41}$$

so from (8.39a)

$$i_t(x) \Delta x = (V(x - \Delta x) - V(x))/(r_i \, \Delta x) - (V(x) - V(x + \Delta x))/(r_i \, \Delta x) \tag{8.42}$$

$$i_t(x) \Delta x = (1/r_i)[(-V(x) + V(x - \Delta x))/\Delta x + (V(x + \Delta x) - V(x))/\Delta x] \tag{8.43}$$

or

$$i_i(x) = (1/r_i)[[(-V(x) + V(x - \Delta x))/\Delta x + (V(x + \Delta x) - V(x))/\Delta x]/\Delta x]$$

(8.44)

In the limit when $\Delta x \to 0$

$$\frac{V(x) - V(x - \Delta x)}{\Delta x} \to (d/dx)(V(x - \Delta x))$$

(8.45)

However, with this annulus approach it is more difficult to imagine the three-dimensional flow of the current (Figure 8.7c) and so in most textbooks current is graphically represented as flowing in two dimensions (i.e. along the axon and out across the membrane), and the radial flow of current, although assumed, is neither displayed nor analysed.

Equation (8.39) describes the current flow across a membrane annulus (of unit length) at any instant of time (t) and any point (x) along the axon. This current (i_i) can either be applied locally to the axon, by means of a voltage- or current-clamp, or it might flow into a membrane annulus as the result of endogenous electrical activity that takes place either locally or elsewhere.

In order to describe the flow of current through the whole axon membrane we cut up the axon into small cylindrical elements of length Δx (Figure 8.8a) and examine the current that flows across the axoplasm and through the surface membrane. For each element we can draw, for the reasons discussed above, an equivalent circuit of the type shown in Figure 8.6 (see Figure 8.8b).

Fig.8.8

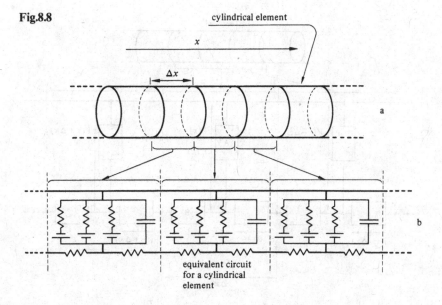

cylindrical element

equivalent circuit
for a cylindrical
element

Figure 8.8 can be further simplified, and this is shown in Figure 8.9. Block A is assumed to contain the membrane equivalent circuit of Figure 8.8b, and block B is half the axoplasmic resistance of the cylindrical element.

Derivation of the cable equation

The membrane current ($i_t(x)$) flowing across each element is (from Kirchhoff's Law (see Appendix 15))

$$i_t(x)\,\Delta x = i(x) - i(x + \Delta x) \tag{8.39a}$$

and

$$(V(x + \Delta x) - V(x))/\Delta x \rightarrow (d/dx)(V(x)) \tag{8.46}$$

If we substitute (8.45) and (8.46) into (8.44) and rearrange, we obtain for the right-hand side within the square brackets

$$(d/dx)(V) - (d/dx)(V(x - \Delta x))/\Delta x$$

when $\Delta x \rightarrow 0$, that is

$$\lim_{\Delta x \rightarrow 0} (d/dx)(V) - (d/dx)(V(x - \Delta x))/\Delta x = (d/dx)^2(V(x)) \tag{8.47}$$

hence

$$i_t = \frac{1}{r_i}(\partial/\partial x)^2(V(x)) \tag{8.48}$$

However,

$$i_t = c_m(\partial/\partial t)(V) + i_i \tag{8.49}$$

Fig.8.9

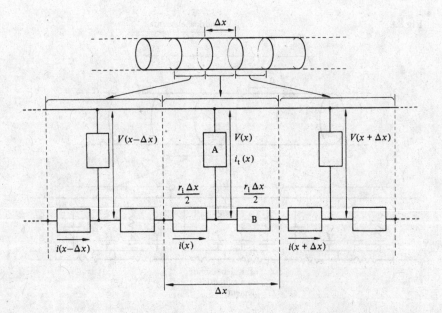

where i_i is the total ionic membrane current (per unit length), so

$$c_m(\partial/\partial t)(V(x,t)) - i_i = 1/r_i(\partial/\partial x)^2(V(x,t)) \tag{8.50}$$

This is a second-order partial differential equation in x and t. The solutions of these types of equations are discussed in Appendix 19.

If we rearrange equation (7.6a) and express the membrane current and the membrane resistance (r_m) for a unit *length* of axon membrane, we obtain an expression for i_i in equation (8.52). From equation (7.6a)

$$V = i_i r_m + V_{oc} \quad \text{(from equation (7.6a))} \tag{8.51}$$

(the units of r_m are $\Omega \cdot cm$: remember resistance is the reciprocal of conductance, and if conductance is expressed per unit length, that is, cm^{-1}, so the dimensions of r_m are $\Omega \cdot cm$). Therefore

$$i_i = V/r_m - V_{oc}/r_m \tag{8.52}$$

In an axon 'at rest' i_i is negligible. (An axon is said to be at rest when the membrane potential is not being displaced by the application of a current, or a voltage, or it is going through regenerative activity.) This is because the current that flows through g_{Na} is small (as g_{Na} is very small), and both E_K and E_L are almost equal to the membrane resting potential (V_{rp}). So we can write

$$V_{rp} \approx V_{oc}$$

If $V(x)$ is the membrane potential at any point relative to the resting membrane potential, then from equation (8.52) i_i will be given by

$$i_i = (V(x) + V_{rp})/r_m - V_{oc}/r_m$$
$$= V(x)/r_m + (V_{rp}/r_m - V_{oc}/r_m)$$

Since $V_{rp}/r_m \approx V_{oc}/r_m$, then

$$i_i = V(x)/r_m \tag{8.53}$$

If we substitute for i_i from equation (8.53) into equation (8.50), we now obtain

$$c_m(\partial/\partial t)(V(x,t)) + V(x)/r_m = (1/r_i)(\partial/\partial x)^2(V(x,t)) \tag{8.54}$$

Multiplying throughout by r_m gives

$$r_m c_m(\partial/\partial t)(V(x,t)) + V(x) = (r_m/r_i)(\partial/\partial x)^2(V(x,t)) \tag{8.55}$$

The dimensions of $r_m/r_i = \Omega \cdot cm/\Omega \cdot cm^{-1} = cm^2$. If we multiply c_m by r_m we obtain $(\Omega \cdot cm)(F \cdot cm^{-1}) = \Omega \cdot F$. But this is

$$\text{(volts/current)} \cdot \text{(charge/volts)} = \text{charge/(charge/time)} = \text{time}$$

If we substitute τ_m for $r_m c_m$ and λ^2 for r_m/r_i in (8.55), it becomes

$$\tau_m(\partial/\partial t)(V(x,t) + V(x,t)) = \lambda^2(\partial/\partial x)^2(V(x,t)) \tag{8.56}$$

We should note that $V(c)$ is also a function of time (t) as well as distance x and is written as $V(x,t)$, in order to keep the dimensions in equation (8.56) correct.

Solutions of the cable equation

Equation (8.56) is sometimes known as the *cable equation* where τ_m is the *membrane time constant* and λ is the *space constant*. This equation was originally derived by Kelvin to describe the transmission of electrical signals along underwater telephone cables and was later applied by Hodgkin and Rushton to axons. It is a second-order partial differential equation which, when solved, gives the value of $V(x, t)$ as a function of both time and distance.

Steady-state solution

The cable equation was derived in order to give an analytical description of the curves shown in Figure 8.1. Those curves were obtained at steady-state following and during the injection of a constant current into the middle of an axon. Because we are dealing with a steady-state situation, this means that the term $\partial(V(x, t))/\partial t$ in the *cable equation* is zero and this equation will now reduce to

$$V(x) = \lambda^2 (d/dx)^2 V(x) \tag{8.57}$$

where $V(x)$ is now only a function of distance. Equation (8.57) is an ordinary second-order differential equation, and the solutions of equations of this type (see Appendix 16) are of the general form

$$V(x) = A \exp(-kx) + B \exp(kx) \tag{8.58}$$

If we define the voltage at the current injection site ($x = 0$), as

$$V(x) = V(0) \quad \text{and} \quad e^0 = 1$$
$$V(0) = A + B \tag{8.59}$$

Also from Figure 8.1 when x, the distance away from the injection site is large, that is

$$x \to \infty \tag{8.60a}$$

then the voltage has decayed almost to zero

$$V(x) \to 0 \tag{8.60b}$$

so B must be equal to zero. (If B is different from zero, $\exp(kx)$ becomes larger and larger as $x \to \infty$ and we know that this is not the case.)

When $x = 0$ (at the current-injection site), $\exp(-kx)$ is zero (from (8.59)) which implies, from equation (8.58), that

$$A = V(0) = V_0$$

If we substitute for A and B in equation (8.58) we obtain

$$V(x) = V_0 \exp(-kx) \tag{8.61}$$

We can now substitute this solution into equation (8.57). Since

$$(d/dx)(V) = -kV_0 \exp(-kx) \tag{8.62}$$

and
$$(\mathrm{d}/\mathrm{d}x)^2(V(x)) = k^2 V_0 \exp(-kx) \tag{8.63}$$
then
$$V_0 \exp(-kx) = \lambda^2 k^2 V_0 \exp(-kx) \tag{8.64}$$

The space constant

Dividing both sides of equation (8.64) by $V_0 \exp(-kx)$ we obtain
$$1 = \lambda^2 k^2 \tag{8.65}$$
(If the solution $V(x) = V_{(0)} \exp(kx)$ is substituted into equation (8.57), the same result for $x < 0$ as equation (8.65) is obtained.) Thus
$$k^2 = 1/\lambda^2 \tag{8.66}$$
$$k = 1/\lambda \tag{8.67}$$
and
$$V(x) = V_0 \exp(-x/\lambda) \tag{8.68}$$

This equation is an analytical description of the curves shown in Figure 8.1. The spread of the voltage away from the injection site is determined by λ, the space constant.

The higher the membrane resistance the greater the spread of the potential. The solution described by equation (8.68) is valid only if the potential decays to zero, that is, if the axon length is much greater than the space constant. If this is not so, a different solution to equation (8.57) is obtained (see Appendix 20).

Non-steady-state solution

It should be remembered that equation (8.68) is not the complete solution of the cable equation and applies only in the steady-state (see Figure 8.1). When the cable equation is solved for *non-steady-state* conditions (for both distance (x) and time (t), we obtain (see Appendix 20)
$$V(X, T) = (I_0 (r_i r_m)^{1/2}/4)(\exp(-X)(1 - \mathrm{erf}((X/2\sqrt{T}) - \sqrt{T}))$$
$$- (\exp(X)(1 - \mathrm{erf}((X/2\sqrt{T}) + \sqrt{T})) \tag{8.69}$$
where
$$X = x/\lambda \tag{8.70}$$
and
$$T = t/\tau_m \tag{8.71}$$
and I_0 is the constant current injected at $x = 0$. In Figure 8.10, curve $(T = 0.01)$ describes the voltage spread in an axon just after a constant current has been applied, and it is possible to draw a curve for any instant of time (Figure 8.10 shows five specific examples). In Figure 8.10 the quantity

plotted in the y axis is

$$V(X, T)/(I_0(r_i r_m)^{1/2}/4)$$

Thus for a specific axon $V(X, T)$ is obtained by multiplying the values of y in Figure 8.10 by $I_0(r_i r_m)^{1/2}/4$.

In the steady-state ($T \to \infty$), equation (8.69) becomes

$$V(X, \infty) = (I_0(r_m r_i)^{1/2}/2) \exp(-X/\lambda) \tag{8.72}$$

This is because $\mathrm{erf}(X/2\sqrt{T} - \sqrt{T})$ when $T \to \infty$ becomes -1 as can be seen from tables of the values $\mathrm{erf}(1)$.

The input resistance

This is also the steady-state solution and by comparison with equation (8.61) we can see that

$$V_0 = I_0(r_i r_m)^{1/2}/2 \tag{8.73}$$

Equation (8.73) enables us to define the input resistance (R_{In}) as

$$R_{In} = V_0/I_0 = (r_i r_m)^{1/2}/2 \tag{8.74}$$

The input resistance (R_{In}) is very easy to measure since I_0 is known and V_0 can be measured at the current-injection site. In practice the voltage-recording electrode is difficult to insert exactly at the injection site, but it can be inserted close to the current electrode (by close, we mean that the

Fig.8.10

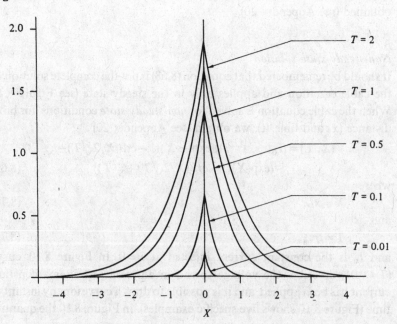

distance between electrodes should be negligible when compared with the space constant (λ)).

The membrane time constant

With a voltage electrode placed near to the current-injection site, it is also easy to measure the membrane time constant (τ_m). When $X = 0$, equation (8.69) reduces to

$$V(0, T) = I_0(r_i r_m)^{1/2} \, \text{erf}(\sqrt{T})/2 \qquad (8.75)$$

Where, from above,

$$T = t/\tau_m$$

When $t = \tau_m$, $T = 1$, so

$$\text{erf}(\sqrt{T}) = \text{erf}(1) = 0.84 \qquad (8.76)$$

Also, when $t \rightarrow \infty$

$$\text{erf}(\infty) = 1 \qquad (8.77)$$

so equation (8.75) becomes

$$V(0, \infty) = I_0(r_i r_m)^{1/2}/2 \qquad (8.78)$$

where $V(0, \infty)$ is the steady-state value of the voltage measured at the current injection site ($X = 0$).

If equations (8.76) and (8.78) are substituted into (8.75) we obtain, after rearranging,

$$V(0, \tau_m)/V(0, \infty) = 0.84 \qquad (8.79)$$

This means that the time taken for the voltage to reach 84% of its final value is equal to τ_m, the membrane time constant. This value may be compared with the value obtained from spherical cells or in axons where the current density is the same along the axon for any instant of time. Here, τ_m is the time taken for the voltage to reach about 63% of its final value.

Non-infinite cables

Equation (8.72) is the steady-state solution of the cable equation (8.56) for the special case of an axon where the length (l) is much larger than the space constant (λ). In this case, the axon is known as an 'infinite cable'. In this situation the fraction of the current injected at $x = 0$ that flows outwards across the axon membrane at $x = l$ is virtually zero.

We can also solve the cable equation for the case where the cable length is short compared with λ. This case is for a cable of finite length, and an example of this is short twitch muscle fibres of the snake. We start with the general solution (equation (8.58))

$$V(x) = A \exp(-kx) + B \exp(kx) \qquad (8.58)$$

Current injection in the middle of the fibre

Let us consider the case of a muscle fibre of length $2l$ and current injected at $x=0$ in the middle of the fibre. Let us assume that the resistance of the membrane at both ends is very large ($\rightarrow\infty$) so that no current will flow across the ends of the fibre. This means that the voltage profile is constant near $x=l$ and $x=-l$. Since the system is symmetrical we will derive the solution for $x \geqslant 0$, so

$$(d/dx)(V)=0 \quad \text{when } x=l$$

From equation (8.58)

$$dV/dx = Bk \exp(kx) - Ak \exp(-kx)$$

At $x=l$

$$Bk \exp(kl) - Ak \exp(-kl) = 0$$

or

$$B \exp(kl) - A \exp(-kl) = 0$$

so

$$A = B \exp(2kl) \tag{8.80}$$

If we substitute (8.80) in (8.58) we obtain

$$V(x) = B \exp(kx) + B \exp(2kl) \exp(-kx)$$
$$= B(\exp(kx) + \exp(2kl) \exp(-kx)) \tag{8.81}$$

So

$$V(0) = B(1 + \exp(2kl)) = V_0$$
$$B = V_0/(1 + \exp(2kl)) \tag{8.82}$$

From (8.81) and (8.82)

$$V(x) = V_0[(\exp(kx) + \exp(2kl) \exp(-kx))/(1 + \exp(2kl))] \tag{8.83}$$

If we multiply top and bottom of (8.83) by $\exp(-kl)$ we obtain

$$V(x) = V_0[(\exp(k(x-l)) + \exp(-k(x-l)))/(\exp(-kl) + \exp(kl))]$$

The function $(\exp(x) + \exp(-x))/2$ is known as the hyperbolic cosine of x and is symbolically written as:

$$\cosh(x) = (\exp(x) + \exp(-x))/2$$

So

$$V(x) = V(0)[\cosh(k(x-l))/\cosh(kl)]$$

Since $k = 1/\lambda$

$$V(x) = V(0)[\cosh((x-l)/\lambda)/\cosh(l/\lambda)] \tag{8.84}$$

Current input at one end of the fibre

Another situation which provides a solution similar to equation (8.84) is when we inject current near the end of a nerve or muscle fibre. The space constant may now be small when compared with the length of the fibre, and we shall consider current injected into the fibre near the naturally occurring high-resistance membrane terminations. If current is injected at l and the fibre terminates at $x=0$, then, because of the high resistance at $x=0$, $dV/dx=0$.

Starting with equation (8.58) and exactly the same conditions as (8.30), and with the same reasoning as used above, we write

$$dV/dx = Bk \exp(kx) - Ak \exp(-kx)$$

As

$$k = 1/\lambda$$

$$dV/dx = (B/\lambda) \exp(x/\lambda) - (A/\lambda) \exp(-x/\lambda)$$

But at $x=0$, $dV/dx=0$, so

$$0 = B/\lambda - A/\lambda$$

Thus

$$B = A$$

From equation (8.58) we can write

$$V(x) = B(\exp(x/\lambda) + \exp(-x/\lambda)) \tag{8.85}$$

But at the end of the fibre $x=0$ and if we define the voltage there as V_0 equation (8.85) becomes, at $x=0$,

$$V_0 = 2B$$

So

$$V_0/2 = B$$

Substituting in (8.85) for B

$$V(x) = (V_0/2)(\exp(x/\lambda) + \exp(-x/\lambda))$$

So

$$V(x) = V_0 \cosh(x/\lambda) \tag{8.86}$$

Space-clamping

In Chapter 8 we showed that by inserting a wire down the inside of an axon we were able to voltage clamp the whole of an axon membrane at any given potential and measure time-dependent membrane currents. The reason for this internal longitudinal electrode was that, as shown in this chapter, the potential is not uniform along the length of the nerve fibre and the wire effectively reduces the internal resistance to zero. This effectively makes the space constant (r_m/r_i) infinitely large, and so the membrane potential becomes uniform along the length of the fibre. Applied potentials also decay with distance in muscle fibres and, since inserting a wire along the inside of many types of muscle fibres is often very difficult (as the fibres are small and fragile), alternative means of voltage clamping these tissues have had to be devised.

Point-clamp techniques

These voltage-clamp techniques are known as point-clamp techniques and involve, in their simplest form, two microelectrodes – a current electrode and a voltage electrode. With a two-microelectrode voltage clamp it is possible to clamp the end-plate region of a muscle fibre and this is discussed in some detail in Chapter 9.

If the total length of the muscle fibre is small when compared with its space constant, then the steady-state potential change along the length of the fibre will be small if a current electrode is placed in the centre of the fibre (see Figure 8.11a). The actual potential decay can be calculated with equation (8.84). If we plot the ratio $V(x)/V_0$ (where $V(x)$ is the voltage at distance x and V_0 is the voltage at the current injection site (maximum voltage)) versus $(l - x)/l$, we obtain the alternative form of the voltage as a function of x. In Figure 8.12 we can see that, for a fibre which is *ten* times longer than the space constant, the potential decays much faster with

Fig.8.11

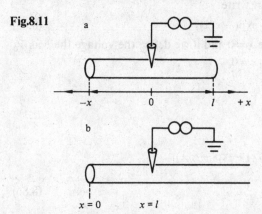

Fig.8.12

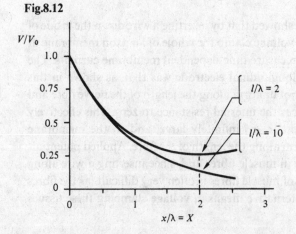

distance, when compared with a fibre which is *twice* as long as the space constant. Under certain experimental conditions the potential changes at the centre of the fibre, brought about by a point clamp, may not differ markedly from the potential changes at the end of the fibre. Under these conditions it may be assumed that the whole membrane is at one potential and the cell is then said to be *effectively* space-clamped.

End of the fibre voltage-clamp technique

It is possible to voltage-clamp a muscle fibre at its end region by using a point-clamp technique with an additional microelectrode. In this situation the muscle fibre is not space clamped and the additional electrode allows the membrane current, when the membrane is point voltage-clamped, to be computed. This arrangement is shown in Figure 8.13. Let us assume that the membrane current i'_m corresponds to the current flowing across the membrane between $x=0$ and $x=3l/2$. Since no current is flowing at $x=0$

$$i'_m \approx (V_2 - V_1)/(r_i l) \tag{8.87}$$

The right-hand side of equation (8.87) corresponds to the current flowing

Fig.8.13

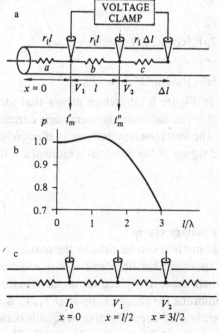

(Drawings not to scale in a and c)

inside the cell across element b. The current flowing per unit length ($i_m(l)$) of membrane is thus

$$i_m(l) = i'_m/(3l/2) \tag{8.88}$$

If we now substitute (8.87) into (8.88) we obtain

$$i_m(l) \approx 2(V_2 - V_1)/3r_i l^2 \tag{8.89}$$

This expression is an approximation since (8.87) is only an approximate equation because it assumes that all the current flowing across the first $3l/2$ cm flows out at point 2 when, in fact, current is flowing across the whole length of the $3l/2$ cm. From equation (8.86)

$$V(2l) = V_2 = V_0 \cosh(2l/\lambda)$$

and

$$V(l) = V_1 = V_0 \cosh(l/\lambda)$$

so

$$V_2 - V_1 = V_0(\cosh(2l/\lambda) - \cosh(l/\lambda)) \tag{8.90}$$

The current flowing at point l ($i_m(l)$) is from Ohm's Law

$$i_m(l) = V_1/r_m$$
$$= (V_0 \cosh(l/\lambda))/r_m \tag{8.91}$$

We can now introduce a correction factor p in (8.89) so that the equation now becomes exact. So

$$i_m(l) = 2p(V_2 - V_1)/3r_i l^2 \tag{8.92}$$

From (8.90), (8.91) and (8.92)

$$(V_0 \cosh(l/\lambda))/r_m = 2pV_0[\cosh(2l/\lambda) - \cosh(l/\lambda)]/3r_i l^2 \tag{8.93}$$

We can now solve (8.93) for

$$p = [3l^2 r_i/2r_m][\cosh(l/\lambda)/(\cosh(2l/\lambda) - \cosh(l/\lambda))] \tag{8.94}$$

Equation (8.94) is plotted in Figure 8.13b, which shows that for values $(l/\lambda) < 2$ the error in using (8.89) to calculate the membrane current is less than 5%. This means that the voltage-clamp circuit is effectively space-clamping the fibre in the end region, as the potential is more or less the same between $x = 0$ and $x = 2l$.

Middle of the fibre voltage clamp

The three-electrode method can be used in the middle of a fibre with the advantage that an accessible fibre end is not required. It is described in Figure 8.13c where the current electrode is placed in the middle of the fibre ($x = 0$). The membrane is voltage clamped at V_1, V_2 is another recording electrode. The membrane current (I_0) divides equally between the two halves of the fibre. The current flowing into V_1 is $I_0/2$. The current flowing out at V_1 is

$$(V_1 - V_2)/(r_i l)$$

Thus, the membrane current per unit length can be calculated approximately by

$$i_m \approx (1/l)[I_0/2 - (V_1 - V_2)/(r_i l)] \tag{8.95}$$

The general solution (8.59) is a steady-state solution to the cable equation. Equations (8.72), (8.94), (8.99) are also special cases of the general solution of the cable equation. Above we have shown how steady-state solutions may be used to measure time-dependent current changes. Although equations (8.89) and (8.95) were derived for a steady-state situation, they are the basis of voltage-clamp techniques in which the membrane current is measured as function of *time*. The mathematical basis for these clamping techniques is discussed more fully in the original papers (see Adrian, Chandler & Hodgkin; Adrian & Marshall).

Calculation of the propagated action potential: derivation of the wave equation

We have yet to consider the case where a local potential transient can generate a propagated action potential along the axon. Hodgkin and Huxley solved this case of the propagated action potential by first considering equation (7.3).

$$\bar{I}_t = \bar{C}_m \, dV/dt + \bar{G}_{Na}(V - E_{Na}) + \bar{G}_K(V - E_K) + \bar{G}_L(V - E_L) \tag{7.3}$$

where $\bar{I}_t$ is the total membrane current density $(A \cdot cm^{-2})$. In equation (8.48) we showed that the total membrane current per unit length $(A \cdot cm^{-1})$ is

$$i_t = (1/r_i)(d/dx)^2(V(x)) \tag{8.48}$$

where r_i is the total resistance of the cytoplasm per unit length $(\Omega \cdot cm^{-1})$. To convert membrane current per unit length (i_t) into membrane current density $(\bar{I}_t)$, the total current (I) across the membrane of an axon of length l and radius a is given by

$$I = \bar{I}_t 2\pi a l$$

But

$$i_t = I/l$$

so

$$\bar{I}_t = i_t/(2\pi a)$$

or

$$i_t = 2\pi a \bar{I}_t \tag{8.96}$$

The total resistance (R) of an axon cylinder of length l and radius a is

$$R = \rho_{In} l/A$$

where ρ_{In} is the specific resistance of the cytoplasm and A is the cross-sectional area given by the expression

$$A = \pi a^2$$

But

$$r_i = R/l = \rho_{In}/A = \rho_{In}/\pi a^2 \qquad (8.97)$$

If we now substitute (8.96) and (8.97) into (8.48) we obtain

$$2\pi a \bar{I}_t = (\pi a^2/\rho_{In})(d/dx)^2(V(x)) \qquad (8.98)$$

So the membrane current density ($\bar{I}_t$) is given by

$$\bar{I}_t = (a/(2\rho_{In}))(d/dx)^2(V(x)) \qquad (8.99)$$

If equation (8.99) is substituted into equation (7.3) we obtain

$$(a/(2\rho_{In}))(\partial/\partial x)^2(V) = \bar{C}_m(\partial/\partial t)(V) + \bar{G}_{Na}m^3h(V - E_{Na})$$
$$+ \bar{G}_K(V - E_K) + \bar{G}_L(V - E_L) \qquad (8.100)$$

We should note that partial differentials have to be used (see Appendix 18) as V is now a function of both distance and time. This is because, as we showed in Chapter 7, $\bar{G}_K$ and $\bar{G}_{Na}$ are functions of time. Since voltage is a function of distance, they will also be functions of distance. In Chapter 7 we showed that

$$\bar{G}_{Na} = \bar{\bar{G}}_{Na}m^3h \qquad (7.57)$$
$$\bar{G}_K = \bar{\bar{G}}_K n^4 \qquad (7.33)$$
$$\bar{G}_L = \bar{\bar{G}}_L \quad \text{(see leak conductance in Chapter 7)}$$

Substituting these equations into (8.100) we obtain

$$(a/(2\rho_{In}))(\partial/\partial x)^2(V) = \bar{C}_m(\partial/\partial t)(V) + \bar{\bar{G}}_{Na}m^3h(V - E_{Na})$$
$$+ \bar{\bar{G}}_K n^4(V - E_K) + \bar{\bar{G}}_L(V - E_L) \qquad (8.101)$$

In this equation, m, h and n are functions of voltage and time (see Chapter 7) and so equation (8.101) is a non-linear partial differential equation (see Appendix 19).

In the beginning of Chapter 7 we considered the waveform travelling at velocity v along an axon and we showed that a moving waveform is a replica of itself displaced in distance. An observer that stands at a distance x' from the point of origin (x) sees the same waveform passing by with a delay t' which is given by

$$t' = x'/v$$

where v is the velocity of propagation. So

$$x' = vt' \qquad (8.102)$$

and the waveforms v (at x) and v' (at $x = x + x'$) are related by

$$v(x, t) = v(x - x', t - t')$$

The right-hand side of this equation is the same function as the left-hand side where x is substituted by $x - x'$ and t by $t - t'$.

If we observe both waveforms at the same time t, then this relationship is $V(x) = V(x - x')$ where $V(x)$ is the voltage at x and $V(x - x')$ is the voltage at x'.

From equation (8.102)

$$V(x) = V(x - vt') \tag{8.103}$$

If we differentiate both sides of this equation in relation to x, we obtain

$$(\partial/\partial x)(V(x)) = (\partial/\partial x)(V(x - vt')) \tag{8.104}$$

But $V(x - vt')$ is a function of a function (see Appendix 2), that is

$$y = x - vt'$$

so

$$V(x - vt') = V(y)$$

Then

$$(\partial/\partial x)(V(x) - vt') = (\partial/\partial y)(V(y))(\partial/\partial x)(x - vt')$$
$$= (\partial/\partial y)(V(y))$$

So

$$(\partial/\partial x)(V(x)) = (\partial/\partial y)(V(y))$$

If we differentiate this equation again, by the same arguments

$$(\partial/\partial x)^2(V(x)) = (\partial/\partial y)^2(V(y)) \tag{8.105}$$

If we differentiate (8.103) in relation to t, we obtain

$$(\partial/\partial t)(V(x)) = (\partial/\partial t)(V(x - vt'))$$
$$= (\partial/\partial y)(V(y))(\partial/\partial t)(-vt)$$
$$= -v(\partial/\partial y)(V(y)) \tag{8.106}$$

Again differentiating (8.106) in relation to t

$$(\partial/\partial t)^2(V(x)) = v^2(\partial/\partial y)(V(y)) \tag{8.107}$$

or

$$(\partial/\partial y)^2(V(y)) = \frac{1}{v^2}(\partial/\partial t)^2(V(x)) \tag{8.108}$$

The one-dimensional wave equation

If we substitute (8.108) into (8.105) we obtain

$$(\partial/\partial x)^2(V(x)) = (1/v^2)(\partial/\partial t)^2(V(x))$$

or more generally

$$(\partial/\partial x)^2(V(x, t)) = (1/v^2)(\partial/\partial t)^2(V(x, t)) \tag{8.109}$$

This is the so-called one-dimensional wave equation and can be used to solve equation (8.101). Substituting (8.109) into (8.101) we obtain

$$(a/(2\rho_{In}v^2))(d/dt)^2(V) = \bar{C}_m(d/dt)(v) + \bar{G}_{Na}m^3h(V - E_{Na})$$
$$+ \bar{G}_K n^4(V - E_K) + \bar{G}_L(V - E_L) \tag{8.110}$$

Solution of the wave equation: the propagated action potential

Equation (8.110) is now a second-order differential equation in $V(t)$ which can be solved. This equation has to be solved numerically and there is a complication that the propagation velocity is not known beforehand. The procedure for solving the equation is to guess a value of v, then compute the action potential and see whether or not a final solution is obtained. Successive guesses of v are usually required before a correct solution is found. In Figure 8.14 we show a propagated action potential calculated according to this procedure, with different values of v.

Distributed model of the axon to solve the propagating action potential

An alternative way of solving this equation is not to assume a value of v (the uniform longitudinal propagation velocity). If the axoplasm is considered to be purely resistive, and if this resistance is split up into a number of stations each Δx centimetres apart, the resistance of each segment (Δr_i) is then given by equation (8.97). That is,

$$\Delta r_i = r_i \, \Delta x = \rho_{In} \, \Delta x / \pi a^2$$

where ρ_{In} is the internal resistivity and a is the fibre radius. The equivalent circuit of this model is represented in Figure 8.15. The arrows represent the membrane current ($i_m(j)$) crossing the membrane at each station (j). From Kirchhoff's Law of the currents

$$(V(j+1) - Vj)/(\rho_{In} \, \Delta x / \pi a^2) = i_m(j) + (V(j) - V(j-1))/(\rho_{In} \, \Delta x / \pi a^2)$$

Fig.8.14

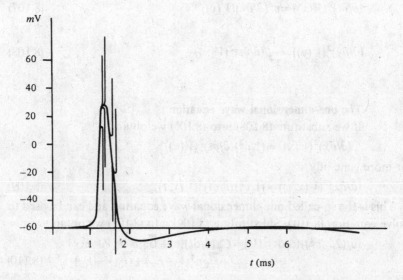

t (ms)

where $V(j)$ is the potential across the membrane at the jth station. Or

$$i_m(j) = (V(j+1) - V(j) - V(j) + V(j+1))/(\rho_{In}\,\Delta x)/(\pi a^2)$$

so

$$i_m(j) = (V(j+1) + V(j-1) - 2V(j))\pi a^2/\rho_{In}\,\Delta x \qquad (8.111)$$

at the nth station, where a constant current $i_{applied}$ is applied,

$$i_{applied} = i_m(n) + (V(n) - V(n-1))/(\rho_{In}\,\Delta x/\pi a^2)$$

or

$$i_m(n) = i_{applied} - (V(n) - V(n-1))\pi a^2/\rho_{In}\,\Delta x \qquad (8.112)$$

At station 1

$$i_m(1) = (V(2) - V(1))\pi a^2/\rho_{In}\,\Delta x \qquad (8.113)$$

At the j station

$$i_m(j) = i_i(j) + i_c(j)$$

$$i_m(j) = i_i(j) + c_m(d/dt)(V(j)) \qquad (8.114)$$

where $i_m(j)$ is the total membrane current at station j and $i_i(j)$ and $c_m(d/dt)$ $(V(j))$ are the ionic (i_i) and capacitative currents (i_c) (expressed per unit length) at the same station. We can now substitute (8.111), (8.112), (8.113) into (8.114) to obtain

$$(d/dt)(V(j)) = (1/c_m)[(V(j+1) + V(j-1) - 2(Vj))\pi a^2/\Delta x\rho_{In} - i_i(j)]$$
$$(8.115)$$

$$(d/dt)(V(n)) = (1/c_m)[(V(n) - V(n-1))\pi a^2/\Delta x\rho_{In} - i_i(n)] \qquad (8.116)$$

and

$$(d/dt)(V(1)) = (1/c_m)[(V(2) - V(1))\pi a^2/\Delta x\rho_{In} - i_i(1)] \qquad (8.117)$$

In these equations the ionic current $i_i(j)$ (where $j = 1, \ldots, n$) is given by

$$i_i(j) = (1/2\pi a\,\Delta x)[\bar{G}_{Na}m^3(j)h(j)(V(j) - E_{Na})$$
$$+ \bar{G}_K n^4(j)(V(j) - E_K) + \bar{G}_L(V(j) - E_L)] \qquad (8.118)$$

Fig.8.15

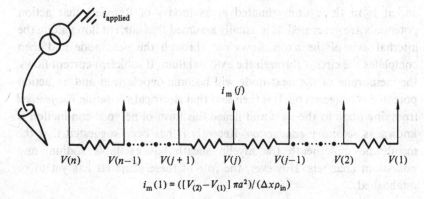

$$i_m(1) = ([V_{(2)} - V_{(1)}]\,\pi a^2)/(\Delta x\rho_{in})$$

In equation (8.118) the values of $m(j)$, $h(j)$ and $n(j)$ are obtained from equations (7.25), (7.43) and (7.47).

For each station we have four differential equations in n, m, h and V which can be solved individually as for a membrane action potential. This technique was described in detail in Chapter 7 and Figure 7.50b.

The system is solved for the case of an applied current at the nth station and the numerical integration of the sets of simultaneous first-order differential equations is started from the first station. This method, although more cumbersome to set up, does not involve the guess of any additional parameters. Furthermore, it allows the conduction velocity to vary along the fibre. Under normal conditions the conduction velocity will vary at the site of initiation and towards the end of the fibre.

Conduction velocity

The conduction velocity of an action potential is a parameter of some physiological importance. For example, neural pathways that are involved in fast responses require fast-conducting axons. Also, as many reflex pathways occur over long distances, long time delays are not acceptable if the skeletal muscle responses are to be fast. Experimentally it was found that the conduction velocity increases with the diameter of the fibre, and for the case of myelinated fibres the conduction velocity is proportional to the fibre diameter. In non-myelinated fibres the relationship is not clearly established, but it has been suggested that the conduction velocity is proportional to the square root of the fibre diameter.

Saltatory conduction

In myelinated axons, potentials are not generated contiguously along the length of the fibre. The myelin sheath, which acts as an electrical isolator, does not surround the axon along the whole length. At regular spaces (which are different for different axons) the myelin sheath is absent and it is in these unmyelinated areas (nodes of Ranvier) that action potentials are generated. It is usually assumed that current flows along the internal axis of the axon, flows out through the next node and then completes the circuit through the external fluid. If sufficient current flows, the membrane of the next node will become depolarized and an action potential is triggered off. It is then said that electrical excitation has *jumped* from one node to the next and hence this form of nervous conduction is known as *saltatory conduction*. Recently it has been suggested that the membrane underneath the myelin sheath has excitable sodium and potassium channels. However, the role of these channels has yet to be established.

9

Synaptic potentials

Introduction

The activity of different cells, tissues and organs in an animal is coordinated by means of specialized communication systems and these systems may be either chemical or electrical. Hormones and neurotransmitters are *chemical* communicators, that is, they act at a point different from that at which they were produced and released. *Electrical* communication is by means of excitable cells and the message is carried by action potentials. Because each excitable cell usually produces action potentials of fixed waveforms, information is transmitted by the *number* of action potentials per unit time (frequency), rather than by the shape of the waveforms. In this chapter we will discuss how these electrical signals are transmitted from one excitable cell to another (Synaptic Transmission) and this is often by a chemical communicator.

The neuromuscular junction

The experimental model used probably most frequently to study synaptic transmission is the nerve-muscle preparation. Electrical stimulation of a nerve results in action potentials being recorded by microelectrodes that are inserted in the muscle fibre. The nerve fibre when it reaches the surface of the muscle fibre splits into a number of different branches, and a recording microelectrode in the muscle fibre in the vicinity of one of these branches shows a slightly unusual action potential in that the action potential has a small hump on its rising edge (see Figure 9.1).

The synapse

If calcium is replaced by magnesium in the bathing fluid stimulation of the nerve will produce action potentials only in the nerve and not in the muscle fibre. If the amount of calcium in the bathing solution is sufficiently reduced, potentials can be recorded in the muscle in an area only near the nerve terminal. These areas are specialized regions of the nerve terminal and the muscle membrane and are known as *synapses*. When examined by electron microscopy their structure is as shown schematically in Figure 9.2. This figure shows, amongst other structures, small vesicles inside the nerve terminal, the presynaptic membrane, a gap known as the synaptic cleft and a postsynaptic (muscle) membrane. The size of the vesicles is around 500 Å and the cleft is about 100–300 Å.

The end-plate potential (EPP)

For a given calcium concentration, stimulation of the nerve in the synaptic region of the muscle fibre gives a potential of the type represented in Figure 9.3a. This potential is a depolarization of the muscle membrane and is called an end-plate potential (EPP). Moving the electrode away from the synaptic region (Figure 9.3b–d) results in potentials recorded being of increasingly smaller sizes. An EPP recorded at the synaptic region is known as a focal EPP and the smaller potentials recorded away from the synapse are due to the electrotonic spread of the focal EPP.

Fig.9.1

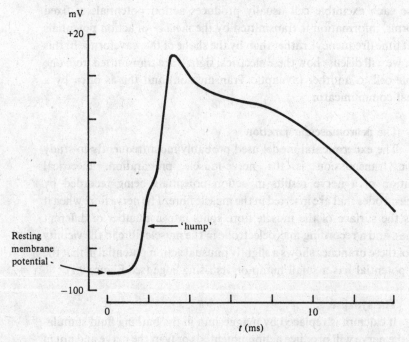

Modified from '*Nerve, muscle and synapse*' by
B. Katz, publisher McGraw-hill, 1966.

When the calcium concentration in the bathing solution is increased, EPPs increase in amplitude until they are sufficiently large to trigger off an action potential. Figure 9.1 shows an EPP (the small hump) triggering off an action potential.

The miniature end-plate potential (MEPP)

In the absence of nerve stimulation, or when calcium is removed

Fig.9.2

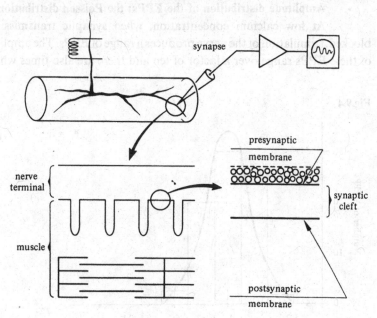

Fig.9.3

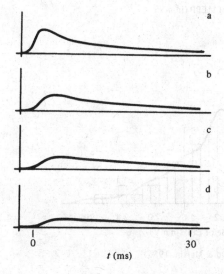

from the bath, miniature EPPs (MEPPs) of amplitude less than 1 mV can be recorded at the end-plate synaptic region. Although the MEPPs are of approximately the same size, if the amplitude of a sufficiently large number of them is measured, a range of amplitudes can be recorded. The MEPPs can be classified according to these amplitudes and a histogram of these classes is shown in Figure 9.4.

Amplitude distribution of the EPPs: the Poisson distribution

At low calcium concentration, when synaptic transmission is blocked, stimulation of the nerve produces a range of EPPs. The amplitudes of these EPPs range over a factor of ten and there are also times when *no*

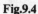

Fig.9.4

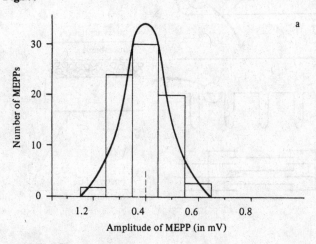

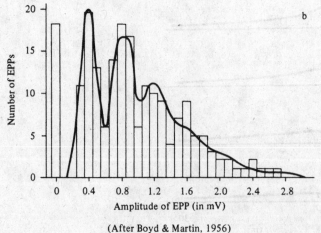

(After Boyd & Martin, 1956)

EPPs can be recorded. The amplitude distribution of the larger EPPs is skewed and shows a number of peaks (see Figure 9.4b), and these peaks occur at amplitudes 1, 2, 3 times the mean amplitude of the MEPP. If we number the EPP peaks from 1, 2, 3, ... through to x the peaks of the distribution follow the expression

$$N_x = NP_x$$

where

$$P_x = (q^x/x!) \exp(-q) \tag{9.1}$$

P_x is the probability of occurrence of an EPP of amplitude x, q is the ratio between the amplitude of the peak of class x and the mean amplitude of the MEPP. The symbol $x!$ (factorial x) is defined in Appendix 2. N is the total number of stimulations of the nerve, and N_x is the number of times that an EPP of class x occurs after N stimulations of the nerve.

The expression (9.1) is known as the *Poisson distribution* and is described in detail in the next chapter (and in Appendix 7) where we consider probabilistic events in excitable cells.

If the generation of EPPs follows the Poisson distribution, we can say the production of an EPP is a random event. We can also say that each of the EPPs is made up of a discrete number of units (MEPPs), all of approximately the same size. Since the chance of a MEPP taking place at any specific moment in time is very low, it can be considered an independent event. However, when the rate of stimulation is high, this is no longer the case.

Presynaptic depolarization

It can be shown that the EPP is not a propagated *electrical* response that crosses the synaptic cleft. For if current is passed through the *pre*synaptic terminal a microelectrode in the synaptic area of the muscle, the *post*synaptic membrane, does not pick up the same presynaptic potential profile, but an EPP is recorded whose onset is later than the start of the presynaptic current injection. In this experiment the sodium and potassium channels of the presynaptic membrane are blocked by Tetrodotoxin (TTX) and tetraethylammonium (TEA) respectively before current is passed and depolarization from the resting membrane potential occurs. For about a 25 mV depolarization no EPPs are recorded. Further increases in presynaptic depolarization then result in a large increase in the amplitude of the EPP until a maximum value is obtained (Figure 9.5), which is not affected by further presynaptic depolarizations.

Synaptic delay

Since the EPP is delayed in time following the current injection, the propagation across the synaptic cleft is much slower than would be expected if it were due to a local current. The explanation for the delay is provided in experiments which show that a chemical (acetylcholine) is released by nerve stimulation, and that local application of this chemical to the synaptic region causes the muscle fibre to depolarize and contract.

The release of acetylcholine (Ach)

The amount of acetylcholine (Ach) released per action potential, determined by perfusing the neuromuscular junction and collecting the perfusate, is of the order of 10^6 molecules. When Ach is topically applied, excitation of the muscle fibre requires more than 10^6 molecules. It thus is likely that not all of the topically applied Ach reaches the active site. Alternatively underestimates may be obtained if, of all the Ach released by nerve stimulation, not all of it is collected. The release of Ach, the diffusion across the synaptic cleft and the interaction with the postsynaptic membrane can be distinguished from one another by means of pharmacological agents.

Effect of curare

The action of Ach on muscle can be markedly reduced and eventually abolished by applying increasingly large doses of the poison curare. Radiolabelled curare can be seen to bind to neuromuscular junctions, and can be only partially washed off. This suggests that the

Fig.9.5

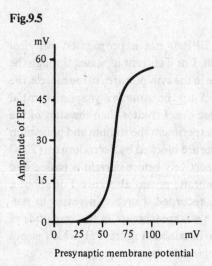

Presynaptic membrane potential

neuromuscular junctions have binding sites for curare and it is likely that curare competes for these with Ach.

Competitive inhibition

When several concentrations of curare are used, the *dose response* of Ach follows competitive inhibition kinetics (see Appendix 28). (By dose response, we mean the value of the EPP (response) as a function of the concentration (dose) of acetylcholine.)

Inhibitors of Ach release

Pharmacological agents, such as botulinum toxin, or a high magnesium concentration, or a low concentration of calcium ions in the bathing fluid, all block the release of Ach from the neuromuscular junction. Since the muscle is still responsive to locally applied Ach, it is assumed that these agents interfere with the release of Ach from the nerve terminal and are thus known as presynaptic blocking agents.

Postsynaptic inhibitors: depolarizing blockers

Another group of substances can bind to the Ach receptor and depolarize the muscle. These agents, such as succinylcholine, have molecular structures similar to Ach and produce a long-lasting depolarization when compared with the effect of Ach. Ach is removed from the receptor partly by being broken down by a locally released enzyme called cholinesterase and partly by diffusing off the receptor site. One of the mechanisms proposed to explain the long-lasting depolarization is that molecules such as succinylcholine are not broken down by this enzyme and so keep the muscle depolarized.

Synaptic vesicles and the role of calcium

Before Ach is released, following nerve stimulation, a number of events takes place at the presynaptic terminal. Morphological studies of the nerve terminals show the presence of small vesicles (~ 500 Å diameter), and the number of these vesicles decreases after nerve stimulation. Morphologists have also shown that the vesicles are able to fuse with the presynaptic terminal membrane. Katz interpreted the events that occur in neuromuscular transmission when he proposed his 'vesicular hypothesis'. In this hypothesis he assumed that the vesicles were packed with Ach and that there was a random movement of vesicles inside the presynaptic terminal. At certain specialized sites they fused with the membrane and discharged their contents into the synaptic cleft, and the chance of this fusing occurring increased when the nerve terminal was depolarized.

Depolarization caused calcium to enter the presynaptic terminal by the voltage switching on (opening) calcium channels. The calcium was then assumed to bind to an internal receptor site and activate (increase the probability of) vesicular fusion with the presynaptic membrane.

Synaptic delay: diffusion over the synaptic cleft

After vesicular release, Ach diffuses across the synaptic cleft. In Chapter 3 we showed that the time (t) taken for a molecule to diffuse over a distance Δx is given by

$$t = \Delta x^2/(2D)$$

where D is the diffusion coefficient. The diffusion coefficient of Ach in the synaptic cleft is unknown. However, if we assume that it is the same as in free solution (around $7.6 \times 10^{-6} \, cm^2 \cdot s^{-1}$), and since Δx is at most 500 Å

$$t = (5 \times 10^{-6})^2/(7.6 \times 10^{-6} \times 2) = 1.6 \times 10^{-6}$$
$$(cm^2)/(cm^2 \cdot s^{-1}) = s$$

The observed synaptic delays that take place are of the order of 5×10^{-4} s, which is much larger than the above calculated diffusional delay. This means that either diffusion through the cleft is not the rate-limiting step or that the diffusion through the synaptic cleft is much slower than in free solution. Some of the delay may also be due to the events that take place in the postsynaptic membrane.

Number of Ach molecules that interact with a receptor site

These events include the binding of one (or two) Ach molecules to a single Ach receptor in the postsynaptic membrane (the number of molecules of Ach that bind to a single receptor can be estimated in a way shown in Appendix 29) and the consequent opening of a 'chemically gated' channel. A 'chemically gated' channel is a channel which is switched on (or off) as a result of a chemical reaction. It can be compared with the voltage-gated channels which are discussed in Chapter 7.

Depolarization induced by 1–2 molecules of Ach

From a study of the voltage fluctuations (see Chapter 10) of the muscle membrane potentials that follows a local application of Ach, Katz and Miledi estimated that the depolarization produced by the interaction of one, or possibly two, molecules of Ach with the muscle membrane is around 0.3 µV.

Number of Ach molecules per vesicle

Since MEPPs are, on average 0.5 mV, about a thousand molecules of Ach are required to produce one MEPP.

Number of vesicles required to trigger an action potential

This number has been interpreted as corresponding to the number of molecules of Ach per vesicle and it has been estimated that for an EPP of 40–50 mV (that is, an EPP that is sufficiently large to trigger off an action potential in muscle), some 300 vesicles discharge their Ach at the presynaptic nerve terminal.

Conductance changes in the postsynaptic membrane

It is clear that Ach interacts with the postsynaptic membrane in such a way as to cause a membrane depolarization. This depolarization must be due to a change in membrane conductance. As discussed in Chapter 7, one of the best ways of examining conductance changes is to voltage-clamp the membrane. Takeuchi and Takeuchi voltage-clamped the postsynaptic muscle membrane at several different voltages by means of a point microelectrode clamp. The voltages at which the muscle membranes were clamped were always more negative than the threshold potential for a muscle action potential. (Below threshold potential had to be used because, although the EPP is not affected by TTX and TEA, since the release of Ach was obtained by nerve stimulation, these drugs could not be added to the bathing fluid.) The amplitudes of the end-plate currents (measured after stimulation of the nerve) are plotted as a function of the clamped-muscle membrane potentials in Figure 9.6.

Fig.9.6

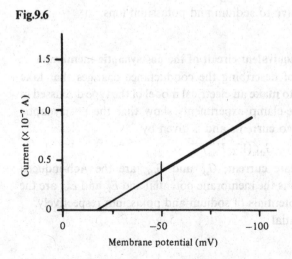

The reversal potential of the postsynaptic membrane in the presence of Ach

The extrapolation of the straight line obtained in Figure 9.6 to the voltage axis gives the potential at zero current (this potential is often called the zero current potential or reversal potential). From the Figure 9.6 it can be seen that the value of the reversal-potential was approximately -15 mV.

Ach-gated channels

The same authors also showed that when the sodium and potassium concentrations in the bathing fluid were reduced, the reversal-potential changed. But the reversal-potential remained unchanged by changes in external chloride concentration. These results indicate that Ach causes the opening of channels that are permeable to potassium and sodium and impermeable to chloride. Under these experimental conditions these channels are voltage-insensitive, for the I/V relationship is linear which means that the conductance is constant and so independent of voltage. Since the sodium and potassium end-plate currents produced by Ach are not blocked by TTX or TEA, this means that the end-plate sodium and potassium channels are specialized channels. They are gated by Ach and are different from the TTX- or TEA-sensitive channels, the voltage-gated sodium and potassium channels, that produce the action potential (see Chapter 7).

Fluctuation analysis of these Ach channels shows that their unit conductances are around 100 pS. This is an order of magnitude greater than the unit conductances of the voltage-sensitive extrajunctional sodium and potassium channels which suggests that the Ach-gated channels are wider and so less selective to sodium and potassium ions.

The electrical equivalent circuit of the postsynaptic membrane

Another way of describing the conductance changes that take place during an EPP is to make an electrical model of the type discussed in Chapter 6. The voltage-clamp experiments show that the postsynaptic current is the sum of two currents and is given by

$$I_s = G_{sK}(V - E_K) + G_{sNa}(V - E_{Na})$$

where I_s is the end-plate current, G_{sK} and G_{sNa} are the Ach-induced conductance changes, V is the membrane potential and E_K and E_{Na} are the equilibrium (Nernst) potentials of sodium and potassium respectively.

At the reversal potential

$$I_s = 0$$

so
$$G_{sK}(V-E_K)+G_{sNa}(V-E_{Na})=0$$
Rearranging
$$G_{sNa}/G_{sK} = -(V-E_K)/(V-E_{Na})$$
If we substitute -15 mV for V, -99 mV for E_K and $+50$ mV for E_{Na} we obtain
$$G_{sNa}/G_{sK} = 1.29$$

Since this ratio is not much greater than one, the changes in sodium and potassium conductance during an EPP are similar. This suggests that Ach channels have almost similar conductances to sodium and potassium ions and thus cannot easily discriminate between the two ions. This result is in agreement with the high unit conductance of the Ach channel found from the fluctuation-analysis experiments.

A simple cable model for the end-plate region: transient analysis
The above analysis is a steady-state analysis in that the total membrane current due to the transmitter interaction is assumed to be zero (i.e. $I_s = 0$). The disadvantage of this type of analysis is that it does not describe the time course of the EPP and so does not consider the charging up of the membrane capacity.

In Figure 9.7a we represent a muscle fibre by a cable similar to the distributed axon model used in Chapter 8. For the sake of simplicity we consider the fibre to be a cylinder and do not include the muscle transverse-tubular system. In the middle of the fibre we represent the postsynaptic membrane by one switchable branch which corresponds to the Ach receptor. In Figure 9.7b we have further simplified the distributed model by lumping the voltage-dependent (triggered) conductances and the chemically gated (synaptic) conductances for each section. The batteries of Figure 9.7b for each section were derived in Chapter 7 and are given by
$$E_{(n)} = (G_{Na}E_{Na}+G_K E_K+G_L E_L)/(G_{Na}+G_K+G_L) \qquad (9.2a)$$
where $E_{(n)}$ is the resting membrane potential of the nth section and G_{Na}, G_K and G_L are the conductances for sodium, potassium and chloride in this section. Likewise,
$$E_s = (G_{sNa}E_{Na}+G_{sK}E_K)/(G_{sNa}+G_{sK}) \qquad (9.2b)$$
where E_s is the open-circuit potential across the postsynaptic membrane when the Ach-gated channels are open.

Before the synaptic branches are switched on by the Ach, E_s is equal to zero. Figure 9.7c is a lumped model of Figure 9.7b where

$$G_m = \sum_{j=1}^{n} G_m(j)$$

$$E_m = \sum_{j=1}^{n} G_m(j) E_m(j) \bigg/ \left(\sum_{j=1}^{n} G_m(j) \right)$$

and

$$C_m = \sum_{j=1}^{n} C_m(j)$$

Fig.9.7

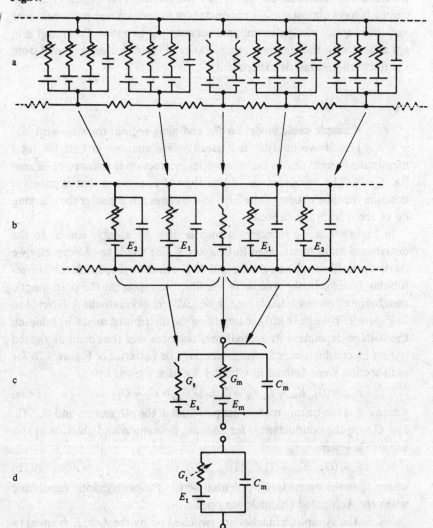

In a lumped model the assumption is that it behaves exactly as the original model. In practice when 'lumping' equivalent circuits the techniques of circuit analysis are used which allow the combination of conductances, capacitors and voltages. These techniques are based on Ohm's and on Kirchhoff's Laws (see Appendix 15). The lumped circuit of Figure 9.7c can only be an adequate representation of Figure 9.7b if the space constant (λ) of the cable is sufficiently large for the membrane potential to be uniform along its length. This means that there is no potential drop across the internal resistance r_i and so r_i can be ignored. We can now write the equation for the currents across the three branches of Figure 9.7c

$$I_t = G_s(V - E_s) + G_m(V - E_m) + C_m(dV/dt) \tag{9.2c}$$

I_t must be zero at all times since no external circuit is injecting or collecting current from the system. Before the Ach–receptor interaction the membrane is at rest, so $I_t = 0$. When this interaction takes place, current flows inwards through G_s and outwards through G_m and C_m. The net current (I_t) across the whole fibre is still zero. If we rearrange equation (9.2c) we obtain for $I_t = 0$

$$V(G_s + G_m) - (G_s E_s + G_m E_m) + C_m(dV/dt) = 0$$

and, dividing by $(G_s + G_m)$,

$$V - \frac{G_s E_s + G_m E_m}{G_s + G_m} + \frac{C_m}{G_s + G_m} \frac{dV}{dt} = 0 \tag{9.3}$$

If we define

$$E_T = \frac{G_s E_s + G_m E_m}{G_s + G_m} \tag{9.4}$$

and

$$\tau_m = \frac{C_m}{G_s + G_m} \tag{9.5}$$

equation (9.3) becomes

$$V - E_T + \tau_m(dV/dt) = 0 \tag{9.6}$$

E_T and τ_m each have two values. Before the Ach–receptor interaction

$$G_s = 0$$

so one set of values is $E_T = E_m$ and $\tau_m = C_m/G_m$. After G_s is switched on by Ach the other set of values for E_T and τ_m is given by (9.4) and (9.5) respectively.

Equation (9.3) describes the behaviour of equivalent circuit Figure 9.7d when G_s, the synaptic conductance, is switched on, so

$$G_T = G_m + G_s$$

When the synaptic conductance is switched off

$$G_T = G_m$$

τ_m is the time constant of the system (see Chapter 6).

In order to integrate equation (9.6) it can be rearranged as

$$dV/dt = -(1/\tau_m)(V - E_T)$$

and by the technique of separation of variables (see Appendix 9) we can write

$$dV/(V - E_T) = -dt/\tau_m \tag{9.7}$$

As discussed in this chapter, the Ach–receptor interaction opens channels for a specific time (τ). Equation (9.7) has to be integrated between the time when the Ach–receptor interaction takes place ($t = 0$) and $t = \tau$ (for channels being open) and between $t = \tau$ and $t \rightarrow \infty$ (when channels are closed again). Between $t = 0$ and $t = \tau$ equations (9.4) and (9.5) apply, after $t = \tau$ equations (9.7), (9.8) and (9.9) apply.

In order to obtain the general solution of equation (9.7) we integrate both sides of equation (9.7) directly

$$\int dV/(V - E_T) = -(1/\tau_m) \int dt$$

So

$$\ln(V - E_T) + B = -(1/\tau_m)t \tag{9.8}$$

where B is the constant of integration. For the 'on' interval between 0 and t at $t = 0$

$$\ln(V_0 - E_T) + B = -(1/\tau_m)0$$

So

$$\ln(V_0 - E_T) = -B \tag{9.9}$$

If we substitute (9.9) in (9.8) we obtain

$$\ln(V - E_T) - \ln(V_0 - E_T) = -t/\tau_m \tag{9.10}$$

where V_0 is the resting muscle membrane potential at $t = 0$. Although G_s is switched on at $t = 0$, the membrane potential does not change instantaneously, therefore its value is the resting value at that instant. E_T is given by equation (9.4), τ_m is given by equation (9.5), and V is the membrane potential at any time up to t.

Equation (9.10) can be rearranged as

$$\ln(V - E_T) - \ln(V_0 - E_T) = \ln((V - E_T)/(V_0 - E_T)) = -t/\tau_m$$

or

$$(V - E_T)/(V_0 - E_T) = \exp(-t/\tau_m) \tag{9.11}$$

If we rearrange equation (9.11) we obtain

$$V = E_T + (V_0 - E_T)\exp(-t/\tau_m) \tag{9.12}$$

Equation (9.12) is plotted in Figure 9.8b. The corresponding conductance G_s is plotted in Figure 9.8a.

Equation (9.8) can also be used to obtain solution for $t > \tau$. At $t = \tau$ the potential will be V and so

$$\ln(V_\tau - E_T) + B = -\tau/\tau_m \tag{9.13}$$

At $t > \tau$

$$\ln(V - E_T) + B = -t/\tau_m \tag{9.14}$$

If we subtract equation (9.13) from (9.14) so as to eliminate B, we obtain

$$\ln(V - E_T) - \ln(V_\tau - E_T) = -t/\tau_m + \tau/\tau_m$$

or

$$V = E_T + (V_\tau - E_T)\exp(-(t - \tau)/\tau_m) \tag{9.15}$$

Fig.9.8

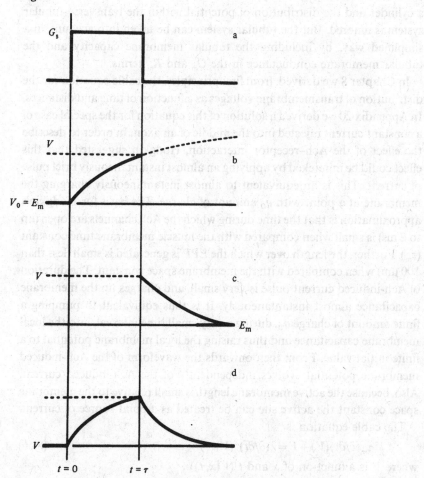

where E_T is given by (9.8) and τ_m is given by (9.9). Equation (9.15) is plotted in Figure 9.8c.

The shape of the EPP

The overall curve is represented in Figure 9.8d and is the approximate representation of the EPP. The equivalent circuits of Figure 9.7c and d (and thus equation (9.2)) do not describe the attenuation with distance of the EPP that is observed experimentally (see Figure 9.3a–d).

Attenuation of the EPP with distance

Mathematically we could have a description of the attenuation of the EPP if we use the cable equation that was described in Chapter 8 for an axon. This would still be an approximation because the muscle is treated as a cylinder and the distribution of potential within the transverse-tubular system is ignored. But the tubular system can be taken into account, in a simplified way, by including the tubular membrane capacity and the tubular membrane conductance in the C_m and R_m terms.

In Chapter 8 we derived, from first principles, the cable equation for the distribution of transmembrane voltages as a function of time and distances. In Appendix 20 we derived a solution of this equation for the special case of a constant current injected into the middle of an axon. In order to describe the effect of the Ach–receptor interaction, Hodgkin suggested that this effect could be mimicked by applying an almost instantaneously brief pulse of current. This is an equivalent to almost instantaneously charging the membrane at a point with q_0 amount of charge. The basis for Hodgkin's approximation is that the time during which the Ach channels are open (up to 2 ms) is small when compared with the muscle membrane time constant (τ_m). Further, the length over which the EPP is generated is small (less than 100 μm) when compared with the membrane space constant. The duration of Ach-induced current pulse is very small, and charges up the membrane capacitance almost instantaneously. It is thus equivalent to pumping a finite amount of charge q_0, during a very small time interval, into the local membrane capacitance and thus raising the local membrane potential to a finite initial value. From then onwards the waveform of the Ach-induced membrane potential evolves independently of the Ach-induced current. Also, because the active membrane length is small relative to the membrane space constant the active site can be treated as a point source of current.

The cable equation is

$$\tau_m(\partial/\partial t)(V) + V = \lambda(\partial/\partial t)^2(V) \tag{8.56}$$

where V is a function of x and t $(V(x, t))$.

The solution for equation (8.56) with the initial conditions of the instantaneous application of a charge (q_0) at $t=0$ and $x=0$ is

$$V = (q_0/2C_m\lambda(\pi t/\tau_m)^{1/2})\exp(-x^2\tau_m/4\lambda^2 t + t/\tau_m) \quad (9.16)$$

(see Appendix 20). Equation (9.16) can be plotted in a general way if we define the variables

$$X = x/\lambda \quad (9.17)$$

and

$$T = t/\tau_m \quad (9.18)$$

This is equivalent to measuring distance as per unit λ and to measuring time per unit τ_m.

If we substitute (9.17) and (9.18) into (9.16) we obtain

$$V(X, T) = (q_0/2C_m\lambda(\pi T)^{1/2})\exp(-(X-4T^2)/4T) \quad (9.19)$$

Equation (9.14) is plotted for various distances in Figure 9.9 and can be shown to be a reasonable description of the experimentally recorded curves. If the current injection takes place at $X = l$, rather than $X = 0$, then equation (9.19) becomes

$$V_l(X, T) = (q_l/2C_m\lambda(\pi T)^{1/2})\exp(-((X-L)^2 + 4T^2)/4T) \quad (9.20)$$

where $L = l/\lambda$.

Spatial summation

If current is injected simultaneously at $x=0$ and $x=l$ (equivalent to q_0 and q_l amounts of charge respectively), this is equivalent to a muscle

Fig.9.9

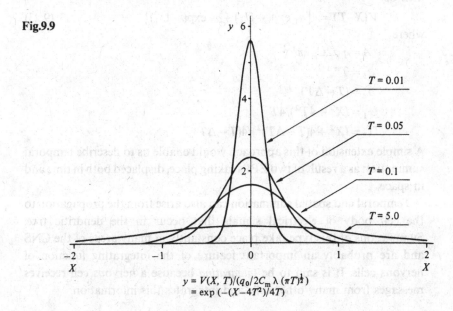

$$y = V(X, T)/(q_0/2C_m\lambda(\pi T)^{\frac{1}{2}})$$
$$= \exp(-(X-4T^2)/4T)$$

fibre receiving simultaneous excitation from two different end-plate regions. This might occur, for example, in non-twitch multiply-innervated muscle fibres. The membrane potential is then the result of the super-position (summation in space) of equations (9.19) and (9.20), that is

$$V(X, T) = (1/2C_m \lambda(\pi T)^{1/2})[q_0 \exp(-U_1) + q_l \exp(-U_2)] \qquad (9.21)$$

where

$$U_1 = (X^2 - 4T^2)/4T \quad \text{and} \quad U_2 = ((X - L)^2 + 4T^2)/4T$$

Spatial summations of this type are an important control feature in the central nervous system (CNS). In addition, spatial summation is important in the control of the graded contractions seen in multiply-innervated muscles.

Temporal summation

Temporal summation (summation in time) occurs when the transmitter–receptor interaction is displaced in time. The simplest case is when the same point on the membrane is stimulated at different intervals in time.

In order for equation (9.19) to show a time delay (Δt) we can write

$$V(X, T) = (q_0/2C_m \lambda[\pi(T - \Delta T)]^{1/2}) \exp(-U) \qquad (9.22)$$

where

$$U = (X^2 + 4(T - \Delta T)^2)/(4(T - \Delta T)) \quad \text{and} \quad \Delta T = \Delta t/\tau_m$$

Equation (9.22) applies only when $T \geqslant \Delta T$, because, for smaller values of T, the second current injection has not taken place. The compound EPP will then be

$$V(X, T) = A[a_1 \exp(-U_1) + a_2 \exp(-U_2)] \qquad (9.23)$$

where

$$A = q_0/2C_m \lambda \pi^{1/2}$$
$$a_1 = T^{-1/2}$$
$$a_2 = (T - \Delta T)^{-1/2}$$
$$U_1 = (X^2 + 4T^2)/4T$$
$$U_2 = (X^2 + 4(T - \Delta T)^2)/4(T - \Delta T)$$

A simple extension of this approach would enable us to describe temporal summation as a result of two EPPs taking place, displaced both in time and in space.

Temporal and spatial summation can also arise from the propagation to the cell body of electrical signals that occur in the dendritic tree. Summations of this type take place constantly in many areas of the CNS and are probably an important feature of the integrating function of nervous cells. It is said to be *integrating* because a nervous cell receives messages from many other cells and integrates this information.

Other synapses

Although the concepts presented so far were developed using the neuromuscular junction as a model, the principles readily apply to other synapses. These synapses include synapses between nerve terminals and cell bodies, nerve terminals of one cell and another, and nerve terminals and axons and multiply-innervated muscle fibres.

Other transmitter substances

The transmitter at synapses is not always Ach, and a number of transmitter substances have been identified, such as biogenic amines (dopamine, norepinephrine, serotonin, histamine) and amino acids (γ-aminobutyric acid (GABA), glycine, glutamate, aspartate). A large number of neuroactive peptides (gut-brain peptides such as vasoactive intestinal polypeptide (VIP), cholecystokinin, substance P, neurotensin, encephalins, insulin, glucagon, hypothalamic releasing hormones, pituitary peptides, angiotensin II, bradykinin, vasopressin, oxytocin, carnosine, bombesin) can cause, when locally applied, excitation or inhibition of nerve cells and can be isolated from CNS. It is not yet well established that these neuroactive peptides are neurotransmitters. In addition, the effect of the transmitter is such that it does not always result in a depolarization of the postsynaptic membrane. The reason for this may be understood if we reconsider the model of the postsynaptic membrane shown in Figure 9.7c. The synaptic conductance (G_s) is, in general, the sum of more than one ionic conductances, so

$$G_s = G_{sNa} + G_{sK} + G_{sCl} + \cdots$$

For Ach at the neuromuscular junction $G_{sCl} = 0$, but in the case of other transmitters this is not always true. The synaptic potential is given by a more general form of equation (9.2b)

$$E_s = (G_{sNa}E_{Na} + G_{sK}E_K + G_{sCl}E_{Cl})/G_s \qquad (9.24)$$

Depolarizing and hyperpolarizing transmitters: EPSPs and IPSPs

A transmitter may activate different ionic channels, which is equivalent to switching on individual conductances or a combination of the conductances of equation (9.24). The effect of switching on one of the conductances of equation (9.24) is to displace the membrane potential towards the equilibrium potential of the corresponding ion. If the transmitter switches on G_{sK} or G_{sCl}, and if the equilibrium potential of these ions (E_K and E_{Cl}) is more negative than the resting membrane potential, the transmitter will hyperpolarize the membrane. This hyperpolarization is known as an inhibitory postsynaptic potential (IPSP) and can be seen, for example, when the transmitters glycine or GABA interact with a number of CNS cells. A transmitter may also cause an IPSP by decreasing G_{Na}. On the other hand, in some cells, EPSPs can result from a decrease in G_K.

Combined effect of EPSPs and IPSPs

Synaptic potentials in CNS that depolarize cell membranes are generally referred to as excitatory postsynaptic potentials (EPSPs). A cell in the CNS may receive terminals from different cells. Some of the terminals come from cells that release inhibitory transmitters and produce IPSPs, while others come from cells that release excitatory transmitters which produce EPSPs. In the sympathetic ganglia, the postsynaptic potentials can be further categorized as either slow or fast. In general, the slow postsynaptic potentials (EPSPs and IPSPs) are due to a decrease in the conductance of the postsynaptic membrane to either potassium or sodium.

The flow of current in the synaptic region

The effect of all transmitters is to cause a local flux of current across a postsynaptic membrane. The local currents associated with the trans-mitter—receptor interaction which results in an EPSP (or an EPP) are shown in Figure 9.10a. The flow of current is inward at the synapse and outward across the surrounding membrane, and the further away a region is from the synaptic area the lower is the current density. The inset in Figure 9.10a shows the equivalent circuit associated with this current flow. Figure 9.10b shows a current flow associated with an IPSP and here the direction of the current flow is reversed.

An inward (positive) current across the postsynaptic membrane will depolarize the surrounding membrane. If this depolarization is large enough, and provided there are voltage-gated sodium and potassium channels in the surrounding membrane, an action potential will be fired off. But this is not always the case, as some synapses are not surrounded by voltage-gated sodium and potassium channels, in which case the spread of the EPSP is not propagated. A generated action potential will contain a depolarization on its rising edge (see Figure 9.1) and propagate away from the synaptic region on either side.

Although we have discussed the transient changes in postsynaptic potential that take place as a result of suddenly switching on the Ach-gated channels, we have yet to consider the kinetics of the underlying Ach–channel interaction. In the following analysis we will examine the effect of transmitter–receptor interaction on the shape of the voltage transients that occur when a population of Ach-channels open.

The mathematical description assumes that there is a sudden rise of Ach concentration near the postsynaptic membrane, which results in the combination of Ach molecules with their receptors. At any instant in time the conductance of the postsynaptic membrane, that is, the number of open Ach-channels is proportional to the concentration of Ach–receptor complexes. As time goes on, the Ach–receptor complexes dissociate because the transmitter diffuses away from the receptor and is also broken down by enzyme action.

Kinetics of the transmitter–receptor interaction

Although chemical transmission may take place through the release of different kinds of transmitters, the overall scheme of chemical transmission is somewhat similar. This scheme is summarized in Figure 9.11a. If we make the reasonable assumption that synaptic conductance G_s is proportional to the concentration of the transmitter–receptor complex, we can analyse the factors that determine the time that G_s is switched on. To

Fig.9.10

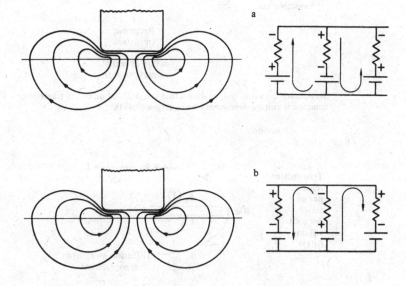

a

b

Fig.9.11

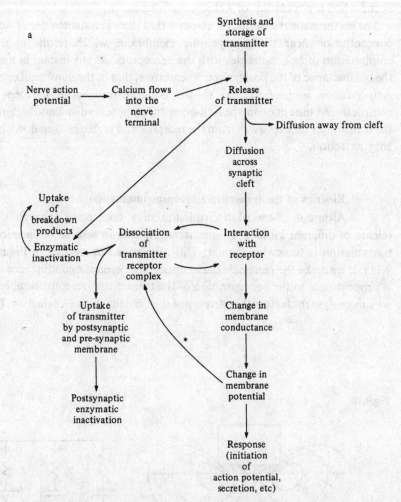

a

Nerve action potential → Calcium flows into the nerve terminal → Release of transmitter

Synthesis and storage of transmitter → Release of transmitter

Release of transmitter → Diffusion away from cleft

Diffusion across synaptic cleft

Uptake of breakdown products

Enzymatic inactivation

Dissociation of transmitter receptor complex ⇄ Interaction with receptor

Uptake of transmitter by postsynaptic and pre-synaptic membrane

Change in membrane conductance

*

Postsynaptic enzymatic inactivation

Change in membrane potential

Response (initiation of action potential, secretion, etc)

* Stevens and co-workers have shown that the dissociation of the transmitter complex is voltage dependent (see equation (9.45)).

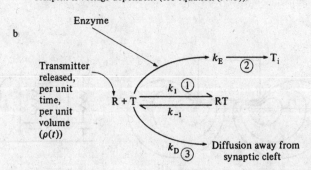

b

Enzyme

Transmitter released, per unit time, per unit volume $(\rho(t))$

$$R + T \underset{k_{-1}}{\overset{k_1 \;\text{①}}{\rightleftarrows}} RT$$

k_E ② → T_i

k_D ③ → Diffusion away from synaptic cleft

do this we extract a simpler kinetic scheme from Figure 9.11a which may be described by the sequence shown in Figure 9.11b.

The kinetic scheme

Here, T_i represents the inactive form of the transmitter (T) which results from the action of the corresponding inactivating enzyme (E). For the sake of simplicity we shall assume that only a small fraction of the receptor population is complexed and that only one transmitter molecule binds to each receptor. We shall also assume that the concentration of transmitter ([T]) surrounding the binding sites is very small so that the *concentration* of enzyme ([E]) is not rate-limiting. This means that the enzyme reaction is well below saturation, so that the rate of breakdown is proportional to the concentration of transmitter that surrounds the binding sites.

The mathematical model

The velocities of reactions (1), (2) and (3) are thus given by

$$v_1 = k_1[R][T] \qquad (9.25)$$
$$v_{-1} = k_{-1}[RT] \qquad (9.26) \quad \text{reaction (1)}$$
$$v_2 = k_E[T] \qquad (9.27) \quad \text{reaction (2)}$$
$$v_3 = k_D[T] \qquad (9.28) \quad \text{reaction (3)}$$

All these velocities have the dimensions $\text{mol} \cdot \text{cm}^{-3} \cdot \text{s}^{-1}$. If the total concentration of receptors ([R_t]) is constant

$$[R_t] = [R] + [RT]$$

so

$$[R] = [R_t] - [RT] \qquad (9.29)$$

If we substitute (9.29) into (9.25) we obtain

$$v_1 = k_1([R_t] - [RT])[T] \qquad (9.30)$$

The rate of increase of the transmitter concentration ($d[T]/dt$) is then given by

$$(d/dt)[T] = v_{-1} - v_1 - v_2 - v_3 + \rho(t) \qquad (9.31)$$

In equation (9.31) the term $\rho(t)$ describes the velocity ($\text{mol} \cdot \text{cm}^{-3} \cdot \text{s}^{-1}$) at which the transmitter is released from the presynaptic membrane. Equation (9.31) states that the rate of increase of transmitter concentration ($d[T]/dt$) is the result of the following processes:

(1) the release from the presynaptic membrane ($\rho(t)$)
(2) the release from the transmitter–receptor complex (v_{-1})
(3) the breakdown of the transmitter complex (v_2)
(4) the association of transmitter with receptor (v_1)
(5) the diffusion away from the synaptic cleft (v_3)

The rate of increase of transmitter–receptor complex is then given by

$$(d/dt)[RT] = v_1 - v_{-1} \tag{9.32}$$

If we substitute equations (9.25) to (9.28) into (9.31) we obtain

$$(d/dt)[T] = k_{-1}[RT] - k_1[R][T] - k_E[T] - k_D[T] + \rho(t) \tag{9.33}$$

But from equation (9.29) as $[R] = [R_t] - [RT]$

$$(d/dt)[T] = k_{-1}[RT] - k_1[R_t][T] + k_1[RT][T] - k_E[T] - k_D[T] + \rho(t)$$

or

$$(d/dt)[T] = k_{-1}[RT] - [T](k_1[R_t] - k_1[RT] + k_E + k_D) + \rho(t) \tag{9.34}$$

If

$$[RT] \ll [R_t] \tag{9.35}$$

equation (9.34) can be simplified to

$$(d/dt)[T] = k_{-1}[RT] - [T](k_1[R_t] + k_E + k_D) + \rho(t) \tag{9.36}$$

If we substitute (9.26) and (9.30) into equation (9.32) we obtain

$$(d/dt)[RT] = k_1([R_t] - [RT])[T] - k_{-1}[RT] \tag{9.37}$$

Because of the assumption made in (9.35), equation (9.37) simplifies to

$$(d/dt)[RT] = k_1[R_t][T] - k_{-1}[RT] \tag{9.38}$$

The solution of the mathematical model

Equations (9.36) and (9.38) constitute a system of two first-order, linear equations in $[T]$ and $[R]$ which must be integrated. In order to simplify the manipulations we will make the following substitutions

$$x = [T]$$
$$Y = [RT]$$
$$A = k_1[R_t] + k_E + k_D$$
$$B = k_1[R_t]$$

Equations (9.36) and (9.38) then become

$$(d/dt)(x) = k_{-1}Y - xA + \rho(t) \tag{9.39}$$
$$(d/dt)(Y) = Bx - k_{-1}Y \tag{9.38a}$$

Since the conductance changes are proportional to the concentration of transmitter-complex ($[RT]$) and thus to Y, we want to find a function which describes Y as a function of time.

In order to eliminate x we differentiate (9.38a) in relation to time, so

$$(d/dt)^2(Y) = B(d/dt)(x) - k_{-1}$$

or

$$(d/dt)^2(Y) + k_{-1}(d/dt)(Y) = B(d/dt)(x) \tag{9.40}$$

If we substitute (9.39) in (9.40) we obtain

$$(d/dt)^2(Y) + k_{-1}(d/dt)(Y) = B(k_{-1}Y - xA + \rho(t))$$
$$= Bk_{-1}Y - ABx + B\rho(t)$$

But from equation (9.38a)

$$Bx = (d/dt)(Y) + k_{-1}Y$$

so

$$(d/dt)^2(Y) + k_{-1}(d/dt)(Y) = Bk_{-1}Y - A(d/dt)(Y) - Ak_{-1}Y + B\rho(t)$$
$$\tag{9.41}$$

If we rearrange equation (9.41) we obtain

$$(d/dt)^2(Y) + (k_{-1} + A)(d/dt)(Y) + k_{-1}(A - B)Y = B\rho(t) \tag{9.42}$$

But

$$k_{-1} + A = k_{-1} + k_1[R_t] + k_E + k_D$$

and

$$A - B = k_1[R_t] + k_E + k_D - k_1[R_t] = k_E + k_D$$

Equation (9.42) thus becomes

$$(d/dt)^2(Y) + (k_{-1} + k_1[R_t] + k_E + k_D)\,dY/dt + k_{-1}(k_E + k_D)Y$$
$$= k_1[R_t]\rho(t) \quad (9.43)$$

Equation (9.43) is a second-order linear differential equation of the type

$$(d/dt)^2(Y) + b(d/dt)(Y) + cY = d\rho(t) \tag{9.43a}$$

The release function ($\rho(t)$) describes the amount of transmitter per unit volume and per unit time, arriving at the postsynaptic membrane. We approximate this function by the profile shown in Figure 9.12 because the time taken for transmitter release and diffusion across the synaptic cleft is very small compared with the duration of the resulting EPP (or EPSP). Thus we can approximate $\rho(t)$ by a function of infinitely small duration but with a finite area under the profile (a so-called *delta function*, see Appendix 14) because there is a finite amount of transmitter substance released. Dimensionally the area is equivalent to a concentration:

$$\text{area} = \text{time} \times \frac{\text{mol}}{\text{cm}^3 \cdot \text{time}} = \text{mol} \cdot \text{cm}^{-3}$$

This approximation means that the synaptic release of transmitter causes an almost instantaneous rise in transmitter concentration near the postsynaptic membrane. The solution of equation (9.43) can be made if we make the assumption that $\rho(t)$ *is* a delta function, and use the Laplace transform technique (see Appendix 14). The function $\rho(t)$ can be defined as

$$\lim Q/\Delta t \quad \text{when } \Delta t \to 0$$

Then

$$Q\,\delta(t)\,\Delta t = \lim_{\Delta t \to 0} [(Q/\Delta T)\,\Delta t] = Q$$

The Laplace transform of $\delta(t)$ (see Appendix 14) is 1. So, if we take the Laplace transform of (9.43a) we obtain

$$Y(p)(p^2+bp+c)=dQ$$

or

$$Y(p)=dQ/(p^2+bp+c)=dQ/((p+a_1)(p+a_2)) \qquad (9.43b)$$

If we expand (9.43b) in partial fractions (Appendix 8) we obtain

$$Y(p)=dQ[B/(p+a_1)+C/(p+a_2)]$$
$$=A[B/(p+a_1)+C/(p+a_2)]$$

where

$$B=1/(a_1-a_2), \quad C=-1/(a_1-a_2)$$

and Q is the sudden increase in concentration of transmitter due to its presynaptic release; a_1 and a_2 are defined by the expressions

$$a_1=-\varepsilon+(\varepsilon^2+\theta)^{1/2} \quad \text{and} \quad a_2=-\varepsilon-(\varepsilon^2+\theta)^{1/2}$$

The equations

$$\varepsilon=(k_{-1}+k_1[R_t]+k_E+k_D)/2 \quad \text{and} \quad \theta=k_F+k_D$$

Fig.9.12

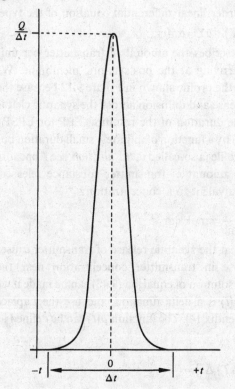

define ε and θ. The concentration of the transmitter–receptor complex as a function of time found from the inverse transform is thus (see Appendix 16):

$$[RT] = (A/(a_1 - a_2))[\exp(-a_1 t) - \exp(-a_2 t)] \tag{9.44}$$

In this way A, a_1 and a_2 of equation (9.44) have been expressed in terms of the parameters (k_1, k_{-1}, k_E, k_D) of the kinetic model and as a function of the total concentration of receptor sites $[R_t]$.

The postsynaptic conductance transient

If we assume that the postsynaptic changes in conductance are proportional to the concentration of receptor–transmitter complex ($[RT]$) (as we did previously), then equation (9.44) should provide a description of the conductance transient which gives rise to the EPP (or EPSP).

However, equation (9.44) contains a number of unknown parameters so to fit this equation to an experimentally obtained EPP (or EPSP) is at present an impossibility. Nevertheless, that equation does predict a conductance that rises and decays as an exponentially rising and decaying conductance. The two-electrode voltage-clamp experiments of Takeuchi and Takeuchi that we described above demonstrated that the peak of the conductance change occurred in about 0.4 ms and that the time of the decline of the conductance was about 1 ms. Furthermore, the declining phase of the experimentally obtained conductance was seen to be an exponential.

The voltage dependence of the conductance change

More recently, it has been found that the end-plate current (epc) decayed exponentially and that the decay constant depended upon the membrane potential. The decay constant (α) was found to depend exponentially on the membrane potential with the following empirical relationship

$$\alpha = B_1 \exp(A_1 V) \tag{9.45}$$

where A_1 and B_1 are constants. The dependence of the epc on voltage can be represented schematically as

$$R + T \underset{k_{-1}}{\overset{k_1}{\rightleftharpoons}} RT_c \underset{\alpha}{\overset{\beta}{\rightleftharpoons}} RT_o \tag{9.46}$$

where the effect of the membrane potential might be to increase the association (k_1) of receptor (R) with the transmitter (T) and at the same time the dissociation (k_{-1}) of the transmitter–receptor complex (RT_c). The overall effect depends on whether the concentration of RT_o increases (effect on β relatively larger than on α) or decreases (effect on α relatively larger than on β).

This model expands the kinetic scheme already proposed above in the following way, where RT_c and RT are equivalent. RT_o (Figure 9.13) represents the formation of an open channel.

Alternatively, the transmitter–receptor complex may not be conducting $((RT_c))$ and, in a model of this type, Stevens and co-workers assumed that (RT_c) was not a conducting channel. A further step is required before (RT_c) becomes conducting (RT_o), and this step has a backward and a forward rate constant (α, β); these are voltage dependent. The empirically derived decay

Fig.9.13

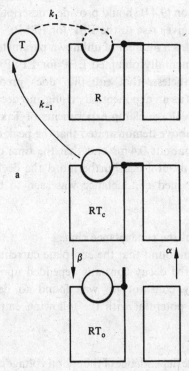

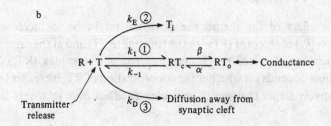

constant (α) of equation (9.45) is the backward rate constant. The forward rate constant (β) can also be obtained experimentally by fitting a mathematical model corresponding to the kinetic scheme described in (9.46). This method of fitting a mathematical model is developed further in the next chapter.

Sensory receptors

We have shown that chemical transmitters are able to produce conductance changes resulting in potentials that may be either depolarizing or hyperpolarizing. However, chemical transmitters are not the only agents capable of producing graded conductance changes and graded potential transients.

Generator and receptor potentials

A number of different types of sensory receptors respond to physical or chemical stimuli in the same way. Although the study of sensory receptors is a very important area of research in electrophysiology, to date, because of technical difficulties associated with this type of research, the progress made has not reached the same level as the advances made in other branches of electrophysiology. However, the basic principles of electrophysiology as presented in this book still seem to apply. That is, stimuli produce conductance changes, which often themselves lead to action potential generation. There seems to be two basic mechanisms responsible for the generation of action potentials in the afferent fibre leaving a sensorial receptor. In the case of receptors such as the retina and the organ of Corti, the stimulus (light or sound) causes a graded change in membrane potential (*receptor potential*) of a specialized receptor cell (cone, hair cell). As a result of this change in potential, the rate at which a chemical transmitter is released by the receptor cell changes in direct proportion to the intensity of the stimulus and thus the rate of firing of the next neuron in the afferent sensory pathway is affected. That is, the action potential is not generated directly in the receptor cell.

In another type of sensory receptor (Pacinian corpuscles, free nerve ending) a stimulus, mechanical for example, produces a local and graded depolarization (*generator potential*) that is proportional to the intensity of the applied stimulus. As a result of the depolarization there is a local flow of current which, if sufficiently large, causes action potentials to fire off in the adjacent section of the nerve membrane. Thus the graded and the action potential are generated in the same cell.

So, sensory receptors have the common property that they transduce the stimuli into graded and stationary (non-propagated) potentials. They differ because they have different physical structures and different receptors respond better to different kinds of stimuli. Moreover, the response may be either a tonic or a phasic discharge.

Tonic and phasic receptors

When the discharges are tonic, there is a maintained response (action potential generation) in the presence of a maintained stimulus. An example of a tonic receptor is the crayfish stretch receptor. When the discharges are phasic, action potentials are generated at the on and at the off of the stimulus. In the presence of a maintained stimulus the frequency of the action potentials rapidly falls. Because of this, phasic receptors are said to be *fast adapting*.

Changes in conductance in receptors

The crayfish stretch receptor is one of the few receptors which, because of its large receptor cells, can be examined by conventional electrophysiological techniques. With two microelectrodes inserted into a receptor cell it is possible to displace the membrane potential by injecting a constant current through one of the microelectrodes and simultaneously record the membrane potential with the other. Under these conditions, and for a given stretch, the change in membrane potential obtained is smaller, the higher the constant current-induced depolarization. When the membrane potential is set at zero millivolts, there is no stretch-induced potential change. This experiment can be compared with the two-microelectrode voltage-clamp experiments carried out by Takeuchi and Takeuchi on the neuromuscular junction and described above. Because the equilibrium potential for the stretched cell is zero, it seems that the generator potential for a stretch receptor is the result of a non-specific change in membrane conductance. Since the membrane potential is depolarized by stretching, there is probably an increase in the sodium conductance, but there must also be other conductance changes if the conductance change is not specific to any one ion species.

Biological transducers

Sensory receptors are also known as biological transducers, because mechanical, electromagnetic, chemical or thermal stimuli induce an electrical response which may be either a receptor potential or a generator potential.

Frequency coding

E. D. Adrian was the first to realize that coding in the sensory pathways was in the frequency of the action potentials generated in the afferent nerve. In this coding the intensity of the stimulus is related to the frequency of the action potential generation.

There are two ways in which the stimulus can modulate the frequency of action potentials in the afferent fibre. In the case of the receptor potential, the release of transmitter by the receptor cell is controlled by its membrane potential. As more transmitter is released the membrane potential in the next neuron in the sensory pathway approaches threshold so that any additional transmitter released will fire off action potentials.

In the case of the generator potential, the potential of the adjacent membrane is also displaced towards threshold. Once an action potential is fired the membrane has to go through a refractory period before it returns to threshold again. Although this mechanism, proposed by Adrian, seems plausible in the light of our present knowledge on the ionic basis of action potential generation, it has yet to be tested.

In Figure 9.14 we present a schematic overview of the concepts presented in Chapters 7, 8 and 9. E. D. Adrian's frequency coding is the link between the transduction process that takes place in receptors and the synaptic transmission and propagation that occur in the nervous system.

Fig.9.14

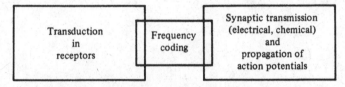

Electrical synapses

Finally, we will end this chapter by mentioning that electrical signals can be transmitted from one cell to another by means of electrical coupling and this electrical transmission is said to occur across an *electrical synapse*. Although electrical coupling between adjacent cells is possible across the extracellular fluid, generally the coupling occurs across specialized junctions that exist between cells, and these junctions are known as gap junctions.

Gap junctions

Gap junctions have been demonstrated in closely adjacent neurons and smooth muscle cells, for example, by using electron microscopy. Also, intracellular dyes have been seen to cross between these cells and it is thought that the route is via these gap junctions.

It has been suggested that in these junctions a large number of bridges occur between adjacent cell membranes, and that these bridges are repeated at intervals of about 100 Å. The bridges are about 30 Å wide and contain a central cytoplasmic core of about 10 Å diameter and are surrounded by a lipid membrane.

One way of testing for an electrical synapse is to use microelectrodes to inject current into one cell and to record the voltage from the other cell. If connections exist, current flows from one cell to another via the junctions. The resistance in these junctions to this current flow is often called the coupling resistance (R_c). When making electrical models of coupled cells the membrane capacitance at the coupling site is often ignored (this is because the opposing cell membranes are in series and so the capacitance is reduced). Because of the physical nature of these electrical synapses the transmission delays that occur when molecules diffuse across synaptic clefts in chemical synapses are absent and lack of delay is often taken as evidence for an electrical synapse.

There is some experimental evidence to suggest that some gap junctions are able to behave in a non-linear (rectifying) way and that some might be unidirectional and inhibitory.

10

Membrane noise

Introduction

In the previous chapter we showed that acetylcholine (Ach) is released in discrete packets (quanta) in an all-or-none way from the presynaptic nerve terminal. In this chapter we derive a statistical model of quantal release that occurs in synaptic transmission. Since the release of transmitter is probabilistic, the postsynaptic membrane potential *randomly* fluctuates around a mean value. These fluctuations, or membrane noise, will be analysed in some detail in the latter part of the chapter and used as an example of the way in which membrane noise can be studied more generally.

A probabilistic model of quantal release

It was seen in the last chapter that the actual number of quanta released is not an exact constant and, in fact, the number changes in a random way with every action potential that invades the nerve terminal. (The average number of released quanta per action potential depends on factors such as the calcium or the magnesium concentrations in the bathing fluid. Under normal conditions the average number of quanta released is around 1000. If the calcium is replaced by magnesium the average number of quanta released per action potential may be quite small. It is this situation that we shall be analysing.) Since the exact number of quanta released is not constant, this means that it is possible (although unlikely) that some action potentials may not release any quanta, while others will release one, or two, or more, quanta. With a small amount of calcium in the bathing fluid it is possible to *classify* the number of quanta released per action potential. Thus out of M action potentials, x_0 action potentials might release no quanta, x_1 might release one quantum, and so on. This classification is thus based upon the frequency of release of $0, 1, \ldots, n$

quanta per action potential. The frequencies $(f_0, f_1, \ldots, f_n)$ can be defined as

$$f_0 = x_0/M, \quad f_1 = x_1/M, \quad \ldots, \quad f_n = x_n/M$$

If we repeat this experiment many times, that is, when M becomes very large, $f_0, f_1, \ldots, f_n$ will approach the probabilities $P_0, P_1, \ldots, P_n$, of 0, 1, 2, $\ldots, n$ quanta being released per action potential. (The probability of an event occurring is assumed here to be the ratio of the number of events of that class $(x_0, \ldots, x_n)$ over the total number of trials (M) when the total number of trials is very large. Probability is thus a number between zero and one. The probability of a *certain* event is one and the probability of an *impossible* event is zero (see Appendix 7).)

When the bathing fluid has a high magnesium and a low calcium content the amplitude of the EPPs is reduced. A reduced EPP is due to the summation of a small number of MEPPs and, as shown in the previous chapter, each MEPP is considered to result from the discharge of one quantum of Ach from the presynaptic terminal. The amplitudes of the EPPs observed over a time period (t) can be sorted according to their frequency. The resulting experimental histogram is shown in Figure 10.1b.

Setting up the model

In an attempt to describe quantal release we can make the following model and fit a theoretical histogram to the experimental one. If the theoretical model fits the experimental data we can then assume that the model is a reasonable one. In this model of an idealized nerve–muscle junction (see Figure 10.1d), we make the following assumptions:

(1) The synapse contains a large number (N) of vesicles.
(2) Each action potential releases $0, 1, 2, \ldots, x, \ldots$ of these vesicles (quanta) during a period of observation t, following an action potential (which we shall assume to be of very short duration relative to the duration of the release process). Thus at $t = 0$ the action potential sets the release process in motion. This release process may go on after time t.
(3) For a large number of action potentials (M) we obtain the following classes of events:

n_0 = number of occasions where action potentials do not release any quanta,

n_1 = number of occasions where action potentials release one quantum,

$\vdots$

n_x = number of occasions when action potentials release x quanta.

Fig.10.1

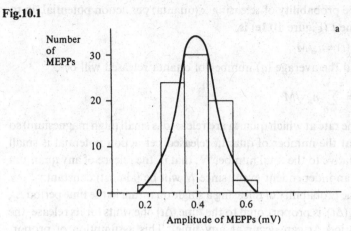

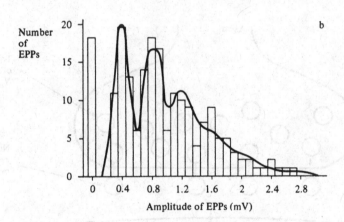

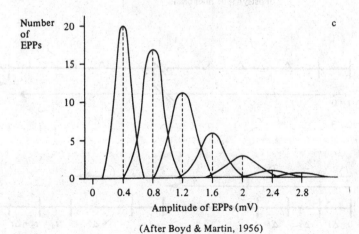

(After Boyd & Martin, 1956)

(4) The probability of releasing x (quanta) per action potential up to time t (Figure 10.1e) is:

$P_x(t) = n_x/M$

and the average (q) number of quanta released will be

$$q = \sum_{x=0}^{x=\infty} n_x x/M$$

(5) The rate at which quanta are released is small (high magnesium) so that the number of quanta released per action potential is small relative to the total number N; that is, the release of any quantum is an independent event since N will be (almost) constant.

(6) The probability of releasing a single quantum in the time period Δt, $P_1(\Delta t)$, is proportional to the time (Δt) one waits for its release (the period Δt can occur at any time). This assumption of propor-

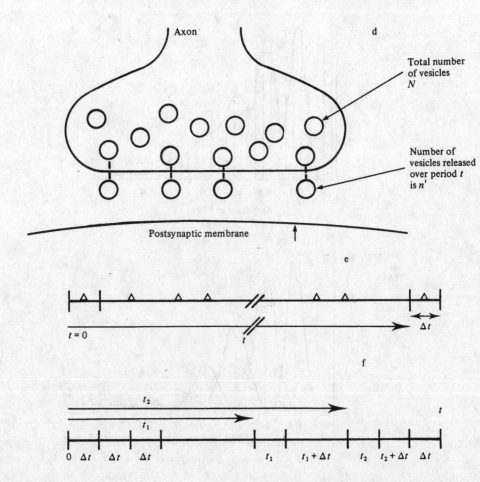

tionality is an important one and not really unreasonable. Mathematically we write this as

$$P_1(\Delta t) \propto \Delta t$$

or

$$P_1(\Delta t) = \alpha_r \Delta t \tag{10.1}$$

where α_r is the proportionality constant. From (10.1) we see that α_r must have the dimensions of probability per unit time since the two sides of the equation have to balance dimensionally.

The probability of *no* quanta being released during Δt ($P_0(\Delta t)$) is given by

$$P_0(\Delta t) = 1 - P_1(\Delta t) = 1 - \alpha_r \Delta t \tag{10.2}$$

This is so because *only* one of two events can occur during time Δt. Either one quantum is released or no quantum is released.

We can also say that the probability of more than one quantum being released during the period of time Δt ($P_x(\Delta t)$) is zero, or

$$P_x(\Delta t) = 0 \tag{10.3}$$

for $x > 1$.

The release of x quanta during a time period of observation $(t + \Delta t)$ (Figure 10.1e) may be the outcome of two events: x quanta may be released during a period of time t and *no* quantum released in the following Δt, or $x - 1$ quanta may be released during time t and *one* quantum released in the following Δt. In the first case we have to compute the *joint probability* of two events which are *independent* of one another; that is, the release of one quantum does *not* affect (is independent of) the release of another quantum (this is because the number of quanta released is a very small fraction of the total number of quanta available for release). From Appendix 7, the laws of probability (multiplication rule) allow us to write

$$P_x^{(1)}(t + \Delta t) = P_x(t)(1 - \alpha_r \Delta t) \tag{10.4}$$

Probability of x quanta being released up to time t. First case. Probability of zero quanta being released in the next Δt. ($P_0(\Delta t)$).

In the second case, from similar reasoning, we write

$$P_x^{(2)}(t + \Delta t) = P_{x-1}(t)\alpha_r \Delta t \tag{10.5}$$

Probability of x − 1 quanta being released up to time t. Second case. Probability of one quantum being released in the next Δt. ($P_1(\Delta t)$).

Note. We have assumed that both ways of producing the release of x quanta of Ach, during a period $(t + \Delta t)$ (equations (10.4) and (10.5)), are mutually exclusive. Since both lead to the same event, the probability of the event occurring (that is, of x quanta being released up to $t + \Delta t$) is the *sum* of the probabilities given by equations (10.4) and (10.5). So (from Appendix 7) we write

$$P_x(t + \Delta t) = P_x(t)(1 - \alpha_r \, \Delta t) + P_{x-1}(t)\alpha_r \, \Delta t$$
$$= P_x^{(1)}(t + \Delta t) + P_x^{(2)}(t + \Delta t) \tag{10.6}$$

Equation (10.6) can be rearranged as

$$P_x(t + \Delta t) = P_x(t) - \alpha_r \, \Delta t P_x(t) + P_{x-1}(t)\alpha_r \, \Delta t$$

or

$$(P_x(t + \Delta t) - P_x(t))/\Delta t = -\alpha_r(P_x(t) - P_{x-1}(t)) \tag{10.7}$$

For small Δt, equation (10.7) becomes a differential equation in $P_x(t)$, that is,

$$(d/dt)(P_x(t)) = -\alpha_r(P_x(t) - P_{x-1}(t))$$

or

$$(d/dt)(P_x(t)) + \alpha_r P_x(t) = \alpha_r P_{x-1}(t) \tag{10.8}$$

Analytical solution of the model

Equation (10.8) has to be solved for the different values of x. For $x = 0$ and, since we are considering quanta released for $t \geqslant 0$, then $P_{-1}(t) = 0$.
Equation (10.8) reduces to

$$(d/dt)(P_0(t)) + \alpha_r \, P_0(t) = 0 \tag{10.9}$$

Equation (10.9) can be integrated using the integrating factor (see Appendix 10)

$$\exp\left(\int \alpha_r \, dt \right) = \exp(\alpha_r t)$$

so

$$\exp(-\alpha_r t)(d/dt)(\exp(\alpha_r t)P_0(t)) = 0$$

or

$$(d/dt)(exp(\alpha_r t)P_0(t)) = 0$$

or

$$\exp(\alpha_r t)P_0(t) = C$$

where C is an integration constant. At $t = 0$

$$P_0(0) = C$$

But the probability of no event taking place at time 0 is a certainty and thus equal to one, so

$$C = 1$$

The solution of (10.9) is thus (dividing through by $\exp(\alpha_r t)$)

$$P_0(t) = \exp(-\alpha_r t) \tag{10.10}$$

For $n=1$, substituting in (10.8) and using (10.10),

$$(d/dt)(P_1(t))+\alpha_r P_1(t)=\alpha_r P_0(t)=\alpha_r \exp(-\alpha_r t) \tag{10.11}$$

the integrating factor of equation (10.11) is again

$$\exp(\alpha_r t)$$

so

$$\exp(-\alpha_r t)(d/dt)(\exp(\alpha_r t)P_1(t))=\alpha_r \exp(-\alpha_r t)$$

or

$$(d/dt)(\exp(\alpha_r t)P_1(t))=\alpha_r$$

which on integration gives

$$\exp(\alpha_r t)P_1(t)=\alpha_r t+C \tag{10.12}$$

At $t=0$

$$P_1(0)=C$$

But it is impossible for a quantum to be released exactly at time zero, so the probability of one event (or x events for $x \neq 0$) taking place at time zero is zero, so

$$C=0$$

and

$$P_1(t)=\alpha_r t \exp(-\alpha_r t) \tag{10.13}$$

If we go through the same procedure for $x=2$ we obtain

$$\exp(-\alpha_r t)(d/dt)(\exp(\alpha_r t)P_2(t))=\alpha_r P_1(t)=\alpha_r^2 t \exp(-\alpha_r t)$$

or

$$(d/dt)(\exp(\alpha_r t)P_2(t))=\alpha_r^2 t$$

On integration

$$\exp(\alpha_r t)P_2(t)=(\alpha_r t)^2/2+C$$

but since, from the above reasoning,

$$P_2(0)=0$$

then

$$C=0$$

and

$$P_2(t)=((\alpha_r t)^2/2)\exp(-\alpha_r t)$$

If we continue the integration for $x=3$ we obtain

$$(d/dt)(\exp(\alpha_r t)P_3(t))=(\alpha_r^3 t^2)/2!$$

which on integration gives

$$\exp(\alpha_r t)P_3(t)=(\alpha_r^3 t^3)/3!$$

For $x=4$

$$\exp(\alpha_r t)P_4(t)=(\alpha_r^4 t^4)/4!$$

and so on, until we can write the general expression

$$P_x(t)=((\alpha_r t)^x/x!)\exp(-\alpha_r t) \tag{10.14}$$

where $x!$ is $(x(x-1)(x-2)\ldots 1)$.

Since α_r is the probability of releasing one quantum in the time period Δt, per unit time, and as we are dealing with independent events, the probability of releasing one quantum between, for instance, t_1 and $t_1 + \Delta t$, is independent of the probability of releasing one quantum between t_2 and $t_2 + \Delta t$ (Figure 10.1f). Over a period of time, which can be thought of as the sum of L successive Δt intervals (Figure 10.1f), the average number of quanta released (q) will be

$$q = P_1(\Delta t_1) + P_1(\Delta t_2) + \cdots + P_1(\Delta t_L)$$

$$= \sum_{i=1}^{i=L} P_1(\Delta t_i)$$

But

$$P_1(\Delta t_1) = P_1(\Delta t_2) = \cdots = P_1(\Delta t_L)$$

so

$$q = LP_1(\Delta t)$$

If $\Delta t_1 = \Delta t_2 = \cdots = \Delta t_L = \Delta t$ then $t/\Delta t = L$ and $q = (t/\Delta t)P_1(\Delta t) = tP_1(\Delta t)/\Delta t$. But from equation (10.1)

$$P_1(\Delta t)/\Delta t = \alpha_r$$

so

$$q = t\alpha_r$$

($\alpha_r = q/t =$ average number of quanta released during
time t/t

$=$ average rate of release of quanta)

then equation (10.14) becomes

$$P_x(q^x/x!) \exp(-q) \tag{10.15}$$

Amplitude distribution of the MEPPs

As pointed out in Chapter 9, expression (10.15) is the Poisson distribution. However, this distribution cannot be *directly* applied to the experimental results because the amplitudes of MEPPs, which are the unit events, are not always constant. It was also shown in Chapter 9 that the MEPPs amplitudes distribute themselves in the way shown in Figure 10.1a. The smooth curve fitted through the histogram is a normal distribution. The normal distribution is described by the curve

$$P(v) = (1/(2\pi\sigma^2)^{1/2}) \exp(-((v - \bar{u})/(v\sigma))^2)$$

where $P(v)$ is the probability of obtaining a MEPP of amplitude v, $\bar{u}$ is the mean value of all the amplitudes (0.4 mV) and σ the standard deviation of the MEPPs. The choice of fitting a normal distribution through the histogram is purely arbitrary, except that it seems to be a good fit to the experimental data.

Since quantal release is an independent event when two quanta are released we should expect the amplitude of the corresponding EPP to be, on average, double the average amplitude of a MEPP. As we are dealing with independent events, this means that we should also expect the variance of the amplitude to be double the variance of the MEPP amplitudes. Because of this we should be able to scale up any curves fitted through any amplitude distribution curves. To do this we scale up $\bar{u}$ and σ^2 in the normal distribution curve.

In order to compute the continuous line of Figure 10.1b the different classes (corresponding to the release of one, two, ..., x, quanta) are first computed from the Poisson distribution. Each class, corresponding to the release of x quanta, is then distributed according to a normal distribution of mean $x\bar{u}$ and variance xs^2_{MEPP}, where $\bar{u}$ is the average amplitude of a MEPP and s^2_{MEPP} is the variance of the MEPP amplitudes. All the curves obtained in this way (Figure 10.1c) are then summed to give a continuous distribution. Figure 10.1b shows that the continuous (theoretical) distribution is a good fit to the experimental data. We can thus conclude that the quantal release of Ach follows a Poisson distribution, which means that the initial assumptions we made when we set up the model were reasonable. When the average rate of release (α_r) is very high a better description is provided by a normal distribution (see Appendix 7 on Binomial versus Poisson distribution). With the Poisson distribution it is possible to predict the frequency of failures ($n = 0$). From equation (10.10),

$$P_0(t) = \exp(-\alpha_r t) \tag{10.10}$$

But $\alpha_r t$ is the mean number of quanta released (q) over the period t. By dividing the mean amplitude of the EPPs ($\bar{V}_{\text{EPP}}$) by the mean amplitude of the MEPPs ($\bar{v}$), q can be estimated experimentally, so that

$$q = \bar{V}_{\text{EPP}}/\bar{v} = \alpha_r t \tag{10.16}$$

If the Poisson distribution applies the P_0 obtained from equations (10.10) and (10.16) should be the same as the frequency of failures in quantal release. It was shown by Castillo and Katz that this was the case, and this is taken as further proof that quantal release is a random process well described by the Poisson distribution.

Postsynaptic membrane noise

Since quantal release is a statistical event an implication of this is that there should be detectable fluctuations of the postsynaptic membrane potentials. These fluctuations should represent the random interaction of molecules of Ach with the receptor sites in the postsynaptic membrane. Katz and Miledi observed these phenomena when they applied acetylcholine continuously to the postsynaptic membrane from a micropipette. The Ach caused steady depolarization and increased voltage noise. The amplitude of the depolarization depended upon the Ach concentration and was of the order of millivolts. The noise consisted of fluctuations around the mean value of the membrane potential. These fluctuations were in the microvolt range and should *not* be confused with MEPPs which are the summation of thousands of microscopic potential transients, each of them resulting from the interaction of one or two molecules of Ach with the postsynaptic receptor.

Figure 10.2a is a schematic description of an experiment to record voltage noise. The upper trace shows the membrane potential recorded through a high-gain amplifier in the absence of Ach and an MEPP can be observed as a large upward deflection of the trace. The lower trace shows the membrane potential in the presence of Ach and also shows an MEPP. In both cases, on top of steady membrane potential (d.c. level) there are minute fluctuations of potential which are much larger in the presence of the transmitter. These fluctuations are known as Ach voltage noise, and Katz and Miledi found that this noise associated with the local application of Ach could not be reproduced by other means (such as local current injections). Later, we will show that it is possible to describe noise quantitatively and that the noise produced by Ach is different from that produced by other analogues. As noise results from the opening and closing of conducting channels it must reflect the kinetic properties of these channels, so noise analysis should thus provide some insight into the mechanisms of ion conductance changes at molecular level.

Measurement of synaptic noise

One of the simplest ways of measuring noise is to measure its peak-to-peak amplitude (see Figure 10.2b) because this amplitude increases with increasing amounts of drug–receptor interaction. However, when we use peak-to-peak values we are taking measurements only at the peaks and missing out the rest of the record. If we want to take into account the whole record, the simplest measurement we can obtain is the variance (s^2) of the noise. (Variance is defined in Appendix 7.)

Variance and time average of a time signal

The variance of any quantity which varies with time (time signal) is

$$s^2 = \frac{1}{T} \int_0^T (f(t) - \bar{f})^2 \, dt \tag{10.17}$$

where $f(t)$ is the value of the signal at any time (t), $\bar{f}$ is the *average value* of the signal $f(t)$ (time average) and is defined as

$$\bar{f} = \frac{1}{T} \int_0^T f(t)\, dt \qquad (10.18)$$

where T is the duration of the record.

In order to understand why equation (10.18) is the signal average we can

Fig.10.2

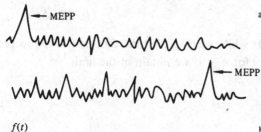

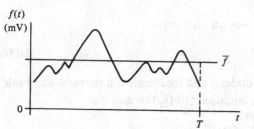

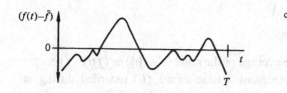

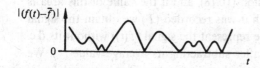

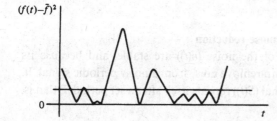

think of a time signal as being made up of rectangles of width Δt and height $f(t)$. If, for example, the average height of this population of rectangles is given by

$$(f_1 + f_2 + f_3 + f_4 + f_5 + f_6 + \cdots + f_{12})/12$$

and if we multiply top and bottom by Δt we obtain

$$(f_1 \, \Delta t + f_2 \, \Delta t + f_3 \, \Delta t + \cdots + f_{12} \, \Delta t)/12 \, \Delta t = \sum_{i=1}^{12} (f_i \Delta t)/12 \, \Delta t$$

$$= \sum_{i=1}^{n} (f_i \, \Delta t)/n \, \Delta t$$

If we reduce the width Δt while keeping the total duration of the record $(n \, \Delta t)$ constant, as $\Delta t \to 0$ for $n \to \infty$ we obtain in the limit

$$\int_0^T (f(t) \, \mathrm{d}t)/T = \bar{f}$$

since $n \, \Delta t = T$.

From equation (10.18) we can also write

$$\bar{f}T = \int_0^T f(t) \, \mathrm{d}t \qquad (10.18a)$$

Since $\bar{f}T$ is the total area under $\bar{f}$ and the integral on the right-hand side is the total area under $f(t)$, equation (10.18a) means that

$$\bar{f}T = \int_0^T \bar{f} \, \mathrm{d}t = \int_0^T f(t) \, \mathrm{d}t$$

so

$$\int_0^T (\bar{f} - f(t)) \, \mathrm{d}t = 0$$

This means that the time average of the noise $(\bar{f} - f(t))$ or $(f(t) - \bar{f})$ is zero.

In Figure 10.2b we represent a time signal $f(t)$ recorded during an interval of time 0 to T. The area under the curve is, by definition, the value of the definite integral in expression (10.18), and if the value of this area is divided by the time over which it was recorded (T) we obtain the signal average $(\bar{f})$. In Figure 10.2c we represent the signal $(f(t))$ without its d.c. component $(f(t) - \bar{f})$, that is, after subtracting its average value $(\bar{f})$. We shall call this signal $(n(t) = f(t) - \bar{f})$ the noise of $f(t)$. The average value of the noise $(n(t))$ is zero.

Signal averaging, noise reduction

If the properties of the noise $(n(t))$ are stable, and because its average value is zero, we can remove noise from a noisy periodic signal. If, for example, a periodic signal $(S(t))$ repeats itself after a set period T, that is,

$$S(t) = S(t + kT)$$

where k can be $0, 1, \ldots, k$, the *noisy* signal, which we shall call $f(t)$, is thus

$$f(t) = S(t + kT) + n(t)$$

If we repeatedly sum consecutive records, each of duration T, we obtain Z so that

$$Z = S(t) + n(t) + S(t+T) + n(t) + S(t+2T) + n(t) + \cdots + S(t+NT) + n(t)$$

since $S(t) \equiv S(t + NT)$, then

$$Z = \sum_1^N S(t) + \sum_1^N n(t) = NS(t) + \sum_1^N n(t)$$

If we now calculate the average

$$(NS(t))/N + \underbrace{\sum n(t)/N}_{\text{is zero}} = S(t) = Z$$

since the average of $n(t)$ is zero. This is the basis of signal averaging.

Analysis of noise

However, although useful for signal averaging, as the average value of the noise $(n(t))$ is zero we square $n(t)$ if we wish to analyse noise, so that the whole record now has positive value. We can think of the squaring procedure in two steps. In the first step (Figure 10.2d) the absolute value of the noise $(|n(t)|)$ is computed. Then the resulting signal is squared (Figure 10.2e). It would be possible to use the absolute value of the signal; however, for mathematical convenience, we use the squared signal. The variance (s^2) given by equation (10.17) is the area under the $n(t)^2$ curve divided by the record duration (T).

Relationship between postsynaptic membrane noise and postsynaptic membrane depolarization

Since the postsynaptic membrane depolarization is due to the Ach–receptor interaction, the larger the depolarization the greater the number of receptors activated and the larger the membrane voltage noise. This is represented in the following sequence of steps

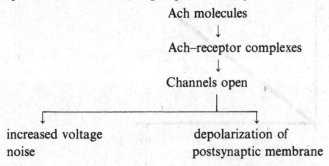

The relationship between postsynaptic membrane noise and postsynaptic membrane depolarization was shown by Katz and Miledi and is represented schematically in Figure 10.3.

Relationship between synaptic noise and the molecular events of synaptic transmission

In order to relate the variance (s^2) to the molecular events responsible for the noise we need to postulate a model for the molecular events. With this model we shall derive an analytical expression which relates some property of the noise, its variance for example, with the underlying molecular mechanism. The analysis is based upon that given by Katz and Miledi, who assumed that the potential transient 'blip' ($b(t)$), associated with the Ach–receptor reaction, was a scaled-down version of an MEPP. That is,

$$b(t) = a \exp(-t/\tau)$$

where τ is the time constant of the decay of the microscopic voltage signal (see Figure 10.4a). These blips ($b(t)$) are produced at an average frequency of Z per second and are spaced apart in time on the average $1/Z$ seconds ($\bar{\theta}$) (see Figure 10.4b). If the average time between the onset of consecutive blips ($\bar{\theta}$) is much larger than the time constant of the decay (τ) this means that each blip will effectively decay to zero before the next one appears. The train of blips is a *time signal* described by the expression

$$B(t) = \sum_{i=1}^{n} b(t_i)$$

Fig.10.3

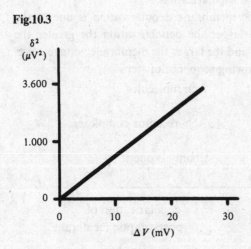

where $t_i = -(t - \theta_i)$, and t_i does not exist for $t_i < t$. So

$$B(t) = b(t_0) + b(t_1) + b(t_2) + \cdots + b(t_i) \ldots \qquad (10.19)$$

1st blip   2nd blip   3rd blip ... ith blip ...

where t_i is given by the expression

$$t_i = t - (\theta_1 + \theta_2 + \theta_3 + \cdots + \theta_i) \qquad (10.19a)$$

t is the lapsed time from zero time, t_i is some elapsed time from the onset of each blip (i) and θ_i is the time between the onsets of blips $i-1$ and i.

Expressions (10.19) and (10.19a) mean that the time signal $B(t)$ is the sum of i blips displaced in time. That is, as the first blip does not exist for $t < 0$, the second blip only appears for $t \geqslant \theta_1$ and so on; in general we say that

$$t_i \geqslant \theta_i$$

The time average $\bar{V}$ of the time signal (10.19) is then given by

$$\bar{V} = \frac{1}{T} \int_0^T B(t)\, \mathrm{d}t$$

or

$$\bar{V} = \frac{1}{T} \int_0^T (b(t_1) + b(t_2) + \cdots + b(t_i))\, \mathrm{d}t \qquad (10.19b)$$

If we substitute (10.19a) into (10.19b) we obtain

$$\bar{V} = \frac{1}{T} \int_0^T (b(t) + b(t - \theta_1) + b(t - (\theta_1 + \theta_2)) + \cdots)\, \mathrm{d}t$$

or

$$\bar{V} = \frac{1}{T} \left(\int_0^T b(t)\, \mathrm{d}t + \int_0^T b(t - \theta_1)\, \mathrm{d}t + \int_0^T b(t - (\theta_1 - \theta_2))\, \mathrm{d}t + \cdots \right)$$

$$(10.20)$$

Since all the blips have the same waveform they must also have the same

Fig.10.4

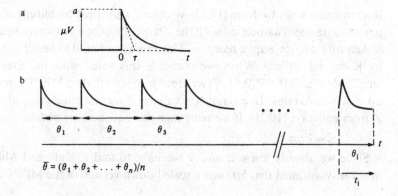

area; that is, their integrals are equal ($a\tau$), so

$$\int_0^T b(t)\,\mathrm{d}t = \int_0^T b(t-\theta_1)\,\mathrm{d}t = \cdots$$

The proof that the area under the function $b(t_i)$ is the same for all blips is obtained as follows:

The integral of $b(t)$ is

$$\int_0^T b(t)\,\mathrm{d}t = \int_0^T a\exp(-t/\tau)\,\mathrm{d}t = a\int_0^T \exp(-t/\tau)\,\mathrm{d}t$$
$$= a\tau[\exp(-t/\tau)]_0^T$$
$$= -a\tau[\exp(-T/\tau)-1]$$

Since $T\gg\tau$

$$\exp(-T/\tau)\approx 0$$

so

$$\int_0^T b(t)\,\mathrm{d}t = a\tau$$

Expression (10.20) becomes

$$\bar{V}=\frac{i}{T}\int_0^T b(t)\,\mathrm{d}t$$

where i is the number of blips during the period of time T. Then i/T is the average frequency of the blips (Z) so

$$\bar{V}=Z\int_0^T b(t)\,\mathrm{d}t = Za\tau \qquad (10.21)$$

By similar reasoning the variance (s^2) of $B(t)$ is

$$s^2 = Z\int_0^T b(t)^2\,\mathrm{d}t = (Za^2\tau)/2 \qquad (10.22)$$

If we substitute (10.21) into (10.22) we obtain

$$s^2 = \bar{V}a/2 \qquad (10.23)$$

If we measure s^2 and $\bar{V}$ from (10.23) we obtain a, the peak amplitude of the potential transient associated with the interaction of one or two molecules of Ach with a postsynaptic receptor. This value was found to be 0.2–0.5 μV by Katz and Miledi. When we compare this value with the average amplitude of an MEPP (0.4 mV) we are able to infer that an MEPP is made up of 800–2000 blips. To estimate the value of Z we first obtain the value of Z from equation (10.21). If we rearrange this equation we obtain

$$Z = \bar{V}/a\tau$$

Since we already know a and $\bar{V}$ we have to find τ. Katz and Miledi arbitrarily assumed that $b(t)$ was a scaled-down version of the MEPP and the value of τ for $b(t)$ was taken to be the same value (10 ms) as the time constant of decay of the MEPP.

For an Ach-induced depolarization ($\bar{V}$) of 10 mV, and assuming an average value for a of 0.35 μV, the value of Z is

$$Z = \bar{V}/a\tau = \frac{10^{-2}\ \text{V}}{3.5 \times 10^{-7} \times \text{V}\,10^{-2}\ \text{s}} \simeq 3 \times 10^{6}\ \text{s}^{-1}$$

Thus 3×10^{6} blips per second cause a depolarization ($\bar{V}$) of 10 mV.

Model dependency of the analysis

This analysis allows us to obtain the amplitude (a) and the frequency (Z) of the blips. However, it was necessary to postulate a waveform with two unknown characteristics a and τ. Thus the information obtained by this analysis is *dependent* upon the information we supplied, that is, the analysis is *model* dependent.

A model encoding the receptor–transmitter interaction

To have an improved description of the noise structure we need to analyse a more complex model proposed by Anderson and Stevens. This model was introduced in Chapter 9 and is now reproduced here

$$n\text{T} + \text{R} \underset{k_{-1}}{\overset{k_1}{\rightleftharpoons}} \text{RT}_c^n \underset{\alpha}{\overset{\beta}{\rightleftharpoons}} \text{RT}_o^n \tag{10.24}$$

where T is the transmitter (Ach), n the number of molecules of transmitter that react with a postsynaptic receptor and R is a postsynaptic receptor. RT_c^n and RT_o^n are transmitter–receptor complexes in their closed and open states respectively. Although noise results from the flipping backwards and forward of the following reaction,

$$\text{RT}_c^n \underset{\alpha}{\overset{\beta}{\rightleftharpoons}} \text{RT}_o^n \tag{10.24a}$$

An expression for the concentration of transmitter–receptor complex

The structure of the noise will be dependent on the overall kinetic scheme shown in (10.24). The first step in the derivation is to obtain an expression for the amount of the transmitter–receptor complex. If the rate constants of the transmitter–receptor association and dissociation (k_1 and k_{-1}) are very large when compared with α and β, the amount of transmitter–receptor complex will depend upon the transmitter concentration. This is because the concentration of RT_c^n will be in equilibrium with the concentrations of T and R. Since R is fixed, the concentration of RT_c^n will be a function of the concentration of T only when this concentration is small (that is, when most receptor sites are unbound). The rate of formation of the transmitter–receptor complex (RT_c^n) is the result of the balance between two processes: the association–dissociation of the complex itself (RT_c^n) and the interconversion between the closed (RT_c^n) and the open (RT_o^n) forms of the complex. The first process is described by two velocities given by the equations

$$v_1 = k_1[T]^n[R] \quad \text{and} \quad v_{-1} = k_{-1}[RT_c^n] \tag{10.24b}$$

The second process is also described by two similar equations, that is,

$$v_\beta = \beta[RT_c^n] \quad \text{and} \quad v_\alpha = \alpha[RT_o^n] \tag{10.24c}$$

The rate of formation $(d/dt)([RT_c^n])$ of the complex RT_c^n is then given by

$$(d/dt)([RT_c^n]) = v_1 - v_{-1} - v_\beta + v_\alpha$$

so

$$(d/dt)([RT_c^n]) = k_1[T]^n[R] - k_{-1}[RT_c^n] - \beta[RT_c^n] + \alpha[RT_o^n]$$

Rate of formation of complex from T and R	Rate of dissociation of complex	Rate of conversion of closed into open complex	Rate of conversion of open into closed complex

At steady state, when all the concentrations are constant

$$(d/dt)([RT_c^n]) = 0$$

so

$$0 = k_1[T]^n[R] - (k_{-1} + \beta)[RT_c^n] + \alpha[RT_o^n] \tag{10.25}$$

Since in our original model it was assumed that $k_1 \gg \alpha$ and $k_{-1} \gg \beta$, equation (10.25) then simplifies to

$$0 = k_1[T]^n[R] - k_{-1}[RT_c^n]$$

or

$$k_{-1}[RT_c^n] = k_1[T]^n[R] \tag{10.26}$$

Dividing both sides of equation (10.26) by k_{-1} and $[R]$ we obtain

$$[RT_c^n]/[R] = (k_1/k_{-1})[T]^n \tag{10.27}$$

The total concentrations of receptors $[R_t]$ is given by

$$[R_t] = [R] + [RT_c^n] + [RT_o^n] \tag{10.28}$$

Since it was assumed that the transmitter concentration is very low the concentration of receptor–transmitter complex is also very low, so

$$[R] > ([RT_c^n] + [RT_o^n])$$

and equation (10.28) becomes

$$[R_t] \approx [R] \tag{10.29}$$

If we substitute (10.29) into (10.27) we obtain

$$[RT_c^n]/[R_t] = (k_1/k_{-1})[T]^n = K[T]^n \tag{10.30}$$

This means that the fraction of the receptor complexed is proportional to (and thus depends on) $[T]^n$ and K, where K is the *binding* or *association* constant. We shall now consider the kinetics of the flipping of the transmitter–receptor complex between the closed and the open states.

Probabilities of the closing and opening of the transmitter–receptor complex

An analysis based on the assumption which led to equation (10.30) allows us to use the simplified kinetic scheme that was described in (10.24a) to describe the noise structure. Since the flipping described by this equation is a random process we have to use probability theory in our kinetic analysis. If we select a time interval (Δt) short enough so that only one channel can be either closed or open, it is not an unreasonable assumption that the probability of closing one channel during Δt $(P_c(\Delta t))$ is given by

$$P_{1,c}(\Delta t) = \alpha \, \Delta t$$

or, more simply,

$$P_c(\Delta t) = \alpha \, \Delta t \qquad (10.31)$$

where α is the average rate of conversion of open into closed channels. This analysis is identical to that previously given in our derivation of the statistics of quantal release.

In equation (10.31) we assume that any one open channel can be closed and that the closing of this channel is an independent event. Expression (10.31) means that for a small Δt, the larger its duration the greater is the probability of closing a single channel; α is the fraction of the open channels that close per unit time, and has the dimensions of t^{-1}. So $\alpha \, \Delta t$ is the probability of one channel closing during time Δt.

By a similar argument the probability of opening a single closed channel during the time interval Δt is given by

$$P_o(\Delta t) = (\beta[RT_c^n]/[R_t]) \, \Delta t \qquad (10.32)$$

where $[RT_c^n]/[R_t]$ is the fraction of the receptor concentration $[R_t]$ which is complexed and can thus be opened. Since it is a ratio between two concentrations it is a dimensionless quantity. If we substitute (10.30) into (10.32) we obtain

$$P_o(\Delta t) = \beta K[T]^n \, \Delta t \qquad (10.33)$$

The probability of the channel being open at time t is by definition $P_o(t)$.

From (10.33) the probability of *not* opening the channel $(\bar{P}_o(\Delta t))$ during a period of time Δt is then

$$\bar{P}_o(\Delta t) = 1 - P_o(\Delta t) = 1 - \beta K^n[T]^n \, \Delta t \qquad (10.34)$$

(This is because the probability of either opening *or not* opening the channel is unity. So $P_o(\Delta t) + \bar{P}_o(\Delta t) = 1$.)

Similarly the probability of not closing the channel during a period of time Δt $(\bar{P}_c(\Delta t))$ is given by

$$\bar{P}_c(\Delta t) = 1 - P_c(\Delta t) \tag{10.35}$$

If we substitute (10.31) into (10.35) we obtain

$$\bar{P}_c(\Delta t) = 1 - \alpha \, \Delta t \tag{10.36}$$

The opening of a given channel over a period of $t + \Delta t$ can be achieved in two ways. By the channel being open at time t and not closing in the following Δt, or by the channel being closed at time t and then opening in the next Δt. So we can write

$$\underbrace{P_o(t+\Delta t)}_{\substack{\text{Probability}\\\text{of the}\\\text{channel}\\\text{being open}\\\text{at time}\\ t+\Delta t}} = \underbrace{P_o(t)}_{\substack{\text{Probability}\\\text{of the}\\\text{channel}\\\text{being open}\\\text{at time } t}} \times \underbrace{(1-\alpha\,\Delta t)}_{\substack{\text{Probability}\\\text{of the}\\\text{channel}\\\textit{not}\text{ closing}\\\text{in the}\\\text{next }\Delta t\\(\bar{P}_c(\Delta t))}} + \underbrace{(1-P_o(t))}_{\substack{\text{Probability}\\\text{of the}\\\text{channel}\\\textit{not}\text{ being}\\\text{open at}\\\text{time } t\\(\bar{P}_o(t))}} \times \underbrace{(K[\text{T}]^n\beta\,\Delta t)}_{\substack{\text{Probability}\\\text{of the}\\\text{channel}\\\text{opening}\\\text{during the}\\\text{following}\\\Delta t\,(P_o(\Delta t))}} \tag{10.37}$$

Joint probability of the two events $(P_o(t)$ and $\bar{P}_c(\Delta t))$ Joint probability of the two events $(\bar{P}_o(t)$ and $P_o(\Delta t))$

If we rearrange equation (10.37) we obtain

$$P_o(t+\Delta t) = P_o(t) - \Delta t\{(\alpha + K[\text{T}]^n\beta)P_o(t) + K[\text{T}]^n\beta\}$$

or $\quad (P_o(t+\Delta t) - P_o(t))/\Delta t = -(\alpha + K[\text{T}]^n\beta)P_o(t) + K[\text{T}]^n\beta \tag{10.38}$

As Δt is very small, equation (10.38) becomes

$$(d/dt)(P_o(t)) = -(\alpha + K[\text{T}]^n\beta)P_o(t) + K[\text{T}]^n\beta \tag{10.39}$$

Since one of our assumptions is that only a small number of channels (of the total number of channels) are open at any one instant of time, from (10.24b, c) we can write for the steady-state

$$v_1 = v_{-1} \quad \text{and} \quad v_\beta = v_\alpha$$

that is

$$k_1[\text{T}]^n[\text{R}] = k_{-1}[\text{RT}_c^n] \quad \text{and} \quad \beta[\text{RT}_c^n] = \alpha[\text{RT}_o^n]$$

From (10.29) $[\text{R}_t] \approx [\text{R}]$ and since $K = k_1/k_{-1}$ we can write

$$K[\text{T}]^n[\text{R}_t] = [\text{RT}_c^n]$$

or

$$K = [\text{RT}_c^n]/([\text{T}]^n[\text{R}_t])$$

and

$$\alpha = \beta[\text{RT}_c^n]/[\text{RT}_o^n]$$

so

$$K[T]^n \beta = ([RT_c^n]/([T]^n[R_t]))[T]^n \beta = ([RT_c^n]/[R_t])\beta$$

Since for very small [T],

$$[R_t] \gg [RT_c^n]$$

then

$$\alpha \gg K[T]^n \beta \tag{10.40}$$

Relation (10.40) implies that

$$\alpha + K[T]^n \beta \approx \alpha \tag{10.41}$$

If we substitute (10.41) into (10.39) we obtain

$$(d/dt)(P_o(t)) = -\alpha P_o(t) + K[T]^n \beta \tag{10.42}$$

If we rearrange (10.42) we obtain

$$(d/dt)(P_o(t)) + \alpha P_o(t) = K[T]^n \beta \tag{10.43}$$

Equation (10.43) can be integrated by using the integrating factor (see Appendix 10)

$$\exp\left(\int \alpha \, dt\right) = \exp(\alpha t) \tag{10.44}$$

so

$$\exp(-\alpha t)(d/dt)[P_o(t)\exp(\alpha t)] = K[T]^n \beta$$

or

$$(d/dt)[P_o(t)\exp(\alpha t)] = K\beta[T]^n \exp(\alpha t) \tag{10.45}$$

The integration of (10.45) is then

$$\int (d/dt)[P_o(t)\exp(\alpha t)] \, dt = K\beta \int [T]^n \exp(\alpha t) \, dt + C \tag{10.46}$$

where C is the constant of integration. So

$$P_o(t)\exp(\alpha t) = K\beta \int [T]^n \exp(\alpha t) \, dt + C \tag{10.47}$$

The concentration of transmitter as a delta function

In order to integrate (10.47) we need to know the value of $[T]^n$ as a function of t. In Chapter 9 we showed that the release of transmitter and the diffusion across the cleft are fast, so that $[T]^n$ can be treated as a very short pulse which can be approximated by a delta function (see Appendix 14) of strength $[T]^{n'}$. That is

$$[T]^n \approx [T]^{n'} \delta(t)$$

In Figure 10.5 we show that the function to be integrated (10.5c) is the product of an exponential (10.5a) and a delta function centred at zero time and of strength $[T]^n$ (10.5b). Since the integral of an impulse function of strength A is just A

$$\int [T]^n \exp(\alpha t) \, dt = [T]^{n'}$$

Equation (10.47) becomes
$$P_o(t) \exp(\alpha t) = K\beta[T]^{n'} + C$$
At $t = 0$, $P_o(0) = 0$ and $[T]^{n'} = 0$, so
$$C = 0$$

The solution
The final solution is thus
$$P_o(t) = K\beta[T]^{n'} \exp(-\alpha t) \qquad (10.48)$$

Fluctuations of conductance at the end-plate region
In (10.48) $P_o(t)$ is the probability of the channel being *open* at time t. The conductance changes at the end-plate region are due to the opening of channels. Equation (10.48) describes the probability of the channel being open. So in order to calculate the average end-plate conductance $g(t)$ we multiply $P_o(t)$ by the total number of available channels (N) and by the

Fig.10.5

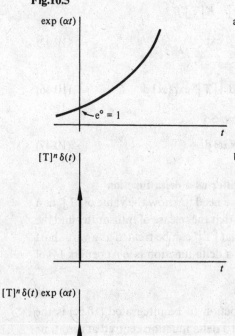

average conductance of each channel (G_{ch}). So

$$g(t) = \underbrace{P_o(t)N}_{\substack{\text{Fraction} \\ \text{of the} \\ \text{total} \\ \text{number} \\ \text{of chan-} \\ \text{nels open}}} \underbrace{G_{ch}}_{\substack{\text{Conductance} \\ \text{per} \\ \text{channel}}} \qquad (10.49)$$

or for one channel

$$g_1(t) = P_o(t)G_{ch} \qquad (10.49a)$$

If we substitute (10.48) into (10.49a) we obtain, for $t \geqslant 0$,

$$g_1(t) = K\beta[T]^{n'} \exp(-\alpha t)G_{ch} \qquad (10.50)$$

(The only time function in (10.50) is $\exp(-\alpha t)$, since $[T]^{n'}$ is a constant.)

The end-plate current

In order to obtain the end-plate current (I_{1Pc}) *per channel*, we compute

$$I_{1Pc} = (V - E_{eq})g_1(t) \qquad (10.51)$$

where V is the end-plate potential and E_{eq} is the equilibrium potential across the postsynaptic membrane in the presence of Ach. So

$$I_{1Pc} = (V - E_{eq})K\beta[T]^{n'} \exp(-\alpha t)G_{ch} \qquad (10.52)$$

Under voltage-clamp V is constant. If we define

$$U = (V - E_{eq})K\beta G_{ch}[T]^{n'}$$

then (10.52) becomes

$$I_{1Pc} = U \exp(-\alpha t) \qquad (10.53)$$

The constant U relates the current waveform to a number of model-dependent parameters (K, β, G_{ch}, α, n). Equation (10.53) describes the end-plate current that occurs when the postsynaptic membrane is hit by a very short pulse of Ach (approximated by a delta function). Next we shall consider the case when the Ach concentration is small but constant (a continuous perfusion). The model is the same as was used for the pulse of Ach.

Postsynaptic current noise under voltage-clamp and continuous perfusion with Ach

We should recall that the model of equation (10.24) describes the interaction between n molecules of transmitter (T) with one molecule of receptor (R), and then the conversion of the closed form of the transmitter–receptor complex (RT_c^n) to the open form (RT_o^n). This second step is considered to be much slower than the first and is thus rate limiting. RT_c^n is thus assumed to be at equilibrium with T and R and [T], the concentration of T, is assumed to be so small that

$$[RT_c^n] \ll [R]$$

With these assumptions we derived equation (10.47)

$$P_o(t) \exp(\alpha t) = K\beta \int [T]^n \exp(\alpha t)\, dt + C \tag{10.54}$$

which can be rearranged as

$$P_o(t) = \exp(-\alpha t)\left\{ K\beta \int [T]^n \exp(\alpha t)\, dt + C \right\} \tag{10.55}$$

With conventional voltage-clamp techniques (which hold the potential constant across relatively large areas of membrane) it is difficult to record single channel events. This is because many channels are being switched on and off and the currents associated with each of these events are small. Recently 'patch-clamp' techniques have been developed and allow us to isolate small membrane areas and to study the electrical activity of a few channels.

Nevertheless, it is still possible to analyse the fluctuations of current or voltage associated with numbers of channels and infer some basic properties of the molecular events.

The way in which this analysis is carried out is to use the model of the elementary event, the opening and closing of a channel, that was previously developed. We start with equation (10.55) where $P_o(t)$ is the probability of a given channel being open at time t when it was in a given state (open, or closed) at time zero. K is the transmitter–receptor binding constant and α and β are rate constants. α is the rate constant for closing channels and β (the opening rate constant) is the rate at which the fraction of the transmitter–receptor complexes $(K[T]^n)$ are opened; C is a constant of integration. If the concentration of transmitter ([T]) is kept constant, (10.55) becomes

$$P_o(t) = \exp(-\alpha t)\left\{ K\beta[T]^n \int \exp(\alpha t)\, dt + C \right\}$$

or

$$P_o(t) = \exp(-\alpha t)\{(K\beta[T]^n/\alpha) \exp(\alpha t) + C\}$$

We shall now consider the case when the channel is open at time zero. The probability that a given channel is open at time t when it was open at time zero is written symbolically as $P_o(o/t)$ and

$$P_o(o/t) = \exp(-\alpha t)\{(K\beta[T]^n/\alpha) \exp(\alpha t) + C\}$$

At time zero, that is, when $t = 0$,

$$P_o(o/0) = K\beta[T]^n/\alpha + C$$

but the probability of the channel being open at time zero when it is open at time zero ($P_o(o/0)$) is obviously unity so the constant of integration (C) is

$$C = 1 - K\beta[T]^n/\alpha$$

So

$$P_o(o, t) = \exp(-\alpha t)\{(K\beta[T]^n/\alpha)\exp(\alpha t) + 1 - K\beta[T]^n/\alpha\}$$

or

$$P_o(o, t) = K\beta[T]^n/\alpha + (1 - K\beta[T]^n/\alpha)\exp(-\alpha t) \qquad (10.56)$$

The probability of a channel being open at time t when it was closed at time zero is

$$P_o(c/t) = \exp(-\alpha t)\{(K\beta[T]^n/\alpha)\exp(\alpha t) + C\} \qquad (10.57)$$

Since the probability of a channel being open at time zero when it was closed at time zero is obviously zero, then

$$0 = K\beta[T]^n/\alpha + C$$

or

$$C = -K\beta[T]^n/\alpha \qquad (10.58)$$

If we substitute (10.58) into (10.57) we obtain

$$P_o(c/t) = \exp(-\alpha t)\{(K\beta[T]^n/\alpha)(\exp(\alpha t) - 1)\}$$

or

$$P_o(c/t) = (K\beta[T]^n/\alpha)(1 - \exp(-\alpha t)) \qquad (10.59)$$

From (10.56) and (10.59) we can calculate the probability that a channel is open when $t \to \infty$, when it was open at time zero ($P_o(o/\infty)$), and when it was closed at time zero ($P_o(c/\infty)$). Since when $t \to \infty$, $\exp(-\alpha t) \to 0$, then

$$P_o(o/\infty) = K\beta[T]^n/\alpha \quad \text{and} \quad P_o(c/\infty) = K\beta[T]^n/\alpha$$

that is,

$$P_o(o/\infty) = P_o(c/\infty) = P_o(\infty) \qquad (10.60)$$

Equation (10.60) means that the state of a channel at time $t \to \infty$ is independent of its state at time zero. So $P_o(o/\infty)$ and $P_o(c/\infty)$ are not joint probabilities but absolute probabilities,

$$P_o(\infty) = P_o(c/\infty) \qquad (10.61)$$

where $P_o(\infty)$ is the probability of a channel being open when $t \to \infty$. Since [T] is constant and the system is thus in a steady-state

$$P_o(0) = P_o(\infty) \qquad (10.62)$$

In a steady-state $P_o(t)$ is equal to $P_o(0)$ only for sufficiently large t, that is, when sufficient time has evolved that the events can be considered to be independent of one another.

The conductance of a channel

Equations (10.56) and (10.59) can now be used to compute the conductance of channel at any time t.

The mean conductance of a channel at time t is given by

$$\dot{G}_{ch}(t) = P_o(t)G_{ch} \tag{10.63}$$

where $P_o(t)$ is the probability that a channel is open at time t regardless of its state at time zero. $P_o(t)$ is thus an absolute probability (see Appendix 7). The meaning of $P_o(t)$ is the following: if we observe N identical channels that are opening and closing we expect to find n channels open at time t. So

$$P_o(t) = n/N$$

for very large N.

In (10.63), $\dot{G}_{ch}(t)$ is the conductance of a channel when it is open. Since there are two possible and independent ways in which a channel can be open at time t, that is, the channel might have been open or closed at time zero, then

$$P_o(t) \;\; = \;\; P_o(0) \;\; \times \;\; P_o(0/t) \;\; + \;\; P_c(0) \;\; \times \;\; P_o(c/t) \tag{10.64}$$

Probability of the channel being open at time t	Probability of the channel being open at time zero	Probability of the channel being open at time t when it was open at time zero	Probability of the channel being closed at time zero	Probability of the channel being open at time t when it was closed at time zero

Under voltage clamp the channel end-plate current is given by

$$\dot{I}_{ch}(t) = (V - E_{eq})\dot{G}_{ch}(t) \quad \text{and} \quad \dot{G}_{ch}(t) = G_{ch}P_o(t) \tag{10.65}$$

This equation is written assuming that $\dot{G}_{ch}(t)$ is an ohmic conductance, but an equivalent expression could just as easily be written for a constant-field channel. Equations (10.63) and (10.65) describe the channel conductance and the channel end-plate current respectively as functions of time. Both the time functions ($\dot{G}_{ch}(t)$ and $\dot{I}_{ch}(t)$) contain temporal information about the switching *on* and *off* of a channel. This switching is a random event and so cannot be analytically defined in the time domain. However, from the definition of probability (see Appendix 7), $P(t)$ in equation (10.64) is also the fraction of an ensemble of channels that is open at time t (see Appendix 13). If there are N channels per square centimetre of membrane then at time t there will be $n(t)$ channels open where $n(t)$ is given by the expression

$$n(t) = P_o(t)N \tag{10.66}$$

Under voltage clamp the ionic current $\dot{I}(t)$ that flows through the n channels is obtained from the equation

$$\dot{I}(t) = n(t)G_{ch}(V - E_{eq})$$
$$= NP_o(t)G_{ch}(V - E_{eq})$$

But from (10.65) $\dot{I}_{ch}(t) = P_o(t)G_{ch}(t)(V - E_{eq})$, so

$$\dot{I}(t) = N\dot{I}_{ch}(t) \tag{10.67}$$

$\dot{I}(t)$ is thus the average value of the current that flows through N channels which are distributed in an area of membrane of one square centimetre. Of these N channels, $n(t)$ channels are open at time t. In practice we cannot measure $\dot{I}(t)$. We measure, instead, the instantaneous value of the current density $(\bar{I}(t))$, which is given by

$$\bar{I}(t) = \sum_{i=1}^{N} I_{chi}(t) \tag{10.68}$$

where $I_{chi}(t)$ is the current that flows through channel i. Of the N channels, only n are actually open at time t, so $I_{chi}(t)$ is zero for $N - n$ channels at time t. However, the time average of $\bar{I}(t)$ is, by definition (see Appendix 13),

$$\left(\frac{1}{T}\right) \int_0^T I(t)\, dt$$

or

$$\left(\frac{1}{T}\right) \int_0^T \left(\sum_{i=1}^{N} I_{chi}(t) \right) dt = \sum_{i=1}^{N} \left(\frac{1}{T}\right) \int_0^T I_{chi}(t)\, dt \tag{10.69}$$

For an ergodic ensemble (see Appendix 13) the time average of one of the members of the ensemble, $(I_{chi}(t))$, is equal to the ensemble average $\bar{I}_{ch}(t)$, that is,

$$\left(\frac{1}{T}\right) \int_0^T I_{chi}(t)\, dt = \dot{I}_{ch}(t) \tag{10.70}$$

So

$$\left(\frac{1}{T}\right) \int_0^T \bar{I}(t)\, dt = \sum_{i=1}^{N} \dot{I}_{ch}(t)$$
$$= N\dot{I}_{ch}(t)$$
$$= \dot{I}(t) \tag{10.70a}$$

This expression relates the time average of the signal $\bar{I}(t)$ to the ensemble average $\dot{I}_{ch}(t)$. With this relationship we can compute the average current that flows through a population of N channels, by observing the total current flowing through one of these channels over a period of time T.

However, since the fluctuations of the signal in which we are interested have zero as their mean value, time averaging the signal *removes* the noise component! In order to analyse this component, further manipulations are required, that is, we have to introduce the autocovariance function defined by the expression shown below (see also Appendix 13).

$$C(\tau) = \left(\frac{1}{T}\right) \int_0^T I_{ch}(t) I_{ch}(t+\tau)\, dt - \left(\frac{1}{T}\right) \int_0^T I_{ch}^2(t)\, dt \tag{10.71}$$

The product of $I_{ch}(t)$ by itself displaced in time (Figure 10.6b) is $I_{ch}(t)$ multiplied by $I_{ch}(t+\tau)$. The second term on the right-hand side of equation (10.71) is the time average of the square of the current that flows through a channel, while the first term on the right-hand side of equation (10.71) is the autocorrelation of the current that flows through a channel (see Appendix 13 for a definition of autocorrelation and autocovariance).

The autocovariance of the channel current

In Appendix 13 we also show that the autocovariance can be obtained from the ensemble average of the channel currents. That is,

$$C(\tau) = \dot{I}_{ch}(t)\dot{I}_{ch}(t+\tau) - \dot{I}_{ch}^2(0) \tag{10.72}$$

where $\dot{I}_{ch}(t)$ is the average of the currents through an ensemble of identical channels and where $\dot{I}_{ch}(0)$ is the current ensemble average at time zero. By comparing equations (10.71) and (10.72) we can write

$$\left(\frac{1}{T}\right)\int_0^T I_{ch}(t)I_{ch}(t+\tau)\,\mathrm{d}t - \left(\frac{1}{T}\right)\int_0^T I_{ch}^2(t)\,\mathrm{d}t$$

$$= \dot{I}_{ch}(t)\dot{I}_{ch}(t+\tau) - \dot{I}_{ch}^2(0) \quad (10.73)$$

If we could record the current that flows through a single channel, the left-hand side of equation (10.73) could be obtained by sampling $I_{ch}(t)$ in the time domain and by numerically computing its autocovariance function (see Appendix 13). However, this is not possible as we can only record the current that flows through a *population* of channels. If we amalgamate equations (10.64) and (10.65) we obtain

$$\dot{I}_{ch}(t) = (V - E_{eq})G_{ch}\{P_o(0)P_o(0/t) + P_c(0)P_o(c/t)\}$$

Fig.10.6

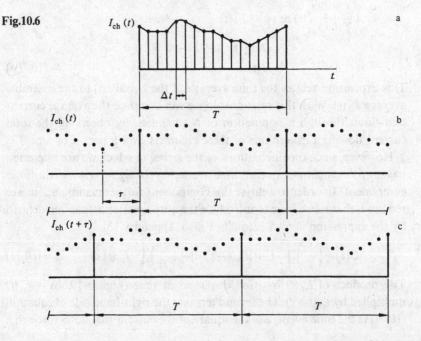

or for $t+\tau$

$$\dot{I}_{ch}(t+\tau)=(V-E_{eq})G_{ch}\{P_o(0)P_o(0/(t+\tau))+P_c(0)P_o(c/(t+\tau))\}$$
(10.74)

and for $t=0$

$$\dot{I}_{ch}(0)=(V-E_{eq})G_{ch}\{P_o(0)P_o(0/0)+P_c(0)P_o(c/0)\}$$
$$=(V-E_{eq})G_{ch}P_o(0)$$

The expressions for $\dot{I}_{ch}(t)$, $\dot{I}_{ch}(t+\tau)$ and $\dot{I}_{ch}(0)$ can now be used to obtain an analytical expression for the autocovariance of the current through a single channel $(C_1(\tau))$

$$C_1(\tau)=(V-E_{eq})G_{ch}\{P_o(0)P_o(o/t)+P_c(0)P_o(c/t)\}$$
$$\times(V-E_{eq})G_{ch}\{P_o(0)P_o(o/(t+\tau))+P_c(0)P_o(c/(t+\tau))\}$$
$$-(V-E_{eq})^2G_{ch}^2P_o^2(0)$$

On rearranging

$$C_1(\tau)=(V-E_{eq})^2G_{ch}^2[\{P_o(0)P_o(o/t)+P_c(0)P_o(c/t)\}$$
$$\times\{P_o(0)P_o(o/(t+\tau))+P_c(0)P_o(c/(t+\tau))\}]$$
$$-(V-E_{eq})^2G_{ch}^2P_o^2(0)$$
(10.75)

or

$$C_1(\tau)=(V-E_{eq})^2G_{ch}^2(Q(\tau)-P_o^2(0))$$
(10.76)

where

$$Q(\tau)=\{P_o(0)P_o(o/t)+P_c(0)P_o(c/t)\}$$
$$\times\{P_o(0)P_o(o/(t+\tau))+P_c(0)P_o(c/(t+\tau))\}$$

On expansion

$$Q(\tau)=P_o(0)^2P_o(o/t)P_o(o/(t+\tau))$$
$$+P_o(0)P_o(o/t)P_c(0)P_o(c/(t+\tau))$$
$$+P_c(0)P_o(c/t)P_o(0)P_o(o/(t+\tau))$$
$$+P_c(0)P_o(c/t)P_c(0)P_o(c/(t+\tau))$$

The second and third terms of the right-hand side are zero, as the product $P_c(0)P_o(0)$ is zero; this is because a channel cannot be simultaneously open and closed. Since we are dealing with stationary processes t may have any value. So for $t=0$

$$Q(\tau)=P_o(0)^2P_o(o/0)P_o(o/\tau)+P_c(0)P_o(c/0)P_c(0)P_o(c/\tau)$$

The second term of the right-hand side is zero since, logically, a channel cannot be open and closed at the same time $(P_o(c/0))$. So

$$Q(\tau)=\underbrace{P_o(0)P_o(o/0)}\ \underbrace{P_o(0)P_o(o/\tau)}$$
(10.77)

| Probability of the channel being open at time zero when it was open at time zero $(=1)$ | Probability of a channel being open at time τ when it was open at time zero |

If we substitute (10.77) in (10.76) we obtain

$$C_1(\tau) = (V - E_{cq})^2 G_{ch}^2 \{P_o(0)P_o(o/\tau) - P_o^2(0)\} \qquad (10.78)$$

But from (10.56)

$$P_o(o/\tau) = K\beta[T]^n/\alpha + \{1 - K\beta[T]^n/\alpha\} \exp(-\alpha\tau)$$

From (10.40)

$$\alpha \gg K[T]^n\beta$$

so

$$1 \gg K[T]^n\beta/\alpha$$

and

$$1 - K[T]^n\beta/\alpha \approx 1$$

Equation (10.56) can thus be simplified to

$$P_o(o/\tau) = K\beta[T]^n/\alpha + \exp(-\alpha\tau) \qquad (10.79)$$

For a stationary process the probability of a channel being open at $t \to \infty$ is the same regardless of whether the channel was open or closed at time zero and is also the same as the probability of a channel being open at time zero. So

$$P_o(0) = P_o(\infty)$$

and from equation (10.79)

$$P_o(\infty) = K\beta[T]^n/\alpha \qquad (10.80)$$

If we now substitute equations (10.79) and (10.80) into equation (10.78) we obtain

$$C_1(\tau) = (V - E_{cq})^2 G_{ch}^2$$
$$\times \{(K\beta[T]^n/\alpha)((K\beta[T]^n)/\alpha) + \exp(-\alpha\tau)) - (K\beta[T]^n/\alpha)^2\}$$
$$C_1(\tau) = (V - E_{cq})^2 G_{ch}^2 (K\beta[T]^n/\alpha) \exp(-\alpha\tau) \qquad (10.81)$$

As shown in Appendix 13, if we Fourier transform the autocovariance function $(C_1(\tau))$ we obtain the power density spectrum $(F(\omega))$ of the fluctuations around the mean value. If we define H as

$$H = (V - E_{cq})^2 G_{ch}^2 (K\beta[T]^n/\alpha) \qquad (10.82)$$

then

$$C_1(\tau) = H \exp(-\alpha\tau)$$

The final step in our analysis is the Fourier transform of $(C_1(t))$:

$$F(\omega) = \int_0^\infty C_1(\tau) \exp(-j\omega\tau) \, d\tau = H \int_0^\infty \exp(-\alpha\tau) \exp(-j\omega\tau) \, d\tau$$

$$= H \int_0^\infty \exp(-(\alpha + j\omega)\tau) \, d\tau \qquad (10.83)$$

So

$$F(\omega) = (H/(\alpha + j\omega))(-1)[\exp(-(\alpha + j\omega)\tau)]_0^\infty$$

or

$$F(\omega) = (H/(\alpha + j\omega))(-1)[0-1]$$
$$= H/(\alpha + j\omega) \tag{10.84}$$

The power density spectrum of the synaptic noise

Since the autocorrelation function is an even function (as shown in Appendix 13), we are only interested in the *real* part of $F(\omega)$. This is because we are dealing with an even function so only the cosine terms need to be included, or, that is, we only deal with the real part of $F(\omega)$. If we multiply top and bottom of (10.84) by $(\alpha - j\omega)$ (the complex conjugate of $\alpha + j\omega$ – see Appendix 2) we obtain

$$H[(\alpha/(\alpha^2 + \omega^2)) - j(\omega/(\alpha^2 + \omega^2))]$$

so the real part is

$$H\alpha/(\alpha^2 + \omega^2) \tag{10.85}$$

But (10.85) is only half of the spectrum (corresponding to the positive value of ω – see Appendix 13), so

$$F(\omega) = 2H\alpha/(\alpha^2 + \omega^2) \tag{10.86}$$

If we substitute (10.82) into (10.86) we obtain

$$F(\omega) = 2(V - E_{eq})^2 G_{ch}^2 (K\beta[T]^n/\alpha)(\alpha/(\alpha^2 + \omega^2))$$

or

$$F(\omega) = 2(V - E_{eq})^2 G_{ch}^2 K\beta[T]^n (1/(\alpha^2 + \omega^2)) \tag{10.86a}$$

But by definition

$$\omega = 2\pi f$$

so

$$1/(\alpha^2 + \omega^2) = 1/(\alpha^2 + (2\pi f)^2) = (1/\alpha^2)/(1 + (2\pi f/\alpha)^2) \tag{10.87}$$

If we substitute (10.87) into (10.86a) we obtain

$$F(\omega) = 2(V - E_{eq})^2 G_{ch}^2 K\beta[T]^n (1/2^2)/(1 + (2\pi f/\alpha)^2) \tag{10.88}$$

Equation (10.88) shows that the power density spectrum of the current is directly related to the conductance of an open channel, and the kinetic parameters of the interaction between transmitter and its receptor.

If instead of one channel we have N channels, then the resulting power density spectrum is the sum of the power spectra of all the individual channels. If we assume that all the channels are identical, then

$$F(\omega) = 2N(V - E_{eq})^2 G_{ch}^2 K\beta[T]^n (1/\alpha^2)/(1 + (2\pi f/\alpha)^2) \tag{10.89}$$

If we define A as

$$A = 2N(V - E_{eq})^2 G_{ch}^2 K\beta[T]^n (1/\alpha^2) \tag{10.90}$$

equation (10.89) becomes

$$F(\omega) = A/(1 + (2\pi f/\alpha)^2) \tag{10.91}$$

When

$$f/\alpha \ll 1$$

then

$$F(\omega) \approx A \tag{10.92}$$

Also, when

$$f/\alpha \gg 1$$

then

$$F(\omega) = A/(2\pi f/\alpha)^2 \tag{10.93}$$

Because we are dealing with a frequency range of several *decades* it is easier to plot (10.91) as a log–log function, that is,

$$\ln(F(\omega)) = \ln(A/(1 + (2\pi f/\alpha)^2))$$

or

$$\ln(F(\omega)) = \ln(A) - \ln(1 + (2\pi f/\alpha)^2) \tag{10.94}$$

(A frequency *decade* consists of a range of frequencies in which the highest frequency is ten times the lowest frequency. For example, 1–10 Hz, or 10 000–100 000 Hz.) With equation (10.89) (or in a more simplified form in (10.94)) we arrived at the end of the journey. For we are now able to relate measurements made on synaptic membrane noise – the power density spectrum of the noise – with an expression derived from the probabilistic model of the molecular events that take place at the postsynaptic membrane. The parameters of this model are the Ach-gated channel conductance (G_{ch}), the number of channels (N), the equilibrium constant (K) of the Ach–receptors interaction, the rate constants of the opening (β) and closing (α) of the Ach–receptor complex and the stoichiometry of the reaction (n). In order to obtain values for all these parameters the system has to be studied under a variety of experimental conditions (for example, different concentrations of transmitter in the perfusate ([T])). Finally, one point that we should again emphasize is that any conclusions that we make will *always* be dependent upon the model that was used to first set up expressions such as that used in equation (10.89).

APPENDICES

APPENDIX 1. Units and numbers

When electrophysiologists measure currents, voltages cr concentrations they measure physical quantities that are the same physical quantities that a physicist or chemist might deal with. In order to characterize precisely these entities it is necessary to specify two things:

(1) The *quality* of the units, and
(2) The *numerical* size of the units used.

Dimensions

We shall deal first with the quality of physical units and this quality is called the *dimension*. Natural scientists have agreed on a number of different systems of units. The two most widely used systems are the *c.g.s. system* in which the fundamental units are:

(L) length – centimetre
(M) mass – gram
(T) time – second

and then there is the *MKS system* with the fundamental units of:

(L) length – metre
(M) mass – kilogram
(T) time – second

The latter is the so-called *rationalized* MKS system, more closely related to the International System of Units (SI), which is coming steadily into universal use.

In Table 1 we give some physical units that are used in the two systems. More detailed information is available in *Quantities, Units, and Symbols*, a report by the Symbols Committee of the Royal Society, 2nd edn, 1975, and in *Units of Measurement*, Preprint from the Geigy Scientific Tables, 7th edn, 1968 (Basle, Switzerland: Geigy).

On reading the main text of this book it is clear that electrophysiologists (and biophysicists) do not follow *either* the MKS or the CGS systems!

Table 2 shows some of the units that are generally used by electrophysiologists, and therefore found in the relevant literature.

The mole

The new quantity in this table is the mole which is also used by chemists. *A mole* of a substance is an amount that contains Avogadro's number of molecules. Avogadro's number (N_0) is

$$N_0 = 6.0232 \times 10^{23} \text{ molecules} \cdot \text{mol}^{-1}$$

Molal solution

When we dissolve 1 mole of a substance in 1 kilogram of solvent we obtain a solution which is said to be 1 *molal*. If we make up 1 mole of a substance in 1 litre of solution we obtain a solution which is said to be 1 *molar*. The symbol for 1 molar solution is M (capital M). There is no fixed relationship between molality and molarity since 1 kg of the solvent has a volume which depends on the temperature. Although electrophysiologists specify the solutions they use by their molarities, when making calculations of fluxes (see Chapter 3) across membranes they sometimes use concentrations in $\text{mol} \cdot \text{cm}^{-3}$.

A certain number of physical constants are frequently used in electrophysiology and so it is useful to know their values (see Table 3).

Table 1. *The MKS and cgs systems*

Quantity	Symbol	MKS, SI	cgs	Equivalent of 1 MKS unit in cgs
Mass	M	kg	gm	10^3 gram
Length	L	metre	cm	10^2 cm
Force	F	Newton	dyne	10^5 dyne
Work	W	joule	erg	10^7 erg
Charge	Q	coulomb	esu	$\simeq 3 \times 10^9 \text{ esu} \cdot \text{s}^{-1}$
Current	I	ampere	esu/sec	$\simeq 3 \times 10^9$ esu
Electrical potential	V (ψ)	volt	stat. volt	$\simeq 1/300$ stat. volt
Resistance	R	ohm	$\text{cm} \cdot \text{s}^{-1}$	$\simeq 1/30\,000 \text{ stat. volt} \cdot \text{cm}^{-1}$
Temperature	K	kelvin	kelvin	1

From Table 2 we can derive other units. For example, the first law of Fick for diffusion can be used to derive the units of the diffusion coefficient (D):

$$J = -D \, dc/dx$$

$\bar{J}$, the flow of a substance across a unit area, is:

$$\text{moles}/(\text{cm}^2 \cdot \text{second}) = \text{mol} \cdot \text{cm}^{-2} \cdot \text{s}^{-1}$$

c, the concentration, is

$$\text{moles}/\text{cm}^3 = \text{mol} \cdot \text{cm}^{-3}$$

x, the distance, is in cm; so from Fick's Law:

$$\text{mol} \cdot \text{cm}^{-2} \cdot \text{s}^{-1} = D \, \text{mol} \cdot \text{cm}^{-3} \cdot \text{cm}^{-1}$$

Since the left-hand side = right-hand side, we can find the units of D. Thus

$$\text{mol} \cdot \text{cm}^{-2} \cdot \text{s}^{-1} = D \cdot \text{mol} \cdot \text{cm}^{-4}$$

Table 2. *Commonly quoted units*

Quantity	Symbol	Units
Mass	mol	mole
Length	L	cm
Force	F	newton (or dyne)
Work	W	joule (or calorie)
Charge	q	coulomb
Current	I	ampere
Electrical potential	V or ψ	volt
Resistance	R or Ω	ohm ($V \cdot A^{-1}$)
Conductance	S	Siemens ($= \text{ohm}^{-1}$)

Table 3. *Physical constants used in electrophysiology*

Absolute temperature (melting point of water)	273.150 K	
Calorie	4.1840 joule	J
Atmosphere (760 mm of Hg at standard conditions)	$1.013 \times 10^6 \, \text{dyne} \cdot \text{cm}^{-2}$	$\text{dyn} \cdot \text{cm}^{-2}$
Boltzmann gas constant (k)	$1.380 \times 10^{-9} \, \text{joule} \cdot \text{deg K}$	$J \cdot K^{-1}$
Electronic charge (c)	1.602×10^{-19} coulomb	C
Faraday's constant (F)	96 494 coulomb ($\simeq 96.500$) or 23 062 cal $\cdot$ volt$^{-1} \cdot$ g $\cdot$ eq^{-1}	$C \cdot \text{mol}^{-1}$ cal $\cdot V^{-1} \cdot$ gr-eq^{-1}
Molar gas constant (R)	1.987 cal $\cdot$ deg$^{-1} \cdot$ mol^{-1} or 8.315 joule $\cdot$ deg. K$^{-1} \cdot$ mol^{-1} or 82.06 cc. atm $\cdot$ deg. K $\cdot$ mol^{-1}	cal $\cdot K^{-1} \cdot$ mol^{-1} $J \cdot K^{-1} \cdot$ mol^{-1}

so, for the equation to balance,

$$D = cm^2/second$$
$$= cm^2 \cdot s^{-1} \tag{1}$$

(1) is called a *dimensional equation* because the units of a physical quantity are called its *dimensions*. When we write dimensional equations we write equations with literal symbols (letters), this means that we cannot multiply out, for example, cm by seconds or divide moles by cm^3. However, we can multiply by cm in the sense that

$$cm \cdot cm = cm^2$$

or we can divide moles by moles so that

$$mole/mole = dimensionless\ quantity$$

To be consistent when we write dimensional equations the following rules must apply:

(1) When we add or subtract quantities the resulting quantity must have the same dimensions. This means that we cannot add quantities of different dimensions

$$cm + cm = cm$$

but

$$cm + seconds = cm + seconds$$

(2) Two quantities are equal only if they have the same dimensions

$$20\ cm = 20\ cm$$

but

$$20\ seconds \neq 20\ cm$$

(3) The ratio of two quantities with the same dimensions is a dimensionless quantity. Thus

$$40\ seconds/20\ seconds = 2 \quad \text{which is a dimensionless quantity}$$
but
$$40\ seconds/20\ cm = 2\ seconds/cm = 2\ s \cdot cm^{-1}$$

that is, the *ratio* of two quantities with different dimensions is a quantity that must have the appropriate dimensions so that the dimensional equation complies with rule (2).

(4) The numerical value of a physical quantity (magnitude) is independent of its dimensions (we can have 20 cm, 40 cm, etc.).

(5) When a quantity is multiplied by or divided by a dimensionless number it does not change its dimensions

$$2 \times 20\ cm = 40\ cm$$

(6) Exponents, in general, and the arguments of the exponential or the logarithm functions, *cannot* have dimensions.

It is current practice to use a fixed set of symbols to specify dimensions. Some examples of these symbols are:

mass   M

length   L

time   T

temperature Φ

etc.

In this book we follow the practice, frequently adopted by the chemists, of using the symbols of units selected (cm instead of L, for example) because dimensional equations written in this way seem easier to understand.

Numbers

We shall next deal with another aspect of a physical quantity – its numerical value. When specifying the magnitude of physical quantities or when writing down quantitative relationships (equations, for example) we deal with different types of numbers.

We use numbers such as 1, 2, ..., 20, etc., and they are called *integers*. They are frequently used to count or they are used in special operations such as the expansion of a series. For example,

$$\sum_{n=1}^{n} \frac{1}{2^n} = \frac{1}{2} + \frac{1}{2^2} + \frac{1}{2^3} + \cdots + \frac{1}{2^n}$$

The sign $\sum_{n=1}^{n}$ means that we substitute 1 into $1/2^n$ and compute it to obtain the first term. Then we substitute 2, compute the second term, and then *add* it to the first term. Then for $n = 3$ and add this to the first two terms until we compute $1/2^n$ and have added it to the first $n-1$ terms.

We also use numbers which are the ratio between two integers (n/m). They are called *rational numbers*. When we carry out the division operation we obtain either an integer ($4/2 = 2$), or a decimal number with a finite number of significant figures. For example

$\frac{1}{8} = 0.125$ (to three significant figures)

or a decimal number with an infinite number of significant figures that repeat themselves. For example,

$\frac{1}{6} = 0.166666\ldots$ (6 repeats itself indefinitely, i.e. is 'recurring')

A third type of numbers are known as *irrational numbers*. For example,

$\sqrt{2} = 2^{1/2} = 1.4142136\ldots$

the decimal number obtained has an infinite number of significant figures but there is no sequence of numbers that repeats itself. Examples of such numbers are the number e and π where

$e = 2.718281\ldots$ and $\pi = 3.1415927\ldots$

The number e is discussed in Appendix 2 and the number π is the ratio between the length of the circumference of a circle and its diameter.

A set

The set that includes *real* numbers, *rational* numbers and the *irrational* numbers is the set of *real* numbers. (A set is defined as a collection of objects or items which share one or more common properties.)

Complex numbers

There is a fourth group of numbers called *complex numbers*. These numbers were conceived in order to solve a certain type of mathematical problem which is insoluble if only real numbers were used. For example, let us try to solve the quadratic equation

$$ax^2 + bx + c = 0$$

Let us divide the equation by a. So

$$x^2 + (b/a)x + c/a = 0$$

Now we collect the terms with x on one side of the equation

$$x^2 + (b/a)x = -c/a$$

If we add $(b/2a)^2$ to both sides of this equation we obtain

$$x^2 + (b/a)x + (b/2a)^2 = (b/2a)^2 - c/a$$

But

$$(x + b/2a)^2 = x^2 + (b/a)x + (b/2a)^2 \quad \text{(see Appendix 2)}$$

so

$$(x + b/2a)^2 = (b/2a)^2 - c/a$$

or

$$x + b/2a = \pm\sqrt{((b/2a)^2 - c/a)} \tag{2}$$

We use the plus and minus sign on the right-hand side because

$$(N)(N) = N^2$$
$$(-N)(-N) = N^2$$

so

$$\sqrt{(N^2)} = \pm N$$

Let us apply (2) to solve the following equation

$$x + 2x + 4 = 0$$

in which $a = 1$, $b = 2$, and $c = 4$, so

$$b/2a = 1 \quad \text{and} \quad c/a = 4$$

then

$$x = -1 \pm \sqrt{(1 - 4)}$$

or

$$x = -1 \pm \sqrt{(-3)}$$

There is no real number that satisfies this solution. For

$$(\sqrt{(-3)})^2 = -3$$

If $\sqrt{(-3)}$ was a real number N then

$$NN = -3$$

and N can be either positive, that is,

$$NN = N^2 = \text{positive number}$$

or negative, since the product of two negative numbers is also a positive number

$$(-N)(-N) = N^2 = \text{positive number}$$

In order to solve problems of this sort mathematicians invented a different type of number. The number i is defined by

$$i = \sqrt{-1} \tag{3}$$

Because in engineering the symbol i is used for electrical current (and also in electrophysiology) we shall use

$$j = \sqrt{-1} \tag{4}$$

If we use the number j in the solution of the quadratic equation we obtain

$$x = -1 \pm j\sqrt{3}$$

x is now a *complex* number and is made up of a real part: -1; and an imaginary part: $\pm j\sqrt{3}$. The number $j\sqrt{3}$ is called an *imaginary* number. Any complex number (Z) is thus defined as

$$Z = a \pm jb \tag{5}$$

where a is the real part and jb the imaginary part (b is a *real* number).

When we represent real numbers we represent them as distances, as points in a straight line. When we represent a complex number we represent them as points in a complex plane or in an Argand diagram (see Figure A1.1).

When we use (5) we represent the number Z in Cartesian coordinates or Cartesian form since a and b are just the x and y (j) coordinates in the complex plane. The complex number $a + jb$ can be represented in a different form.

From trigonometry (see Appendix 3) and from Figure A1.1,

$$a = A\sin(\theta) \quad \text{and} \quad b = A\cos(\theta)$$

and

$$A = \sqrt{(a^2 + b^2)} \quad \text{and} \quad \theta = \tan^{-1}(b/a)$$

When we represent a complex number by its distance to the origin of the complex plane and by angle θ we use *polar coordinates* and the number is said to be in *polar form*.

The next step is to define the arithmetic operations that can be made with complex numbers.

Addition

If

$$Z_1 = a_1 + jb_1 \quad \text{and} \quad Z_2 = a_2 + jb_2$$

then

$$Z_1 + Z_2 = a_1 + jb_1 + a_2 + jb_2$$
$$= (a_1 + a_2) + j(b_1 + b_2)$$

We just add the real parts and the imaginary parts separately. Similarly for subtraction

$$Z_1 - Z_2 = (a_1 - a_2) + j(b_1 - b_2)$$

Multiplication

To multiply two complex numbers

$$Z_1 Z_2 = (a_1 + jb_1)(a_2 + jb_2) = a_1 a_2 + j(a_2 b_1 + a_1 b_2) + j^2 b_1 b_2$$

But $j^2 = (\sqrt{(-1)})^2 = -1$, so

$$Z_1 Z_2 = (a_1 a_2 - b_1 b_2) + j(a_2 b_1 + a_1 b_2)$$

The powers of j reveal an interesting property

$$j^0 = +1$$
$$j^1 = \sqrt{(-1)}$$
$$j^2 = -1$$
$$j^3 = j^2 j = -j$$

Fig.A1.1

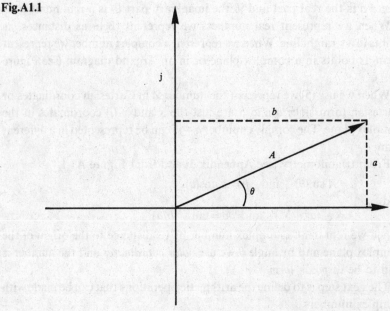

$$j^4 = j^2 j^2 = (-1)^2 = +1$$
$$j^5 = j^4 j = j$$
$$j^6 = j^5 j = -1$$
$$j^7 = j^6 j = -j$$
$$j^8 = j^7 j = 1$$

that is, the powers of j go through $+1$, j, -1, $-j$ in a periodic way.

Division

To divide a complex number $(a_1 + jb_1)$ by the complex number $(a_2 + jb_2)$, that is,

$$(a_1 + jb_1)/(a_2 + jb_2)$$

one multiplies top and bottom by $a_2 - jb_2$. So for the numerator

$$(a_1 + jb_1)(a_2 - jb_2) = a_1 a_2 + j(a_2 b_1 - a_1 b_2) - j^2 b_1 b_2$$

Since $j^2 = -1$

$$(a_1 + jb_1)(a_2 - jb_2) = (a_1 a_2 + b_1 b_2) + j(a_2 b_1 - a_1 b_2)$$

For the denominator

$$(a_2 + jb_2)(a_2 - jb_2) = a_2^2 - j^2 b_2^2 = a_2^2 + b_2^2$$

So

$$(a_1 + jb_1)/(a_2 + jb_2) = (a_1 + jb_1)(a_2 - jb_2)/(a_2 + jb_2)(a_2 - jb_2)$$
$$= ((a_1 a_2 + b_1 b_2) + j(a_2 b_1 - a_1 b_2))/(a_2^2 + b_2^2)$$

or

$$(a_1 + jb_1)/(a_2 + jb_2) = (a_1 a_2 + b_1 b_2)/(a_2^2 + b_2^2) + j(a_2 b_1 - a_1 b_2)/(a_2^2 + b_2^2)$$

The result is also a complex number in which the real part is $(a_1 a_2 + b_1 b_2)/(a_2^2 + b_2^2)$ and the imaginary part is $j(a_2 b_1 - a_1 b_2)/(a_2^2 + b_2^2)$.

If we have a complex number Z given by

$$Z = a_n + jb_n$$

the complex number $\bar{Z}$ is called the *complex conjugate* of Z and is defined as

$$\bar{Z} = a_n - jb_n$$

so

$$Z\bar{Z} = a_n^2 + b_n^2$$

and

$$|Z| = \sqrt{Z\bar{Z}} = \sqrt{(a_n^2 + b_n^2)}$$

is called the *modulus* of Z.

Also

$$Z + \bar{Z} = a_n + jb_n + a_n - jb_n = 2a_n$$

and

$$Z - \bar{Z} = a_n + jb_n - a_n + jb_n = 2jb_n$$

APPENDIX 2. Algebra and calculus – a review

Literal quantities

Quantities can be represented by letters (literal symbols) such as a, or x or β. These literal symbols are called *constants* when they represent a specific number (i.e. π, or F (the Faraday)). Quantities are called *variables* if they represent a *set* of numbers. For example

$$x^2$$

means *any number squared*, unless, of course, we define it otherwise.

We can manipulate literal symbols as if they were numbers, for example,

$$a \cdot a \cdot a \cdots a = a^n \tag{1}$$

is a multiplied by itself n times, and

$$\underset{m \text{ times}}{(a \cdot a \cdot a \cdots a)} \underset{m \text{ times}}{(b \cdot b \cdots b)} = a^m b^m = (ab)^m \tag{2}$$

When we have quantities inside parentheses this means that we compute first what is inside the parentheses.

$$\underset{m \text{ times}}{(a \cdot a \cdot a \cdots a)} \underset{n \text{ times}}{(a \cdot a \cdot a \cdots a)} = (a^m)(a^n)$$

$$= a^{m+n}$$

$$= a^m a^n \tag{3}$$

If instead of multiplying we divide,

$$\underset{m \text{ times}}{} \qquad \underset{n \text{ times}}{}$$

$$(a \cdot a \cdot a \cdot a \cdots a)/(a \cdot a \cdot a \cdot a \cdots a)$$

and if we then split the numerator as follows

$$\frac{a^n a^{m-n}}{a^n} = a^{m-n}$$

So

$$a^m/a^n = a^{m-n} \tag{4}$$

If $m = n$ (for example, 2), then

$$\frac{a \cdot a}{a \cdot a} = \frac{a^2}{a^2} = 1 = a^0 \tag{5}$$

This leads to the general conclusion that any number raised to the power zero is equal to 1.

If $m < n$, for example if $m = 2$ and $n = 4$,

$$(a \cdot a)/(a \cdot a \cdot a \cdot a) = 1/a^2 = a^{2-4} = a^{-2}$$

that is,

$$a^{-m} = 1/a^m \tag{6}$$

Also if

$$B = a^4$$

and

$$A = a^2$$

$$\sqrt{B} = \sqrt{(a^4)} = \sqrt{(a^2 \cdot a^2)} = \sqrt{((a^2)^2)}$$
$$= \sqrt{(A^2)} = A = a^2 = a^{4/2}$$

So, in general,

$$\sqrt[n]{(a^m)} = a^{m/n} \qquad (7)$$

and

$$\sqrt[n]{(a)} = a^{1/n} \qquad (8)$$

and

$$1/(\sqrt[n]{(am)}) = 1/a^{m/n} = a^{-m/n} \qquad (9)$$

From (9) we see that the exponent (x) of any power can be *any rational number*. It can be shown that x can be any *real number*.

We can also have a power of a power

$$\underbrace{(a \cdot a \cdot a \cdots a)}_{m \text{ times}} \underbrace{(a \cdot a \cdot a \cdots a)}_{m \text{ times}} \cdots \underbrace{(a \cdot a \cdot a \cdots a)}_{m \text{ times}}$$

$$\underbrace{}_{\text{'}n\text{ times'}}$$

$$= \underbrace{a^m \cdot a^m \cdots a^m}_{n \text{ times}} = a^{nm} \qquad (10)$$

or

$$(a^m)^n = a^{mn} \qquad (11)$$

Functions

One of the advantages of using literal symbols is that we can always create new symbols to represent a *sub-set* of operations. By sub-set of operations we mean a collection of operations which have in common the properties of the set plus one or more additional properties. For example, if

$$y = a^n \qquad (11)$$

to obtain the value of y we substitute values for a and n. If $a = 2$ and $n = 3$

$$y = 2^3 = 8$$

For the sake of simplicity let us give a a fixed value 2. Then

$$y = 2^n \qquad (12)$$

Since n can be any real number the relation (12) establishes a relationship between n and y. We can think of this relationship as something that establishes the correspondence between two sets of numbers

y	n
1	*0*
2	*1*
4	*2*
8	*3*
$\vdots$	$\vdots$

For each value (member) of the set represented by n there will be a corresponding value (member) of the set represented by y; y is said to be *a function of* n; n is said to be the argument of y and the whole set represented by n is called the *domain* of y.

The domain of a function may be smaller than the set of real numbers. For example

$$y=\sqrt{a}=a^{1/2}$$

the domain of y does not include any negative real number. Let us suppose that $a=-2$. Then

$$y=(-2)^{1/2}$$

then

$$yy=y^2=((-2)^{1/2})^2=-2^1=-2$$

or

$$yy=-2$$

But the square of a number (y) can *never* be a negative number. If y is positive the square is *positive*, if y is *negative* the square is also positive.

Polynomials

A type of function used very frequently is of the form

$$y=a+bx+cx^2+\cdots+px^n \tag{13}$$

where $a, b, c, d, \ldots, p$ are *constants* and the *variable* is x. This function is called a *polynomial* and is the sum of $(n+1)$ terms. Each term is either a constant or the product of a constant and a variable. The constants are called *coefficients*. Some useful functions are the sum of an infinite number of terms of the general type $a_n x^n$. That is,

$$y=a_0+a_1 x^1+a_2 x^2+\cdots+a_n x^n$$

for $n\rightarrow\infty$. Each term can be obtained from the previous one by a specific rule. For example, the rule might be

$$a_{n+1} x^{n+1}=(a_n x^n)(x/(n+1))$$

Let us assume that the first term is 1, that is,

$$a_0 x^0=1 \quad \text{or} \quad a_0=1$$

Since $x^0=1$, the second term is

$$x/1$$

the third

$$(x/1)(x/2) = x^2/(1 \cdot 2)$$

the fourth

$$(x^2/(1 \cdot 2))(x/3) = x^3/(1 \cdot 2 \cdot 3)$$

and so on.

When we have a product of the type

$$1 \cdot 2 \cdot 3 \cdots n$$

we call it

$n!$ or   *n factorial*

so

$$3! = 3 \cdot 2 \cdot 1$$

Power series

The function

$$y = 1 + x + x^2/2! + x^3/3! \ldots \tag{14}$$

is called a *power series*. A power series is thus a sum of an infinite number of terms in which

each term is a power (x^n)

and where

each term is obtained from the previous one by a given
mathematical rule

The power series in (14) arises when we describe a number of natural processes. For example, a function of this type actually describes the growth of a culture of microorganisms. Let us assume that we have a culture, with plenty of nutrients, which at time zero contains N_0 cells. After a time τ, αN_0 new cells are produced where

$$\alpha > 0$$

Let us also assume that, regardless of the number of cells (N) that exist at any time t, at time $t + \tau$ there will always be $N + \alpha N$ cells. That is, the fractional growth (α) of the number of cells (N) is always the same for the same τ.

So, at different times, the following will occur

Time	Number of bacteria
0	N_0
Δt	$N_0 + \alpha N_0 = N_0(1 + \alpha)$
$2\Delta t$	$(N_0 + \alpha N_0) + \alpha(N_0 + \alpha N_0) = N_0(1 + \alpha)^2$
$\vdots$	$\vdots$
$n\Delta t$	$N_0(1 + \alpha)^n$

Let us call $n\Delta t = t$, so

$$n = t/\Delta t$$

If we measure at short Δt then α will also be smaller so we can assume, as an approximation, that for small Δt, α is proportional to t. So

$$\alpha = a\Delta t$$

where a is the proportionality constant, or

$$\Delta t = \alpha/a$$

so

$$n = at/\alpha$$

So the number of bacteria at t is

$$y = N_0(1 + \alpha)^{at/\alpha}$$

For convenience let us define a quantity β such that

$$\beta = 1/\alpha$$

then

$$y = N_0(1 + 1/\beta)^{\beta at} = N_0[(1 + 1/\beta)^\beta]^{at}$$

Because of the reciprocal relationship between β and α when Δt becomes small, α becomes smaller and β becomes larger. When $t \rightarrow 0$ then $\alpha \rightarrow 0$ and $\beta \rightarrow \infty$. As β increases the term inside the bracket, which is

$$Z = (1 + 1/\beta)^\beta$$

will become 1. This is because

$$1/\beta \rightarrow 0$$

However, β in the exponent becomes infinitely large. But we know that

$$1^n = 1$$

for any n, so, intuitively, we expect the function Z to *tend* to a finite value. To actually calculate Z we need to see how $(1 + 1/\beta)^\beta$ behaves as β increases:

β	$(1 + 1/\beta)^\beta$
1	$(1 + 1/\beta)^1 = 1 + 1 = 2$
2	$(1 + 1/\beta)^2 = 1 + 2(1/\beta) + (1/\beta)^2 = 1 + 1 + \frac{1}{4} = 2\frac{1}{4}$
3	$(1 + 1/\beta)^3 = 1 + 3(1/\beta) + 3(1/\beta)^2 + (1/\beta)^3 = 1 + 1 + \frac{3}{9} + \frac{1}{27}$
	$= 2 + \frac{10}{27}$
4	$(1 + 1/\beta)^4 = 1 + 4(1/\beta) + 6(1/\beta)^2 + 4(1/\beta)^3 + (1/\beta)^4$
	$= 1 + \frac{4}{4} + \frac{6}{16} + \frac{4}{64} + \frac{1}{256}$
	$= 2 + \frac{113}{256}$

and so on. Already there are a number of conclusions that we can draw. The first is that

$$(1 + 1/\beta)^3 = 2 + \text{a term that is smaller than 1}$$

The second is that the coefficient of $(1/\beta)^n$ obeys a certain rule

β		coefficients			
1)		1 1			
2)		1 2 1			
3)		1 3 3 1			
4)		1 4 6 4 1			

The binomial expansion

The first and last coefficients are always one. For the inner coefficients each coefficient is equal to the sum of the two adjacent coefficients in the previous row. The coefficients form a triangle which we can expand as far as we like

1)					1 1					
2)				1 2 1						
3)			1 3 3 1							
4)		1 4 6 4 1								
5)	1 5 10 10 5 1									
6)	1 6 15 20 15 6 1									

(This triangle is known as *Pascal's triangle* after the original discoverer.) Instead of constructing a triangle every time we wish to work out a coefficient it is simpler to obtain a rule. Any coefficient can be calculated once we know the power of the binomial. $(1 + 1/\beta)^n$ is a binomial and n is the power (*or order*) of the binomial. Let us select the case where $\beta = 6$. Then from Pascal's triangle the coefficient of $(1/\beta)^2$ is 15. But 15 is also the value of

$$6!/2!\,(6-2)! = (6\cdot5\cdot4\cdot3\cdot2\cdot1)/(2\cdot1\cdot4\cdot3\cdot2\cdot1) = 15$$

In general, the coefficient of the term of order P of a binomial of order n is

$$a_P = n!/P!\,(n-P)!$$

So

$$(1+\alpha)^\beta = 1 + \alpha\beta!/1!\,(\beta-1)! + \alpha^2\beta!/2!\,(\beta-2)! + \alpha^3\beta!/3!\,(\beta-3)!\ldots$$

$$(14)$$

This is called the *binomial expansion*. It can be shown in the same way that if the binomial has the form $(x+\alpha)^\beta$, then the expansion is

$$(x+\alpha)^\beta = x^\beta + \beta!\,x^{\beta-1}\alpha/1!\,(\beta-1)! + \cdots + \beta!\,x^{\beta-P}\alpha^P/P!\,(\beta-P)!\ldots$$

$$(15)$$

The number e

We are now in a position to compute the value

$$Z = (1 + 1/\beta)^\beta$$

If we substitute $1/\beta$ for α in (14) we obtain

$$Z = (1 + 1/\beta)^\beta = 1 + \beta(1/\beta) + (\beta(\beta-1)/2!)(1/\beta)^2$$
$$+ (\beta(\beta-1)(\beta-2)/3!)(1/\beta)^3 + \cdots$$

The coefficients of this expression are easily derived because

$$\beta!/(\beta-P)! = \beta(\beta-1)(\beta-2)\cdots(\beta-P+1)(\beta-P)!/(\beta-P)!$$
$$= \beta(\beta-1)(\beta-2)\cdots(\beta-P+1)$$

so

$$Z = 1 + 1 + (1/2!)(\beta(\beta-1)/\beta^2) + (1/3!)(\beta(\beta-1)(\beta-2)/\beta^3) + \cdots$$
$$+ (1/P!)(\beta(\beta-1)\cdots(\beta-P+1)/\beta^P)$$

When β is *very* large

$$\beta - 1 \simeq \beta$$
$$\beta - 2 \simeq \beta$$
$$\beta - 3 \simeq \beta \quad \text{etc.}$$

So

$$Z = 1 + 1 + 1/2! + 1/3! + \cdots + 1/P!$$
$$= 1 + (1 + 1/2! + 1/3! + \cdots + 1/P!) \tag{16}$$
$$= 1 + U$$

where

$$U = 1 + 1/2! + 1/3! + \cdots$$

The series represented in (16) might tend to a given value as $P \rightarrow \infty$ or it might not. Although each term added to the series is smaller than the previous one, the term is always positive. This means that Z is larger, the larger the value of P. If we could find a number (N), such that regardless of the number of terms (P) that we use to compute Z where

$$N > Z$$

then Z, as $P \rightarrow \infty$, will reach a finite value.

Let us generate another series T such that

$$T = 1 + 1/2 + 1/2^2 + 1/2^3 + \cdots + 1/2^P$$

If we define

$$a = 1/2$$

Then

$$T = 1 + a + a^2 + \cdots + a^P$$

If we compare T with U we can establish a correspondence between the terms of Z and of T

$$T = 1 + 1/2 + 1/(2 \times 2) + 1/(2 \times 2 \times 2) + \cdots$$
$$U = 1 + 1/2 + 1/(2 \times 3) + 1/(2 \times 3 \times 4) + \cdots$$

we can see that for each term U we can generate a term in T and from the third term onwards all the terms of T are larger than the corresponding terms of U. So

$$T > U$$

We can now show that as P tends to infinity, T tends to a finite number. If

$$T = 1 + a + a^2 + a^3 + \cdots + a^P$$

then aT is given by

$$aT = a + a^2 + a^3 + a^4 + \cdots + a^{P+1}$$

If we subtract T from aT we obtain

$$aT - T = T(a-1) = a^{P+1} - 1$$

or

$$T = \frac{a^{P+1} - 1}{a - 1} = \frac{1 - a^{P+1}}{1 - a}$$

when $P \to \infty$, since $a = 1/2$

$$a^{P+1} = (\tfrac{1}{2})^{P+1} \to 0$$

so

$$T = \frac{1}{1-a} = \frac{1}{1 - \frac{1}{2}} = 2$$

$$P \to \infty$$

We can say that *the limit* of T when P *tends to infinity* is 2.

The limit means that if we want to calculate T with an error that is less than a given value (0.001, for example) we can select a value of P such that

$$2 - (1 - a^{P+1})/(1-a) < 0.001$$

Since

$$a = 1/2$$

then

$$2 - 2 + 2a^{P+1} < 0.001$$

or

$$a^{P+1} < 0.0005$$

or

$$(1/2)^{P+1} < 0.0005$$

For $P = 10$

$$(\tfrac{1}{2})^{11} = 0.000488$$

Since we have shown that T is larger than U when P tends to infinity, then

$$U < 2$$

and

$$Z = 1 + U$$

so

$$Z < 1 + T = 3$$

The value of Z, which is an irrational number, is called e. It has been calculated to many decimal figures and is

$$e = 1 + 1 + 1/2! + 1/3! + \cdots + 1/n! \quad (n \to \infty)$$

The exponential

If we now return to the bacterial growth which was described by the formula

$$Y = N_0[(1 + 1/\beta)^{\beta}]^{at}$$

when $\Delta t \to 0$ and $\beta \to \infty$ then

$$Y = N_0 e^{at} = N_0 \exp(at) \tag{17}$$

the function e^{at} which can be written as

$$e^x = \exp(x) \tag{18}$$

is called an *exponential function*. If we substitute (18) into (17) and rearrange, we obtain

$$(Y/N_0) = \exp(x) \tag{19}$$

If we use equation (17)

$$Y = N_0 \exp(at)$$

and make $t = 1$

$$Y = N_0 \exp(a) \quad \text{or} \quad Y/N_0 = \exp(a)$$

then a is known as the fractional growth per unit time and has the dimension time^{-1}. Let us call

$$T = 1/a$$

then

$$Y = N_0 \exp(t/T)$$

and T is called the *time constant*.

The exponential function provides an example where we have an exponent (x) which can be *any real number*. However, we do not as yet know how to deal with numbers like

$$e^{1.3}$$

This means that e is to be multiplied by itself 1.3 times. Let us go back to the original function Y

$$Y = N_0(1 + 1/\beta)^{\beta x}$$

where $x = at$, and expand it following the binomial rule, then

$$Y = N_0[1 + (1/\beta)\beta x + (1/2!)\beta x(\beta x - 1)/\beta^2$$
$$+ (1/3!)\beta x(\beta x - 1)(\beta x - 2)/\beta^3 + \cdots]$$
$$= N_0[1 + (\beta/\beta)x + (1/2!)(\beta/\beta)x((\beta/\beta)x - 1/\beta)$$
$$+ (1/3!)(\beta/\beta)x((\beta/\beta)x - 1/\beta)((\beta/\beta)x - 2/\beta) + \cdots]$$
$$= N_0[1 + x + (1/2!)x(x - 1/\beta) + (1/3!)x(x - 1/\beta)(x - 2/\beta) + \cdots]$$

When $\beta \rightarrow \infty$ all the terms containing β become negligible. So
$$Y = N_0[1 + x + x^2/2! + x^3/3! + \cdots] \tag{20}$$
If we compare (19) with (20) we see that
$$\exp(x) = 1 + x + x^2/2! + x^3/3! + \cdots \tag{21}$$

Relation (21) is an example of a series expansion of a function. With this expansion we can now compute e^x for any value of x since we can compute

$$x^n$$

for any real value of x when n is an integer. The accuracy of the calculation will depend upon the number of terms of the series used in the calculation. Expression (21) was used in the construction of published tables of e^x.

(The exponential function e^x corresponds to the group of *transcendental functions*. In a transcendental function (y) the value of the function *cannot* be calculated from the value of the *argument* (x) by a *finite number of calculations*.)

If we plot the exponential function (e^x) versus the argument (x) (see Figure A2.1a), we see that the function

is always positive

tends to zero when $x \rightarrow -\infty$, and

tends to ∞ when $x \rightarrow \infty$

Fig.A2.1

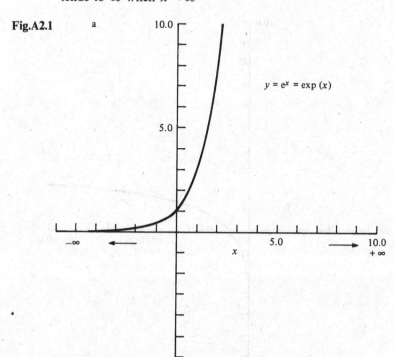

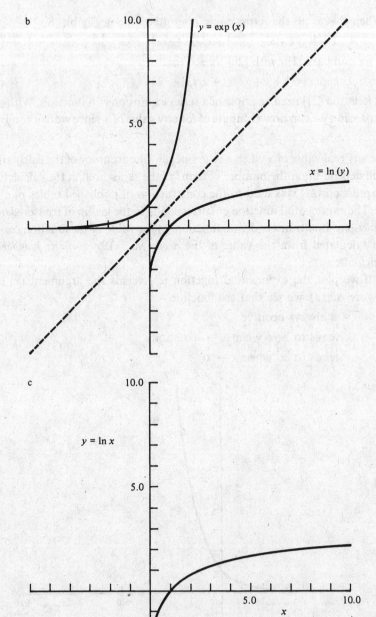

We can now define another function that is related to the exponential function in such a way that

$$x = f(y)$$

The logarithm

This notation means that x is a function of y, in which the y and x of the exponential function have now interchanged their roles. The function f is called the *inverse* function of the *exponential function* and is known as the *natural logarithm*. So if

$$y = \exp(x) \quad \text{then} \quad x = \ln(y)$$

x is thus the value to which e has to be raised so that

$$e^{\ln(y)} = e^x = y$$

Since we normally represent the function by y and the argument by x, the usual way to write the logarithm function is

$$y = \ln(x) \tag{22}$$

In order to plot this ln function, we simply rotate the x and y axes around a line at 45 degrees across the first and the third quadrants (Figure A.21b). Since the exponential can never be negative and recalling that

$$x = \exp(y) \tag{23}$$

the logarithm of a negative number cannot exist. On the other hand, the exponential (x in this case) is zero when the exponent (y) tends to ∞. This means that the logarithm (y) tends to ∞ when $x \to 0$. This is shown in Figure A2.1c where the curve becomes more and more negative as $x \to 0$. Figure A2.1c also shows that $\ln(x)$ is zero when $x = 1$, since

$$\exp(0) = e^0 = 1$$

For values of x smaller than 1, $\ln(x)$ is negative. When y is negative

$$x = e^{-y} = \exp(-y) = 1/\exp(y) < 1$$

From the definition of the logarithm of the number x we see that

$$x = \exp(y) = \exp(\ln(x)) = e^{\ln(x)} \tag{24}$$

That is, any number (x) is equal to e raised to its logarithm ($\ln(x)$). We should now be able to deduce the rules for operating with logarithms. Let us suppose that we have two numbers (x_1, x_2) and their logarithms (y_1, y_2). Then by definition

$$x_1 = \exp(y_1) \quad \text{or} \quad \ln(x_1) = y_1$$
$$x_2 = \exp(y_2) \quad \text{or} \quad \ln(x_2) = y_2$$
$$x_1 x_2 = \exp(y_1)\exp(y_2) = \exp(y_1 + y_2)$$

If we apply logarithms to both sides

$$\ln(x_1 x_2) = y_1 + y_2 = \ln(x_1) + \ln(x_2) \tag{25}$$

That is, the logarithm of a product is equal to the sum of the logarithms.
In general

$$\ln(x_1 \times x_2 \times \cdots \times x_i) = \ln(x_1) + \ln(x_2) + \cdots + \ln(x_i)$$
$$= \sum_{i=1}^{i=n} \ln(x_i)$$

Thus $\sum_{i=1}^{i=n} \ln(x_i)$ is an abbreviated form of saying the sum of n terms in which each of the terms is obtained by substituting for i with $1, 2, \ldots, n$, successively.

The logarithm of a ratio can be obtained in a similar way

$$x_1/x_2 = \exp(y_1)/\exp(y_2) = \exp(y_1 - y_2)$$

or

$$\ln(x_1/x_2) = y_1 - y_2 = \ln(x_1) - \ln(x_2) \tag{26}$$

The logarithm of a power can also be obtained very easily

$$(x)^n = \exp(y)^n = \exp(ny)$$

so

$$\ln(x^n) = ny = n \ln(x) \tag{27}$$

Although we have been using equations (22) and (23) for the definition of the logarithm of a number, it is possible to generalize the definition of a logarithm in the following way. If

$$x = a^y \tag{28}$$

where

$$y = \log_a(x) \tag{29}$$

We say that y is the logarithm of x to the base a. A base which is frequently used is 10. So

$$y = \log_{10}(x) \tag{30}$$

where

$$x = 10^y \tag{31}$$

The symbol log usually means a decimal logarithm. If we know the logarithm (y_1) of a number x in the base a, we can convert it into the logarithm (y_2) of the same number in the base b for

$$x = a^{y_1} = b^{y_2}$$

From (27)

$$\log_a(x) = y_1 = y_2 \log_a(b) = \log_a(b) \log_b(x)$$

or

$$\log_b(x) = y_1 \log_b(a) = \log_b(a) \log_a(x) \tag{32}$$

$\log_a$ functions are transcendental functions, and at least two of them (ln and $\log_{10}$) are tabulated or are available on calculators and thus can readily be used.

Logarithms are useful when we want to compute powers of numbers. For example, if we want to compute N defined by

$$N = 2.5^5$$

we compute

$$y = \log N = 5 \log 2.5$$

since log 2.5 can be obtained from tables, or with a calculator, we calculate the value of $y(\log N)$, which would be approximately 1.1. The antilog of y (that is, 10^y) can then be obtained by reading from the tables or using a calculator.

Log functions can also be used to linearize graphs, that is, to convert curved graphic representation into straight lines. For example, the radioactive decay of isotopes is described by the function

$$Q = Q_0 \exp(-kt)$$

where Q is the amount of radioisotope at time t, and Q_0 is the amount of radioisotope at time zero, and k is a constant (with dimensions of time^{-1}) characteristic for each radioisotope. If we take natural logarithm (ln) of both sides we obtain

$$\underbrace{\ln(Q)}_{y} = \underbrace{\ln(Q_0)}_{a} \underbrace{-kt}_{b}$$

and this is a straight line of the form

$$y = a + bt$$

which is much easier to plot, requiring only two points. Also equations of the form

$$y = x^n$$

can be treated in a similar way. So

$$\underbrace{\ln(y)}_{T} = \underbrace{n \ln(x)}_{U}$$

or

$$T = nU$$

The linearized equation is a straight line through the origin with slope n. If we know the values of x and y (from an experiment) we can obtain n from the graph. When we derived the exponential function we saw that it could be written as

$$y = \exp(at)$$

where a is the fractional rate of change per unit time.

If we apply natural logarithms we obtain

$$\ln(y) = at$$

which is the fractional rate of change of y per unit time, multiplied by t, the time interval. The fractional rate of change of y may be written, approximately, as

$$\frac{\Delta y}{y} \begin{array}{l} \leftarrow\text{change} \\ \leftarrow\text{absolute value} \end{array}\Big\} \begin{array}{l} \text{change as a fraction of} \\ \text{the absolute value} \end{array}$$

The ratio $\Delta y/y$ is only an *approximation* because the value of Δy is obtained from subtracting the value of y (y_2) at some time (t_2), from the value of y (y_1) at some time earlier (t_1) and so the value of y in the denominator is undefined. It might be, for example, y_1, y_2, or some intermediate value. So

$$\Delta y/y \approx \ln(y) = at$$

Derivatives

In Figure A2.2a we represent the function y. We also represent the value of Δy_1 corresponding to t_1, t_2. As we move along the t axis we see that for the same time interval we obtain a larger Δy (Δy_2). That is, although

$$t_2 - t_1 = t_4 - t_3 = \Delta t = \text{constant}$$

$$\Delta y_1 \neq \Delta y_2$$

because the y curve grows steeper as we move along t. If we compute the ratio $\Delta y/\Delta t$ we can have a measure of the *degree* of steepness of the curve. In Figure A2.2b we have magnified the curve in the interval y_1, y_2. The ratio $\Delta y_1/\Delta t$ is the slope (α) of the straight line connecting (y_1, t_1) to (y_2, t_2) where (y_1, t_1) means a point with coordinates y_1 and t_1. If we select a smaller value of Δy $(\Delta y')$ we see from the figure that we also have a different value of α (α'). However, if we keep decreasing the values of Δt and Δy their ratio will tend to a value corresponding to the *tangent* of the curve at $t = t_1$.

To obtain the slope of the tangent let us define y as

$$y = \exp(t)$$

and $y + \Delta y$ as

$$y + \Delta y = \exp(t + \Delta t) = \exp(t)\exp(\Delta t)$$

then

$$y + \Delta y - y = \Delta y = \exp(t + \Delta t) - \exp(t) = \exp(t)(\exp(\Delta t) - 1)$$

so

$$\Delta y/\Delta t = \exp(t)(\exp(\Delta t) - 1)/\Delta t$$

But by (21)

$$\exp(\Delta t) = 1 + \Delta t + (\Delta t)^2/2! + \cdots$$

so

$$\Delta y/\Delta t = \exp(t)[(1 + \Delta t + (\Delta t)^2/2! + \cdots - 1)/\Delta t]$$

so

$$\Delta y/\Delta t = \exp(t)(1 + \Delta t/2! + \Delta t^2/3! + \cdots)$$

But when $\Delta t \to 0$ the right-hand side tends to e^t. That is,

$$\lim(\Delta y/\Delta t) = \exp(t)$$

when

$$\Delta t \to 0$$

This means that although both Δy and Δt tend to zero when $\Delta t \to 0$ the ratio $\Delta y/\Delta t$ tends to e^t, that is, to y. We can think of the calculation of $\Delta y/\Delta t$

Fig.A2.2

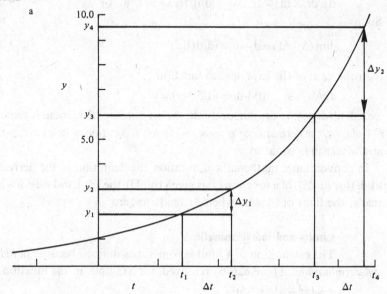

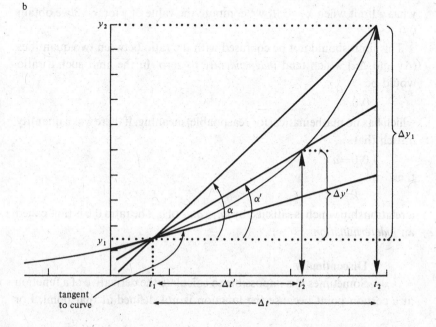

when t tends to zero as *an operation* which is called *differentiation* and is defined as

$$\underset{\substack{\text{limit of}\nearrow \quad \text{when}}}{\lim(\Delta y/\Delta t)_{\Delta t \to 0}}$$

The operation is represented itself by the symbols

$$\mathrm{d}y/\mathrm{d}t, \quad \mathrm{d}(y)/\mathrm{d}t \quad \text{or} \quad (\mathrm{d}/\mathrm{d}t)(y) \quad \text{or} \quad \dot{y} \quad \text{or} \quad y'$$

So

$$\lim_{\Delta t \to 0}(\Delta y/\Delta t) = \mathrm{d}y/\mathrm{d}t = (\mathrm{d}/\mathrm{d}t)(y) \tag{33}$$

In the case of the exponential function

$$\mathrm{d}y/\mathrm{d}t \quad \text{or} \quad \mathrm{d}(y)/\mathrm{d}t = (\mathrm{d}/\mathrm{d}t)(y) = y \tag{34}$$

we call $(\mathrm{d}/\mathrm{d}t)(y)$, or $\mathrm{d}(y)/\mathrm{d}t$, or $\mathrm{d}y/\mathrm{d}t$, the *derivative* of the function y and, as (34) shows, the *derivative of a function is itself a function* since y is a function and $(\mathrm{d}/\mathrm{d}t)(y)$ is equal to y.

In conventional mathematical notation the definition of the derivative $(\mathrm{d}/\mathrm{d}t)$ (or $(\mathrm{d}/\mathrm{d}x)$) of a function (y) is given by (33), the left-hand side of which reads: the limit of $(\Delta y/\Delta t)$ when Δt tends to zero.

Limits and indeterminations

The calculation of a limit is sometimes difficult because of *hidden indeterminations*. These can be removed, for example, in the function

$$y = (x^2 - q)/(x - 3)$$

y has a limit when $x \to 3$. If we compute the value of y for $x = 3$ we obtain $0/0$.

This limit should not be confused with the ratio between two quantities (Δy and Δx) which tend *independently* to zero. In the limit such a ratio would be

$$0/0$$

which has no mathematical (or reasonable) meaning. If there was a quantity a such that

$$0/0 = a$$

then

$$0 = 0a$$

a relationship which is satisfied by *any value* of a. The ratio $0/0$ is thus called an *indetermination*.

Discontinuity

Sometimes it is impossible to calculate the derivative of a function at a certain point because the function is not defined at that point. For example

$$Y=1/(x-2)$$

is not defined at $x=2$ for this

$$Y=1/0 \quad \text{or} \quad 0Y=1$$

But there is no value of Y which multiplied by zero will be equal to one. It is also not possible either to calculate the limit of Y when $x \rightarrow 2$. If we substitute x by values that are slightly smaller or slightly larger than 2 (i.e. 1.99 or 2.01) as these values approach 2 (1.99, 1.999, 1.9999, etc., or 2.01, 2.001, 2.0001, 2.00001, etc.) Y never ceases to increase, that is,

$$\lim_{x \rightarrow 2}(Y) \rightarrow \infty$$

Functions of this type are called *discontinuous*. A discontinuous function may have one discontinuity (2 in the example above) or more, and they cannot be differentiated at their points of discontinuity.

Some rules of differentiation

The *exponential* is the only function which *is equal to its derivative*. The logical steps we followed in order to obtain the derivative of $\exp(t)$ can also be used to obtain the derivative of *any* function. To re-cap, these steps are

(1) we give an increment Δx to the independent variable (x, t, etc.) to obtain:
(2) the new value ($y+\Delta y$) for the function (Y),
(3) we then compute Δy, which is given by $(y+\Delta y)-y$,
(4) then we compute the ratio between the two increments $\Delta y/\Delta x$ or $\Delta y/\Delta t$, and
(5) finally we compute the limit of this ratio when Δx (or Δt) tends to zero, $\Delta y/\Delta x$ or $\Delta y/\Delta t$, that is,

$$\lim_{\Delta x \rightarrow 0}(\Delta y/\Delta x)$$

Let us apply these rules to the differentiation of the derivative of an *inverse function*.

If y is a function of x, that is,

$$y=f(x)$$

then the inverse function $\phi(y)$ will be

$$x=\phi(y)$$

For example

$$y=x^2 \quad \text{and} \quad x=\pm\sqrt{y}$$

From (28) and (29) and when $a = e$

$$y = \ln(x) \tag{28a}$$

and

$$x = \exp(y) \tag{29a}$$

Differentiation of ln(x)

In (29a) x is now the function and y is the independent variable. So if in (34) we substitute dx for dy and dy for dt and x for y we obtain

$$dx/dy = x$$

If in (28a) we give an increment Δx to x we obtain an increment Δy. That is,

$$y + \Delta y = \ln(x + \Delta x)$$

So

$$\Delta y = \ln(x + \Delta x) - \ln(x)$$
$$= \ln((x + \Delta x)/x) = \ln(1 + \Delta x/x)$$

then

$$\Delta y/\Delta x = \ln(1 + \Delta x/x)/\Delta x$$
$$= (1/\Delta x) \ln(1 + \Delta x/x)$$
$$= \ln[(1 + \Delta x/x)^{1/\Delta x}]$$

But from (14) when $\beta = 1/\Delta x$ and $\alpha = \Delta x/x$

$$(1 + \Delta x/x)^{+1/\Delta x} = 1 + [(1/\Delta x)!/(1/\Delta x - 1)!](\Delta x/x)$$
$$+ [(1/\Delta x)!/(2!(1/\Delta x - 2)!)](\Delta x/x)^2 + \cdots$$
$$= 1 + (1/\Delta x)(\Delta x/x) + (1/\Delta x)(1/\Delta x - 1)(\Delta x/x)^2/2 + \cdots$$
$$= 1 + 1/x + [(1 - \Delta x)\Delta x/\Delta x]/(2!)(x^2) + \cdots$$

But when $\Delta x \to 0$

$$(1 - \Delta x) \to 1$$

so

$$\lim[(1 + \Delta x/x)^{1/\Delta x}] = 1 + 1/x + (1/2!)(1/x)^2 + \cdots = \exp(1/x)$$

so

$$\lim_{\Delta x \to 0} (\Delta y/\Delta x) = \lim_{\Delta x \to 0} (\ln(1 + \Delta x/x)/\Delta x)$$

$$= \lim_{\Delta x \to 0} [\ln(1 + \Delta x/x)^{1/\Delta x}]$$

$$= \ln[\exp(1/x)] = 1/x = (d/dx) \ln(x)$$

or

$$d(\ln(x))/dx = 1/x \tag{35}$$

Derivative of an inverse function

This result can be obtained in a more general way for inverse functions. Let us return to (28a) and (29a).

$$y = \ln(x) \tag{28a}$$
$$x = \exp(y) \tag{29a}$$

From (29a) and (34)

$$d(x)/dy = x = \lim_{\Delta x \to 0} (\Delta x / \Delta y)$$

But

$$\Delta y / \Delta x = 1/(\Delta x / \Delta y)$$

then

$$\lim_{\Delta x \to 0} (\Delta y / \Delta x) = \lim_{\Delta x \to 0} (1/(\Delta x / \Delta y))$$

Since when $\Delta y \to 0$, $\Delta x \to 0$ is also given by

$$\lim_{\Delta x \to 0} (\Delta y / \Delta x) = \lim_{\Delta y \to 0} (1/(\Delta x / \Delta y))$$

and the numerator is constant so

$$\lim_{\Delta y \to 0} (\Delta x / \Delta y) = d(x)/dy$$

and

$$\lim_{\Delta x \to 0} (\Delta y / \Delta x) = d(y)/dx = 1/(d(x)/dy)$$

If we know the derivative (dx/dy) of the inverse function (x) of another function (y), the derivative of y is simply the reciprocal of the derivative of the inverse function.

In the case of (28a)

$$d(y)/dx = 1/(d(x)/dy)$$

But from (29a)

$$d(x)/dy = x$$

so

$$d(y)/dx = 1/x = (d/dx)(\ln(x))$$

which is the same result as (35).

The derivative of a constant

The derivative (dy/dx) of a function $y(x)$ at a point (x) of the function is thus the slope of the tangent of the curve at that point. The derivative of a function is also a function of x. The derivative of a constant, that is, the derivative of the function $y = a$, is thus zero, since the slope of the line $y = a$ is zero (see Figure A2.3). So

$$d(y)/dx = d(a)/dx = 0 \tag{36}$$

Let us now apply the steps of differentiation as laid out on page 285 to a number of different functions.

The derivative of powers of x

$y = x$

Steps 1 and 2

$$y + \Delta y = x + \Delta x = y + \Delta x$$

so

$$\Delta y = \Delta x \quad \text{(step 3)}$$

By step 4

$$\Delta y / \Delta x = 1$$

and

$$\lim_{\Delta x \to 0} (\Delta y / \Delta x) = 1$$

so if $y = x$

$$d(y)/dx = 1 \tag{37}$$

$$y = x^2$$

$$y + \Delta y = (x + \Delta x)^2 = x^2 + 2x\,\Delta x + \Delta x^2$$

or

$$y + \Delta y = y + 2x\,\Delta x + \Delta x^2$$

so

$$\Delta y = 2x\,\Delta x + \Delta x^2$$

By step 4

$$\Delta y / \Delta x = 2x + \Delta x$$

When $\Delta x \to 0$ then

$$\lim(\Delta y / \Delta x) = 2x$$

so

$$d(x^2)/dx = 2x \tag{38}$$

$$y = x^3$$

$$y + \Delta y = (x + \Delta x)^3$$

Fig.A2.3

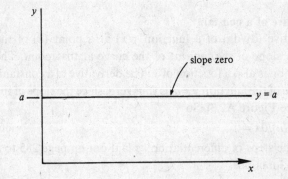

slope zero

$y = a$

a

By the binomial expansion

$$y + \Delta y = x^3 + 3x^2 \, \Delta x + 3x \, \Delta x^2 + \Delta x^3$$
$$= y + 3x^2 \, \Delta x + 3x \, \Delta x^2 + \Delta x^3$$

So

$$\Delta y = 3x^2 \, \Delta x + 3x \, \Delta x^2 + \Delta x^3$$

or

$$\Delta y / \Delta x = 3x^2 + 3x \, \Delta x + \Delta x^2$$

When $\Delta x \rightarrow 0$

$$\lim(\Delta y / \Delta x) = 3x^2$$

or

$$d(x^3)/dx = 3x^2 \tag{39}$$

We can now compare (37), (38) and (39)

$$(d/dx)(x^1) = 1x^0 \tag{37}$$
$$(d/dx)(x^2) = 2x^1 \tag{38}$$
$$(d/dx)(x^3) = 3x^2 \tag{39}$$

and obtain a general rule for differentiation of x raised to the power n

$$(d/dx)(x^n) = nx^{n-1} \tag{40}$$

The derivative of a constant times a function

$$y = ax$$
$$y + \Delta y = a(x + \Delta x)$$
$$= ax + a \, \Delta x$$
$$= y + a \, \Delta x$$

or

$$\Delta y = a \, \Delta x$$

So

$$\Delta y / \Delta x = a$$

and

$$\lim(\Delta y / \Delta x) = a = \underbrace{a1x^0}_{(d/dx)(x^1)}$$

so

$$d(ax)/dx = a \, d(x)/dx$$

or in general

$$d(ay)/dx = a \, d(y)/dx \tag{41}$$

The derivative of the sum of two functions

$$y = x + x^2$$
$$y + \Delta y = x + \Delta x + (x + \Delta x)^2$$
$$= x + \Delta x + x^2 + 2x \, \Delta x + \Delta x^2$$

or
$$\Delta y = \Delta x + 2x\,\Delta x + \Delta x^2$$
so
$$\Delta y/\Delta x = 1 + 2x + \Delta x$$
and
$$\lim_{\Delta x \to 0} (\Delta y/\Delta x) = 1 + 2x = d(x)/dx + d(x^2)/dx$$

In general, if
$$y = f(x) \quad (y \text{ is a function of } x)$$
and
$$z = \phi(x) \quad (z \text{ is also a function of } x)$$
then
$$(d/dx)(y+z) = d(y)/dx + d(z)/dx \qquad (42)$$
the derivative of the sum   sum of the derivatives

Product differentiation

Let us assume that we have a function z which is the product of two functions of x (y and T). That is,
$$y = f(x) \text{ (example: } x^2) \quad \text{and} \quad T = \phi(x) \text{ (example } \exp(x))$$
and so
$$z = yT \quad (\text{or } x^2 \exp(x))$$
If we now make an increment Δx to x, there will be an increment Δy to y and an increment ΔT to T. So
$$z + \Delta z = (y + \Delta y)(T + \Delta T)$$
$$= yT + y\,\Delta T + \Delta y T + \Delta y\,\Delta T$$
$$= z + y\,\Delta T + \Delta y T + \Delta y\,\Delta T$$
or
$$\Delta z = y\,\Delta T + T\,\Delta y + \Delta y\,\Delta T$$
If we now divide both sides of the equation by Δx we obtain
$$\Delta z/\Delta x = y(\Delta T/\Delta x) + T(\Delta y/\Delta x) + \Delta T(\Delta y/\Delta x)$$
When $\Delta x \to 0$, then $\Delta T \to 0$, $\Delta y \to 0$ and $\Delta z \to 0$, so
$$\lim_{\Delta x \to 0} (\Delta z/\Delta x) = d(z)/dx$$
and
$$\lim_{\Delta x \to 0} (\Delta y/\Delta x) = d(y)/dx$$
and
$$\lim_{\Delta x \to 0} (\Delta T/\Delta x) = d(T)/dx$$

However,

$$\lim_{\Delta x \to 0} ((\Delta y/\Delta x)\,\Delta T) = 0$$

$$\downarrow \qquad \downarrow$$

$$\mathrm{d}(y)/\mathrm{d}x \qquad 0$$

so, the rule for the differentiation of a product is

$$\mathrm{d}(z)/\mathrm{d}x = \mathrm{d}(yT)/\mathrm{d}x = y\,\mathrm{d}(T)/\mathrm{d}x + T\,\mathrm{d}(y)/\mathrm{d}x \qquad (43)$$

The chain rule

If we have two functions z and T and

$$z = f(T) \quad \text{and} \quad T = \phi(x)$$

then $z = f(\phi(x))$ is said to be a function (f) of a function (ϕ). For example,

$$z = \exp(T) = f(t) \quad \text{and} \quad T = ax = \phi(x)$$

so when we make an increment to x (Δx) there will be an increment in T (ΔT). For example,

$$T + \Delta T = a(x + \Delta x)$$
$$= ax + a\,\Delta x$$

or

$$\Delta T = a\,\Delta x$$

But corresponding to an increment Δt there is an increment Δz. That is,

$$z + \Delta z = \exp(T + \Delta T) = \exp(T)\exp(\Delta T)$$

or

$$\Delta z = \exp(T)\exp(\Delta T) - z$$
$$= \exp(T)(\exp(\Delta T) - 1)$$

We want to find

$$\lim(\Delta z/\Delta x)$$

when

$$\Delta x \to 0$$

We first form the product

$$(\Delta z/\Delta T)(\Delta T/\Delta x)$$

This product is equal to $\Delta z/\Delta x$, so

$$(\Delta z/\Delta x) = (\Delta z/\Delta T)(\Delta T/\Delta x)$$

or

$$\lim_{\Delta x \to 0} (\Delta z/\Delta x) = \lim_{\Delta x \to 0} ((\Delta z/\Delta T)(\Delta T/\Delta x))$$

But when

$$\Delta x \to 0 \quad \text{then} \quad \Delta T \to 0$$

so

$$\lim_{\Delta x \to 0} (\Delta z/\Delta x) = \lim_{\substack{\Delta x \to 0 \\ \Delta T \to 0}} ((\Delta z/\Delta T)(\Delta T/\Delta x))$$

$$\mathrm{d}(z)/\mathrm{d}T \quad \mathrm{d}(T)/\mathrm{d}x$$

Using an example

$$\Delta z/\Delta x = \exp(T)(\overbrace{(\exp(\Delta T) - 1)/\Delta T)}^{\Delta z/\Delta T} \overbrace{a(\Delta x/\Delta x)}^{\Delta T/\Delta x}$$

If we expand $\exp(\Delta T)$ and cancel $\Delta x/\Delta x$ we obtain

$$= \exp(T)((1 + \Delta T + \Delta T^2/2! + \cdots - 1)/\Delta T)a$$
$$= \exp(T)((\Delta T + \Delta T^2/2! + \cdots)/\Delta T)a$$
$$= \exp(T)(1 + \Delta T/2! + \Delta T^2/3! + \cdots)a$$

then

$$\lim_{\Delta x \to 0} (\Delta z/\Delta x) = \lim_{\substack{\Delta T \to 0 \\ \Delta x \to 0}} [\exp(T)(1 + \Delta T/2! + \Delta T^2/3! + \cdots]a$$

$$0 \qquad 0 \qquad 0$$

$$= \exp(T)a$$
$$= \underbrace{\exp(ax)a}$$

$$\left(\begin{array}{c} \text{derivative of } e^T \\ \text{in relation to } T \end{array} \right) \quad \begin{array}{c} \text{derivative of } T(ax) \\ \text{in relation to } x \end{array}$$

So if

$$z = f(T) \quad \text{and} \quad T = \phi(x)$$
$$\mathrm{d}(z)/\mathrm{d}x = (\mathrm{d}(z)/\mathrm{d}(T))(\mathrm{d}(T)/\mathrm{d}x) \tag{44}$$

Quotient differentiation

Equation (44) describes the so-called 'chain rule'. Along with (40), (43) and (44) we can now derive the derivative of the ratio between any two functions of x. Let us assume that

$$T = f(x) \quad \text{and} \quad y = \phi(x)$$

and that

$$z = T/y$$

By equation (6)

$$z = Ty^{-1}$$

From equation (43)

$$\mathrm{d}(z)/\mathrm{d}x = y^{-1}(\mathrm{d}(T)/\mathrm{d}x) + T(\mathrm{d}(y^{-1})/\mathrm{d}x)$$

By equations (40) and (44)

$$d(y^{-1})/dx = (-1)y^{-2}(d(y)/dx)$$

$$\underbrace{\qquad\qquad\qquad}$$
$$(d(y^{-1})/dy)$$

So

$$d(z)/dx = y^{-1}(d(T)/dx) - Ty^{-2}(d(y)/dx)$$
$$= (d(T)/dx)/y - (T(d(y)/dx))/y^2$$

so

$$d(z)/dx = (d/dx)(T/y) = (y(d(T)/dx) - T(d(y)/dx))/y^2 \qquad (45)$$

Differentiation of implicit functions

Equation (45) can be used to obtain the derivative of an *implicit function* (an *implicit function* is a function where dependent (x) and independent variables (y) are not separated). Let us consider the function

$$y \exp(x) + y^2 x + 3 = 0$$

If we differentiate both sides of this equation we obtain for the right-hand side

$$d(0)/dx = 0 \qquad\qquad \text{derivative of a constant}$$

and for the left-hand side

$$(d/dx)(y \exp(x) + y^2 x + 3) \qquad\qquad \text{derivative of a sum}$$
$$= (d/dx)(y \exp(x)) + (d/dx)(y^2 x) + d(3)/dx$$

But

$$(d/dx)(y \exp(x)) = \exp(x)(d(y)/dx) + y(d/dx)(\exp(x))$$
$$= \exp(x)(d(y)/dx) + y \exp(x)$$
$$\qquad\qquad\qquad \text{derivative of a product}$$
$$(d/dx)(y^2 x) = x(d(y^2)/dx) + y^2(d(x)/dx)$$
$$\qquad\qquad\qquad \text{derivative of a product}$$

But

$$d(y^2)/dx = 2y(d(y)/dx) \qquad\qquad \text{derivatives of a function } (y^2)$$
$$\qquad\qquad\qquad\qquad\qquad \text{of a function } (y)$$

so

$$(d/dx)(y^2 x) = 2xy(d(y)/dx) + y^2$$

Finally

$$d(3)/dx = 0 \qquad\qquad \text{derivative of a constant}$$

So

$$(d/dx)(y \exp(x) + y^2 x + 3)$$
$$= \exp(x)(d(y)/dx) + y \exp(x) + 2x(d(y)/dx) + y^2 = 0$$

If we collect terms in d(y)/dx,

$$(\mathrm{d}(y)/\mathrm{d}x)(\exp(x)+2x)+y\exp(x)+y^2=0$$

or

$$\mathrm{d}(y)/\mathrm{d}x=-(y\exp(x)+y^2)/(\exp(x)+2x)$$

From this example it should be clear that there are no fixed rules that apply to the differentiation of implicit functions. Generally, one applies the rules of differentiation to each of the terms and finally one collects terms with reference to d(y)/dx.

The differential coefficient as a ratio

The differential of a function can be thought of as an *operator*. That is, as something which acts on a function to generate another function.

$$f(x) \xrightarrow{\text{differentiation}} f'(x) \quad (\text{or } \mathrm{d}(f(x))/\mathrm{d}x)$$

In geometrical terms differentiation generates a function ($f'(x)$) which gives the value of the tangent of $f(x)$ for every value of x. Let us consider the function

$$y=x^3$$

Fig.A2.4

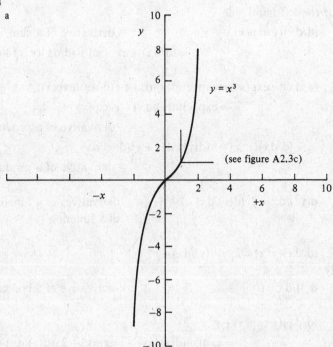

a

$y = x^3$

(see figure A2.3c)

This function is plotted in Figure A2.4a and its derivative (dy/dx) is represented in Figure A2.4b.

$$\mathrm{d}(y)/\mathrm{d}x = 3x^2$$

Differentials

In Figure A2.4c, we have plotted y for x between 1 and 1.5 and dy/dx for $x=1$. For values of $x \geqslant 1$ and near $x=1$ the function can be

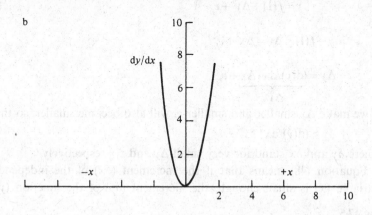

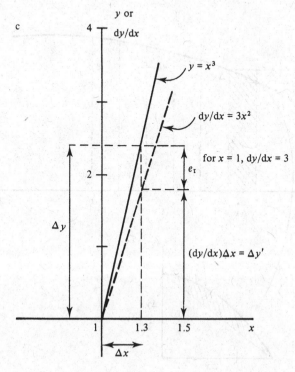

described by

$$y = f(x) = f(1) + \Delta y \tag{46}$$

Where $f(1)$ is the value of the function $(f(x))$ for $x = 1$. We represented in the figure the value of Δy (1.2) when $\Delta x = 0.3$. Figure A2.4c also shows the value of Δy we would obtain $(\Delta y')$ if instead of the function we had used its derivative. That is, if for $x \gg 1$ (and near 1) we approximate the function by a (straight line) tangent to the function. At $x = 1$ we can see that

$$y = f(1) + \Delta y' + e_r \tag{47}$$

So

$$y - f(1) = \Delta y = \Delta y' + e_r$$

or

$$\Delta y = \underbrace{(\mathrm{d}(y)/\mathrm{d}x) \, \Delta x}_{\Delta y'} + e_r$$

If we make Δx smaller and smaller e_r will also become smaller, so that

$$\delta y \approx (\mathrm{d}(y)/\mathrm{d}x) \, \delta x \tag{48}$$

where δy and δx stand for very small Δy and Δx respectively.

Equation (48) means that if the increment (δx) of the independent variable (x) is small enough, the increment (δy) of the function (y) is

Fig.A2.5

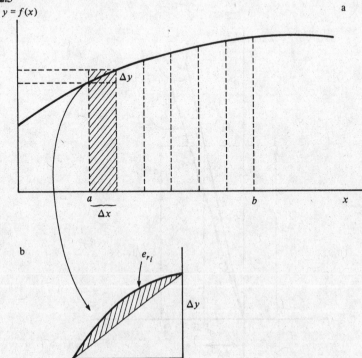

proportional to δx and this proportionality factor is the derivative of the function $(\mathrm{d}(y)/\mathrm{d}x)$ at that point. The relationship may seem trivial but it plays an important role in the calculus. It means that for a small δx we can approximate the function by a *straight line* since (48) is the equation of a straight line. Relationship (48) also means that for small δx we can treat the derivative not only as an operation $(\mathrm{d}/\mathrm{d}x)$ acting on y but also as a ratio

$$\mathrm{d}(y)/\mathrm{d}x$$

That is

$$\mathrm{d}y = f'(x)\,\mathrm{d}x = (\mathrm{d}y/\mathrm{d}x)\,\mathrm{d}x = \mathrm{d}y \tag{49}$$

The δy of equation (48) and $\mathrm{d}y$ of equation (49) are called *differentials* and a differential of y is the product of its derivative by the increment δx (or $\mathrm{d}x$) of the independent variable.

The following is a list of commonly used differentials.

Function:	Differential:
$f(x)$	$f'(x)\mathrm{d}x$ or $(\mathrm{d}(f(x))/\mathrm{d}x)\,\mathrm{d}x$
a (any constant)	0
x^n	nx^{n-1}
$af(x)$	$af'(x)$
$\exp(x)$	$\exp(x)$
$\ln(x)$	$1/x$
$f(\phi(x))$	$f'(\phi(x))\phi'(x)$
$f(x)g(x)$	$g(x)f'(x)+f(x)g'(x)$
$f(x)+g(x)$	$f'(x)+g'(x)$
$f(x)/g(x)$	$(g(x)f'(x)-f(x)g'(x))/g^2(x)$

$$\Big\} \mathrm{d}x \tag{50}$$

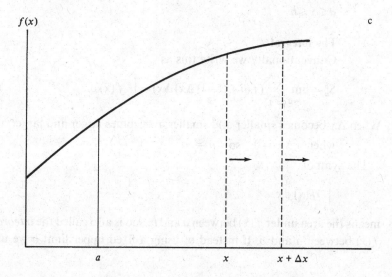

The area under a curve: integrals

One of the applications of equation (49) is in the computation of the area under a curve. In Figure A2.5a we represent a function $f(x)$. The area of the strip bounded by the curve $f(x)$, the x axis and the two vertical lines corresponding to $x=a$ and $x=a+\Delta x$ is given by

$$\Delta S_1 = f(a)\Delta x + \Delta y_1 \Delta x/2 + e_{r_1} \tag{51}$$

The error (e_{r_1}) occurs because the top of the strip (Figure A2.5b) is not a triangle of area $\Delta y_1 \Delta x/2$ as $f(x)$ is, in general, a curve. We can write similar expressions for the next strips, that is,

$$\Delta S_2 = f(a+\Delta x)\Delta x + \Delta y_2 \Delta x/2 + e_{r_2}$$
$$\vdots$$
$$\Delta S_n = f(a+(n-1)\Delta x)\Delta x + \Delta y_n \Delta x/2 + e_{r_n}$$

The area between a and b is the sum, that is,

$$S_a^b = \sum_{i=1}^{i=n} \Delta S_i + (\Delta x/2)\sum_{i=1}^{i=n} \Delta y_i + \sum_{i=1}^{i=n} e_{r_i} \tag{52}$$

$$= \sum_{i=1}^{i=n} f(a+(i-1)\Delta x)\Delta x + (\Delta x/2)\sum_{i=1}^{i=n} \Delta y_i + \sum_{i=1}^{i=n} e_{r_i}$$

If we now make $\Delta x \to 0$ we can observe that:

(i) Each segment of the curve can be approximated by a straight line, so

(ii) As Δx and Δy_i will both tend to zero, so

$$(\Delta x/2)\sum_{i=1}^{i=n} \Delta y_i \to 0$$

(iii) The product $f(a+(i-1)\Delta x)\Delta x$ will tend to $f(x)\,dx$ where $a \leqslant x \leqslant b$

The integral

Conventionally we write this as

$$S_a^b = \lim_{\substack{\Delta x \to 0 \\ n \to \infty}} \sum_{i=1}^{i=n} (f(a+(i-1)\Delta x)\Delta x) = \int_a^b f(x)\,dx \tag{53}$$

When Δx becomes smaller and smaller, n becomes larger and larger, thus

$$\text{when}\quad \Delta x \to 0 \quad \text{so}\quad n \to \infty$$

The symbol

$$\int_a^b f(x)\,dx \tag{54}$$

means the area under $f(x)$ between a and b, and is also called the *integral* of $f(x)$ between a and b. If instead of using a fixed upper limit b we use a variable upper limit, x (see Figure A2.5c), then the area becomes a function of x, $(F(x))$. That is,

$$S_a^x = \int_a^x f(x)\,dx = F(x) \tag{55}$$

or simply

$$S_a^x = \int f(x)\,dx = F(x) \tag{56}$$

The fundamental relationship of calculus

$F(x)$ can be obtained once we know $f(x)$ in the following way. Let us call $F(x)$ the area under the curve $f(x)$ when the upper limit is x. If $F(x + \Delta x)$ is the area under the curve $f(x)$ when the upper limit is now $x + \Delta x$ then

$$F(x + \Delta x) - F(x) = \int_x^{x + \Delta x} f(x)\,dx \tag{57}$$

If we now divide both sides of (57) by Δx

$$\frac{F(x + \Delta x) - F(x)}{\Delta x} = (1/\Delta x)\int_x^{x + \Delta x} f(x)\,dx \tag{58}$$

But

$$\int_x^{x + \Delta x} f(x)\,dx$$

if the *area of a strip* of width Δx between x and $x + \Delta x$ and under $f(x)$. From (51) this area (ΔS) is

$$\Delta S = f(x)\,\Delta x + (\Delta y\,\Delta x)/2 + e_r \tag{59}$$

So, substituting (59) into (58)

$$(F(x + \Delta x) - F(x))/\Delta x = (f(x)\,\Delta x + (\Delta y\,\Delta x)/2 + e_r)/\Delta x$$

For sufficiently small Δx (δx),

$$(F(x + \delta x) - F(x))/\delta x = (f(x)\,\delta x - \delta y\,\delta x/2)/\delta x \tag{60}$$

When $\delta x \to 0$ the left-hand side becomes the derivative of $F(x)$, $(F'(x))$ and the right-hand side becomes simply $f(x)$ or

$$F'(x) = (d/dx)(F(x)) = (d/dx)\left(\int f(x)\,dx\right) = f(x) \tag{61}$$

Equation (61) is the *fundamental rule of calculus*. To understand this further we should remember that we considered two types of integrals. These were:

(a) *The definite integral*

$$\int_a^b f(x)\,dx = \text{constant}$$

The definite integral is a number, and is the area under the curve $f(x)$ between a and b.

(b) *The indefinite integral*

$$\int_a^x f(x)\,dx = \int f(x)\,dx = F(x)$$

This integral is a function of x. Equation (61) means that the derivative is the inverse function of the *integration* of a function, as a *function* of the upper limit of integration. Relation (61) cannot be applied to the definite integral, since

$$(d/dx)\left(\int_a^b f(x)\,dx\right) = (d/dx)(\text{constant}) = 0$$

Application of the fundamental rule of calculus

Let us apply (61) to some examples

Example 1 $f(x) = a = \text{constant}$

So

$$F(x) = \int f(x)\,dx = \int a\,dx$$

Since $F(x)$ is the area under $f(x)$, from Figure A2.6a,

$$F(x) = ax$$

and

$$(d/dx)(F(x)) = (d/dx)(ax) = a = f(x)$$

We should also notice that if we write

$$F(x) = ax + c$$

then

$$(d/dx)(F(x)) = a = f(x)$$

Example 2 $f(x) = x$

From the definition of an integral

$$F(x) = \int f(x)\,dx = (x/2)\,x$$

$$\underset{\substack{\text{base of}\\ \text{a triangle}}}{\nearrow}\qquad \underset{\text{height}}{\nwarrow}\qquad \text{(see Figure A2.5b)}$$

and

$$(d/dx)(F(x)) = (d/dx)(x^2/2) = (d/dx)(x^2/2 + c)$$
$$= (1/2)2x = x$$

It can be shown that in general

$$\int x^n \, dx = x^{n+1}/(n+1) + c$$

If we write (61) in a slightly different way, that is,

$$f(x) = \int f'(x) \, dx \qquad (61a)$$

this means that

$$(d/dx) \int f(x) \, dx = \int (d/dx)(f(x)) \, dx = \int f'(x) \, dx \qquad (62)$$

and we note that we have reversed the order of the two operations (differentiation and integration).

Fig.A2.6

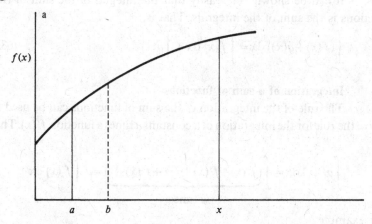

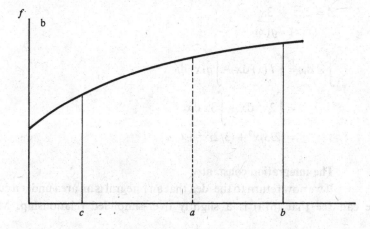

Equation (61a) can be used directly to integrate many functions. If we recall table (50) and invert the order of the two columns we obtain

$f'(x)\,dx$	$f(x)$(integrated functions)
dx	$x+c$
$a\,dx$	$ax+c$
$nx^{n-1}\,dx$ $(x^n\,dx)$	x^n+c $(x^{n+1}/(n+1))+c$
$e^x\,dx$	e^x+c
dx/x	$\ln(x)+c$

$$(63)$$

etc.

There are extensive tables of this type available and these can be found in most books of mathematical data.

The integral of the sum of two functions

It can be shown very easily that the integral of the sum of two functions is the sum of the integrals. That is,

$$\int (f(x)+g(x))\,dx = \int f(x)\,dx + \int g(x)\,dx \tag{63a}$$

Integration of a sum of functions

The rule of the integration of the sum of functions can be used to derive the rule for the integration of a constant a times a function $f'(x)$. That is,

$$\int af'(x)\,dx = \int \underbrace{(f'(x)+f'(x)+\cdots+f'(x)\,dx)}_{a \text{ times}} = a\int f'(x)\,dx$$

For example

$$Z = \underbrace{2x^2}_{f(x)} + \underbrace{3x}_{g(x)}$$

so

$$\int Z\,dx = \int f(x)\,dx + \int g(x)\,dx$$

$$= \int 2x^2\,dx + \int 3x\,dx$$

$$= (2/3)x^3 + (3/2)x^2 + C$$

The integration constant

If we now return to the idea that an integral is an area under a curve we can see that (61a) is a slightly over-simplified relationship. More precisely written, (61a) becomes

$$f(x) = \int_a^x f'(x) \, dx + C \tag{64}$$

where $f(x)$ is the area under the curve $f'(x)$ and between a and x. If instead of a lower limit a we had selected the lower limit b equation (61a) would become

$$f(x) = \int_b^x f'(x) \, dx \tag{65}$$

$f(x)$ defined by (64) (let us call it $f_a(x)$) is different from $f_b(x)$ defined by (65). That is, $f_a(x)$ and $f_b(x)$ correspond to different areas. The difference between the two functions (ΔS_a^b) is the area of the strip under $f'(x)$ and between a and b. That is,

$$f_a(x) - f_b(x) = \Delta S_a^b = \text{constant} \tag{Figure A2.6a}$$

So, in order to define $f(x)$ completely, we have to define the lower limit of integration. But if we change the lower limit of integration $f(x)$ will change by a constant value, so

$$f_a(x) = f_b(x) + \text{constant}$$

We can thus write that, in general,

$$\int f'(x) \, dx = f(x) + C \tag{66}$$

and C is generally called the *constant of integration*. This constant is defined when the lower limit of integration is defined. For example, if we integrate x^2 we obtain

$$\int x^2 \, dx = \tfrac{1}{3}x^3 + C$$

Elimination of the constant of integration

Let us assume that the lower limit of integration is 1 then when $x = 1$ the integral is zero, since the area under $f'(x)$ between the lower limit of integration $(a = 1)$ and the upper limit $(x = 1)$ is zero. Then

$$\tfrac{1}{3} + C = 0 \quad \text{or} \quad C = -\tfrac{1}{3}$$

So

$$\int_1^x = \tfrac{1}{3}(x^3 - 1)$$

To find the area when $x = 2$, we say that, since $f(x) + C$ is the area when the upper limit is x, then

$$f(2) + C$$

is the area for $x=2$. So

$$\int_1^2 = x^2\, dx = \tfrac{1}{3}(2^3-1) = \tfrac{7}{3}$$

If we now return to equation (66) we can derive the expression which will give the area under $f'(x)$ between a and b. For $x=a$

$$\int_d^a f'(x)\, dx = f(a) + C$$

where d is the lower limit of integration, yet undefined. For $x=b$

$$\int_d^b f'(x)\, dx = f(b) + C$$

the area under $f'(x)$ between a and b is the difference between the two areas (see Figure A2.5b). So

$$\int_d^b f'(x)\, dx - \int_d^a f'(x)\, dx = f(b) + C - f(a) - C$$

$$= f(b) - f(a)$$

But this area is also given by the integration of $f'(x)$ between a and b. That is,

$$\int_a^b f'(x)\, dx = f(b) - f(a) \qquad (67)$$

Computation of the definite integral

Equation (67) provides the rule for computing the definite integral, which we can describe as a sequence of three steps:

    (i) first obtain $f(x)$,
    (ii) then compute $f(a)$ and $f(b)$, and
    (iii) finally compute $f(b) - f(a)$.

Symbolically we write this as:

$$\int_a^b f'(x)\, dx = [f(x)]_a^b = f(b) - f(a) \qquad (68)$$

With this rule we can derive two other rules

$$\int_a^b f'(x)\, dx + \int_b^c f'(x)\, dx = f(b) - f(a) + f(c) - f(b)$$

$$= f(c) - f(a) = \int_a^c f'(x)\, dx$$

or

$$\int_a^b f'(x)\, dx + \int_b^c f'(x)\, dx = \int_a^c f'(x)\, dx \qquad (69)$$

and

$$\int_b^a f'(x)\,dx = f(a) - f(b) = -[f(b) - f(a)]$$

$$= -\int_a^b f'(x)\,dx \qquad (69a)$$

That is, to invert the order of integration (to exchange b for a) is equivalent to multiplying the integral by -1.

Integration by parts

In general, it is not easy to identify $f(x)$ once we know $f'(x)$, that is, most functions $f'(x)$ are not tabulated. In such cases we try to transform $f'(x)$ into functions which are tabulated (sometimes these functions are known as standard forms), for example,

$$\int x \exp(x)\,dx \qquad (70)$$

In this case

$$f'(x) = x \exp(x)$$

we can consider that $f'(x)$ is the product of two functions, x and $\exp(x)$. From the derivative of a product of two functions (U and V) we know that

$$(d/dx)(UV) = V(d/dx)(U) + U(d/dx)(V) \text{or rearranging}$$

$$U\,d(V)/dx = (d/dx)(UV) - V(d/dx)(U) \qquad (71)$$

If we now integrate both sides of (71) we obtain

$$\int U(d(V)/dx)\,dx = \int (d(UV)/dx)\,dx - \int (V\,d(U)/dx)\,dx$$

so

$$\int U\,dV = UV - \int V\,dU \qquad (72)$$

Let us assume that in (70)

$$U = x \qquad (73)$$

and

$$dV = \exp(x)\,dx \qquad (74)$$

So

$$\int dV = \int (d(V)/dx)\,dx = \int dV = V = \int \exp(x)\,dx = \exp(x)$$

so

$$V = \exp(x) \qquad (75)$$

and

$$d(V)/dx = dU = (d(x)/dx)\,dx = dx \qquad (76)$$

If we now substitute (73) and (76) into (72) we obtain

$$\int x \exp(x)\, dx = x \exp(x) - \int \exp(x)\, dx$$

$$= x \exp(x) - \exp(x) + C$$

Relation (72) defines the so-called *integration by parts* and converts the integration of function $f'(x)$ into the integrals of functions that can be integrated. The skill in applying this method resides in the appropriate choice of the functions U and V.

If we had defined

$$U = \exp(x) \quad \text{and} \quad dV = x\, dx$$

then

$$dU = \exp(x)\, dx \quad \text{and} \quad V = x^2/2$$

so

$$\int x \exp(x)\, dx = x^2 \exp(x)/2 - \int (x^2 \exp(x)/2)\, dx$$

the second term on the right-hand side is more difficult to integrate than the original $f'(x)$!

Method of substitution

Another method frequently used is *the method of substitution*. We shall apply this method to the integration

$$\int (1/(a+x))\, dx \tag{77}$$

We do not know how to integrate $1/(a+x)$ directly, but we do know how to integrate $1/x$.

Let us define a variable

$$y = a + x \tag{78}$$

then

$$dy/dx = 1$$

or

$$dy = dx \tag{79}$$

We can now substitute (78) and (79) into (77). So

$$\int dy/y = \ln(y) = \ln(a+x) \tag{80}$$

The method involves four steps:

    (i) guess the appropriate substitution ($y = a + x$),
    (ii) obtain the expression for dx ($dx = dy$),
    (iii) substitute the new variable and dx, and
    (iv) finally integrate.

This same method can be applied to the calculation of a definite integral. For example, if we have

$$\int_1^5 dx/(a+x)$$

and we choose the substitution

$$a+x=dy$$
$$dx=dy$$

then when

$$x=1, \quad y=a+1$$

and when

$$x=5, \quad y=a+5$$

So

$$\int_1^5 dx/(a+x) = \int_{a+1}^{a+5} dy/y = [\ln y]_{a+1}^{a+5}$$
$$= \ln(a+5)-\ln(a+1)$$
$$= \ln((a+5)/(a+1))$$

If we are computing the definite integral two more steps have to be included, these are

(v) compute the new limits of integration ($y=a+1$ and $y=a+5$) and
(vi) compute the definite integral ($\ln(a+5)-\ln(a+1)$).

There are other methods of integration, but we shall deal with these when the need arises.

APPENDIX 3. Trigonometric functions

In this appendix we shall deal with a group of transcendental functions (see Appendix 2 for a definition of a transcendental function) that are of special interest to electrophysiologists, and these are the trigonometric functions. These functions describe the relationship between the angles and the sides of a triangle. We shall analyse only triangles with the three sides in the same plane.

The angle
Let us consider an angle A (Figure A3.1a) which results from the rotation of side b anticlockwise around zero. A positive angle results from an anticlockwise rotation and a negative angle results from a clockwise

rotation. We note that an angle can be larger than 360 degrees (Figure A3.1b) when side b rotates around o (the origin) more than 360 degrees.

Degrees

We can measure an angle by dividing the circle into unit sectors and then counting how many of these sectors can be fitted between the two sides of the angle. Conventionally we divide the circle into 360 sectors (degrees) and then each of these sectors into 60 smaller sectors (seconds) and so on. Alternatively we may measure the length of the arc subtended by the two sides. But this method is ambiguous since, for an angle (A), the length of the arc will be larger the greater the radius (a_1, a_2) of the arc (Figure 3.1c). However, the length of the circumference divided by the length of the corresponding radius is a constant value (2π) and the complete circumference corresponds to an angle of 360 degrees.

Fig.A3.1

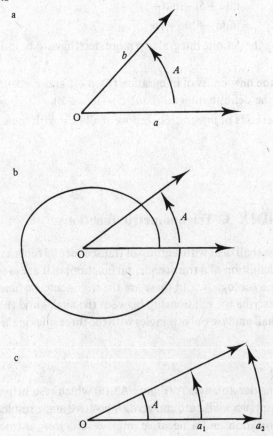

Radians

When the two sides of an angle subtend an arc of length equal to its radius we say that it is an angle of one radian. A radian is thus dimensionless since it is the ratio of two lengths and we can say that 360 degrees are equivalent to 2π radians.

In Figure A3.2 we have drawn two triangles. Sides c and f have the same length. From this figure we can see that the lengths of sides b and a are related to the opposing angles A and B. We can say that for any right-angled triangle the length of any one of its sides is a function of its opposing angle. For the same angle (A) the length of each side is also related to length of the hypotenuse.

The sine and cosine

If we compute the ratio

side/hypotenuse

the relation between this ratio and the opposite angle is now fixed. That is, for each angle (x) there is a specific ratio between the opposing side and the hypotenuse, which we call sin(x). For Figure A3.2b

$$\sin(A) = a/c$$

Fig.A3.2

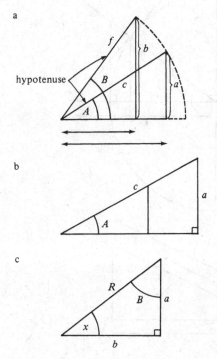

and from Figure A3.2a

$$\sin(B) = b/f$$

We can define in a similar way the relation between an angle (x) and the ratio between the adjacent side and the hypotenuse. Such a ratio is known as the cosine of x, or cosine x, and is written as

$$\cos(x)$$

The sine and the cosine of an angle (x) are related by Pythagoras' theorem (Figure A3.2c), so

$$a^2 + b^2 = R^2$$

dividing both sides by R^2 we obtain

$$(a/R)^2 + (b/R)^2 = 1$$

or

$$\sin^2(x) + \cos^2(x) = 1 \qquad\qquad (1)$$

d

e

From Figure A3.2c we can also see that

$$\sin(B) = b/R = \cos(x)$$

since

$$B = \pi/2 - x$$

$$\sin(\pi/2 - x) = \cos(x) \qquad (2)$$

Similarly

$$\cos(B) = a/R = \sin(x)$$

or

$$\cos(\pi/2 - x) = \sin(x) \qquad (3)$$

Trigonometric functions

Both $\cos(x)$ and $\sin(x)$ are known as trigonometric functions. With these two functions we can define four other trigonometric functions.

$$\tan(x) = \sin(x)/\cos(x) = (a/R)/(b/R) = a/b \qquad (4)$$

(tangent of (x))

$$\cotan(x) = \cos(x)/\sin(x) = b/a \qquad (5)$$

(cotangent of (x))

$$\sec(x) = 1/\cos(x) = R/b \qquad (6)$$

(secant of (x))

$$\cosec(x) = 1/\sin(x) = R/a \qquad (7)$$

(cosecant of (x))

We shall, however, deal only with sines, cosines and tangents. In Figure A3.2d we have drawn a circle of unit radius (R) (trigonometric circle) and a central angle (α). A central angle is the angle formed by two radii of a circle. If we now apply our definitions of the six trigonometric functions we obtain the following relationships.

$$\sin(\alpha) = a/R = a$$
$$\cos(\alpha) = b/R = b$$
$$\tan(\alpha) = a/b = c$$
$$\cotan(\alpha) = b/a = d$$
$$\sec(\alpha) = 1/b = e$$
$$\cosec(\alpha) = 1/a = f$$

All these relationships are derived from the following relationships between two triangles with a common angle (Figure A3.2e).

$$a/c = b/d \quad \text{or} \quad a/b = c/d$$
$$a/e = b/f \quad \text{or} \quad a/b = e/f$$
$$c/e = d/f \quad \text{or} \quad c/d = e/f$$

This means that the lengths of the line segments a to R are numerically equal to the values of $\sin(x), \cos(x), \tan(c), \cot(x)$ and $\csc(x)$ and $\sec(x)$.

In Figure A3.3a we have drawn a trigonometric circle. The lengths of the thick vertical lines drawn inside the circle are the sines of the opposite central angles.

Function $\sin(x)$ is plotted in Figure A3.3b with x measured in radians. $\text{Sin}(x)$ has a maximum value of 1 (for $x = \pi/2$) and a minimum value of -1 (for $x = -\pi/2$). It is positive between 0 and π and negative between π and 2π (or 0).

Fig.A3.3

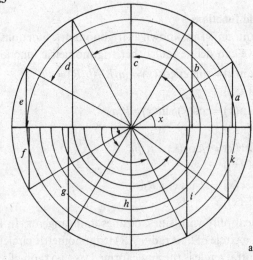

a

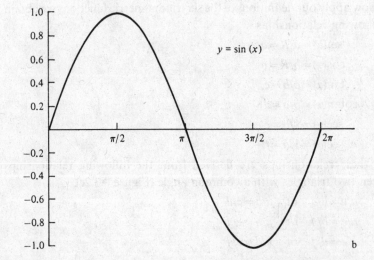

$y = \sin(x)$

b

Another important property of sin(x) is its periodicity. A function is periodic when it repeats itself, that is, when

$$f(x)=f(x+e)=f(x-e)=f(x\pm ke)$$

Here k is an integer, which can be $0, 1, 2, \ldots, k$, and 1 is the *period* of the function.

In the case of sin(x) the period is 360 degrees (or 2π if x is expressed in radians).

or
$$\sin(x)=\sin(x\pm k\cdot 360) \quad (x \text{ in degrees})$$

$$\sin(x)=\sin(x\pm 2k\pi) \quad (x \text{ in radians}) \tag{8}$$

In Figure A3.4a we have drawn a central angle x in a trigonometric circle. The cosine of angle x is the length of segment b since

$$\cos(x)=b/R=b$$

In Figure A3.4b we can see the cosines (thick lines) of a number of angles existing between 0 and 2π.

The values of cos(x), as a function of x (in radians), are plotted in Figure A3.4c.

This graph shows that cos(x) is also a periodic function, so

or
$$\cos(x)=\cos(x\pm k\cdot 360)$$

$$\cos(x)=\cos(x\pm 2\pi k) \tag{9}$$

The function has a maximum value of 1 at

$$x=2k\pi \quad \text{where} \quad k=0, \pm 1, \pm 2,\ldots$$

and a minimum value of -1 when

$$x=(2\cdot k+1)\cdot\pi \quad \text{where} \quad k=0, \pm 1, \pm 2,\ldots$$

Fig.A3.4

a

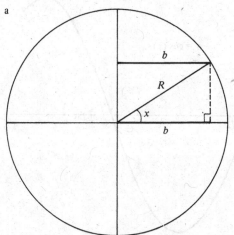

The sine and cosine of the sum of two angles

We shall now derive a very useful relationship, the sine and the cosine of the sum of two angles.

In Figure A3.5 we have drawn the first quadrant of the trigonometric circle and two central angles. Line $\overline{AC}$ is perpendicular to $\overline{OA}$ and line $\overline{CB}$ is perpendicular to $\overline{OB}$.

By definition

$$CA = \sin(\alpha + \beta)$$

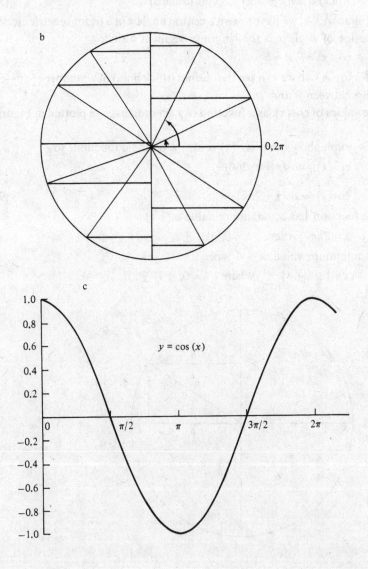

and

> CA = projection of $\overline{OB}$ on the y axis plus the projection of $\overline{BC}$ on the y axis

From Figure A3.5 it can be seen that angle BCA is equal to α. So

> projection $\overline{OB}$ onto $y = \overline{OB}\sin(\alpha)$

and

> projection $\overline{BC}$ onto $y = CB\cos(\alpha)$

so

> $\sin(\alpha + \beta) = \overline{OB}\sin(x)$

but

> $\overline{OB} = \cos(\beta)$ and $\overline{CB} = \sin(\beta)$

so

> $\sin(\alpha + \beta) = \sin(\alpha)\cos(\beta) + \sin(\beta)\cos(\alpha)$ (10)

From the same Figure A3.5

> $\overline{OA} = \cos(\alpha + \beta)$

But

> $\overline{OA} = \overline{OD} - \overline{AD}$

Fig.A3.5

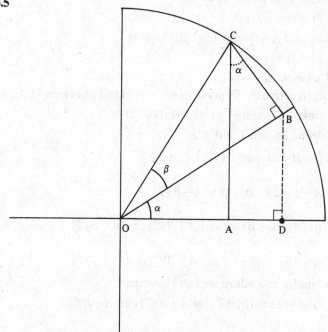

and
$$\overline{OD} = \overline{OB}\cos(\alpha)$$
also
$$\overline{OB} = \cos(\beta)$$
since
$$\overline{AD} = \overline{CB}\sin(\alpha)$$
and
$$\overline{CB} = \sin(\beta)$$
then
$$\cos(\alpha + \beta) = \cos(\alpha)\cos(\beta) - \sin(\alpha)\sin(\beta) \tag{11}$$

With (10) and (11) we can now derive a further set of useful relationships.
From Figures A3.3 and A3.4 we can see that
$$\sin(-\alpha) = -\sin(\alpha) \quad \text{and} \quad \sin(-\beta) = -\sin(\beta)$$
also
$$\cos(-\alpha) = \cos(\alpha) \quad \text{and} \quad \cos(-\beta) = \cos(\beta)$$
so
$$\sin(\alpha - \beta) = \sin(\alpha)\cos(\beta) - \sin(\beta)\cos(\alpha) \tag{12}$$
and
$$\cos(\alpha - \beta) = \cos(\alpha)\cos(\beta) + \sin(\alpha)\sin(\beta) \tag{13}$$

A function such as $\sin(x)$ where
$$f(-x) = -f(x)$$
is called an *odd function*, while $\cos(x)$ where
$$f(-x) = f(x)$$
is called an *even function*.

In order to derive the formula for the sum of two sines we add (10) to (12).
$$\sin(\alpha + \beta) + \sin(\alpha - \beta) = 2\sin(\alpha)\cos(\beta)$$

If we define angles A and B as
$$A + B = 2\alpha \quad \text{or} \quad \alpha = (A + B)/2$$
and
$$A - B = 2\beta \quad \text{or} \quad \beta = (A - B)/2$$
so
$$\sin(A) + \sin(B) = 2\sin((A + B)/2)\cos((A - B)/2) \tag{14}$$
also
$$\sin(A) - \sin(B) = 2\sin((A - B)/2)\cos((A + B)/2) \tag{15}$$

Using a similar procedure we can show that
$$\cos(A) + \cos(B) = 2\cos((A + B)/2)\cos((A - B)/2) \tag{16}$$
and
$$\cos(A) - \cos(B) = 2\sin((A + B)/2)\sin((A - B)/2) \tag{17}$$

If
$$\alpha = \beta = A$$
then (10) becomes
$$\sin(2A) = 2\sin(A)\cos(A) \tag{18}$$
and
$$\cos(2A) = \cos^2(A) - \sin^2(A)$$
Since, from equation (1),
$$\cos^2(A) + \sin^2(A) = 1$$
so
$$\sin^2(A) = 1 - \cos^2(A)$$
or
$$\cos^2(A) = 1 - \sin^2(A)$$
so
$$\cos(2A) = 2\cos^2(A) - 1$$
or
$$\cos^2(A) = 1/2 + 1/2\cos(2A) \tag{19}$$

The derivative of sin(x) and cos(x)

If we examine the graphs of $\sin(x)$ and $\cos(x)$, it is easy to see that both these functions are continuous. We should thus be able to compute the derivative of $\sin(x)$ or of $\cos(x)$ for every value of x.

The derivative of $\sin(x)$ is given by

$$\sin'(x) = \lim_{\Delta x \to 0} [(\sin(x + \Delta x) - \sin(x))/\Delta x]$$

From (10)

$$\sin(x + \Delta x) = \sin(x)\cos(\Delta x) + \sin(\Delta x)\cos(x)$$

so

$$\lim_{\Delta x \to 0} [(\sin(x + \Delta x) - \sin(x))/\Delta x]$$
$$= \lim_{\Delta x \to 0} [\sin(x)\cos(\Delta x) + \sin(\Delta x)\cos(x) - \sin(x)]/\Delta x$$
$$= \lim_{\Delta x \to 0} [(\sin(x)(\cos(\Delta x) - 1) + \sin(\Delta x)\cos(x))/\Delta x]$$
$$= \lim_{\Delta x \to 0} [\sin(x)(\cos(\Delta x) - 1)/\Delta x + \cos(x)\sin(\Delta x)/\Delta x]$$

Since $\sin(x)$ and $\cos(x)$ are independent of Δx we have to find

$$\lim_{\Delta x \to 0} (\cos(\Delta x) - 1)/\Delta x \quad \text{and} \quad \lim_{\Delta x \to 0} \sin(\Delta x)/\Delta x$$

From Figure A3.6 we can see that
$$\sin(\Delta x) < \Delta x < \tan(\Delta x)$$
$$\text{arc}$$

or

$$\sin(\Delta x) < \Delta x < \sin(\Delta x)/\cos(\Delta x)$$

If we divide the three terms by $\sin(\Delta x)$ we obtain

$$1 < \Delta x/\sin(\Delta x) < 1/\cos(\Delta x)$$

But when

$$\Delta x \to 0$$
$$\cos(\Delta x) \to 1$$

so

$$\lim_{\Delta x \to 0} (1/\cos(\Delta x)) = 1$$

and

$$\lim_{\Delta x \to 0} (\Delta x/\sin(\Delta x)) = 1 \qquad (20)$$

or

$$\lim_{\Delta x \to 0} (\sin(\Delta x)/\Delta x) = 1$$

Also

$$
\begin{aligned}
(1 - \cos(\Delta x))/\Delta x &= [(1 - \cos(\Delta x))(1 + \cos(\Delta x))]/[\Delta x(1 + \cos(\Delta x))] \\
&= (1 - \cos^2(\Delta x))/\Delta x(1 + \cos(\Delta x)) \\
&= \sin^2(\Delta x)/\Delta x(1 + \cos(\Delta x)) \\
&= (\sin(\Delta x)/\Delta x)(1/(1 + \cos(\Delta x))) \sin(\Delta x)
\end{aligned}
$$

So

$$\lim_{\Delta x \to 0} [(1 - \cos(\Delta x))/\Delta x]$$

$$= \lim_{\Delta x \to 0} [\sin(\Delta x)/\Delta x] \lim_{\Delta x \to 0} [1/(1 + \cos(\Delta x)] \lim_{\Delta x \to 0} (\sin(\Delta x))$$

The first limit on the right-hand side is 1, the second is $\frac{1}{2}$ $(\cos(0) = 1)$ and the third is zero $(\sin(0) = 0)$; so

$$\lim_{\Delta x \to 0} [(1 - \cos(\Delta x))/\Delta x] = 0 = \lim_{\Delta x \to 0} [(\cos(\Delta x) - 1)/\Delta x]$$

Fig.A3.6

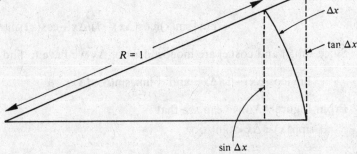

Δx

$\tan \Delta x$

$R = 1$

$\sin \Delta x$

Therefore

$$\lim_{\Delta x \to 0} \left[(\sin(x + \Delta x) - \sin(\Delta x)) / \Delta x \right]$$

$$= \lim_{\Delta x \to 0} \left[\sin(x)(\cos(\Delta x) - 1)/\Delta x \right] + \lim_{\Delta x \to 0} \left[\cos(x)(\sin(\Delta x)/\Delta x) \right]$$

$$= 0 + \cos(x)$$

or

$$(d/dx)(\sin(x)) = \cos(x) \tag{21}$$

For the cosine of x

$$(d/dx)(\cos(x)) = \lim_{\Delta x \to 0} \left[(\cos(x + \Delta x) - \cos(x))/\Delta x \right]$$

using a similar approach as for $\sin(x)$

$$(d/dx)(\cos(x)) = \lim_{\Delta x \to 0} \left[\cos(x)(\cos(\Delta x) - 1)/\Delta x \right]$$
$$\downarrow$$
$$0$$

$$- \lim_{\Delta x \to 0} \left[\sin(x)(\sin(\Delta x)/\Delta x) \right]$$
$$\downarrow$$
$$- \sin(x)$$

so

$$d(\cos(x))/dx = - \sin(x) \tag{22}$$

Since both $\sin(x)$ and $\cos(x)$ can be differentiated and since each time we differentiate them we obtain again a differentiable function we should be able to expand $\sin(x)$ and $\cos(x)$ as a Taylor series (see Appendix 4).

The Taylor series of a function $f(x)$ around $x = 0$ is defined as

$$f(x) = f(0) + f'(0)x + (f''(0)/2!)x^2 + \cdots + (f^n(0)/n!)x^n$$

where $f^n(0)$ is the nth derivative of $f(x)$. At $x = 0$, for $\sin(x)$

$$\sin(0) = (0) = f(0)$$

and

$$f'(x) = \cos(x)$$
$$f''(x) = - \sin(x)$$
$$f'''(x) = - \cos(x)$$
$$f''''(x) = \sin(x)$$
$$\vdots$$

so

$$f'(0) = 1$$
$$f''(0) = 0$$
$$f'''(0) = - 1$$
$$f''''(0) = 0$$
$$\vdots$$

The derivatives of $\sin(x)$ at $x=0$ are thus periodic going through the values

n	0	1	2	3	4	5
$f^n(0)$	0,	1,	0,	-1,	0,	1

so

$$\sin(x)=x-x^3/3!+x^5/5!-x^7/7!+\cdots \tag{23}$$

Application of the same procedure to $\cos(x)$ will show that

$$\cos(x)=1-x^2/2!+x^4/4!-\cdots \tag{24}$$

From the fundamental relation of calculus, that is,

$$f(x)=\int f'(x)\,dx \quad \text{(see Appendix 2)}$$

$$\int \cos(x)\,dx = -\sin(x)+C \tag{25}$$

and

$$\int \sin(x)\,dx = \cos(x)+C \tag{26}$$

From (26) we can also obtain the definite integral of $\cos(x)$.

If we integrate between 0 and 2π, that is, over a period, we obtain

$$\int_0^{2\pi} \cos(x)\,dx = [-\sin(x)]_0^{2\pi} = [-\sin(0)+\sin(2\pi)] = -0+0=0 \tag{27}$$

If we integrate $\sin(x)$ in a similar way

$$\int_0^{2\pi} \sin(x)\,dx = [\cos(x)]_0^{2\pi} = [\cos(2\pi)-\cos(0)] = 1-1=0 \tag{28}$$

This result is also intuitively obvious from our understanding of the integral since the sum of the area under either a sine or a cosine curve is zero.

Average value of a function

At this point we will introduce the important concept of the *average value* of a function (f). We use average value extensively in signal analysis and it is given by:

$$\bar{f}=(1/X)\int_0^X f(x)\,dx \tag{29}$$

where X is the interval of integration. Geometrically the average value is the area under $f(x)$ between 0 and X, divided by X.

From the definition of an integral

$$\int_0^X f(x)\,dx = \lim_{\substack{\Delta x \to 0 \\ n \to \infty}} \sum_{i=1}^{i=n} f(x_i)\,\Delta x_i$$

where $n\,\Delta x = X$.

The average value is thus given by

$$\bar{f} = (1/X) \int_0^X f(x)\,dx = \lim_{n \to \infty} (1/X) \sum_{i=1}^{i=n} f(x_i)\Delta x$$

$$= \lim_{n \to \infty} \sum_{i=1}^{i=n} (f(x_i)\Delta x)/(n\,\Delta x)$$

$$= \lim_{n \to \infty} \sum_{i=1}^{i=n} f(x_i)/n$$

$$= \lim_{n \to \infty} (1/n) \sum_{i=1}^{i=n} f(x_i) \cdot$$

Because of the definition of an average value the average value of $\sin(x)$ or $\cos(x)$ over one period is zero.

Integration of other trigonometric functions

Three other results of the integration of trigonometric functions are very useful in electrophysiology.

Let us consider the integral

$$\int \sin(mx) \sin(nx)\,dx \tag{30}$$

$\mathrm{Sin}(mx)$ and $\sin(nx)$ are two sinusoids with different periods. That is, if we give values to x, $\sin(mx)$ will repeat itself with a period $x = 2\pi/m$ and $\sin(nx)$ with a period $x = 2\pi/n$.

When we write a sinusoid in the form

$$\sin(mx) \quad \text{or} \quad \cos(mx)$$

if L is the period, then

$$m = 2\pi/L$$

In order to integrate (30) we have to rearrange the integrand slightly, as follows.

If $A = mx$ and $B = nx$ from (11)

$$\cos(A+B) = \cos(A)\cos(B) - \sin(A)\sin(B)$$

and

$$\cos(A-B) = \cos(A)\cos(B) + \sin(A)\sin(B)$$

so

$$2\sin(A)\sin(B) = \cos(A-B) - \cos(A+B)$$

$$\sin(A)\sin(B) = \cos(A-B)/2 - \cos(A+B)/2$$

and

$$\sin(nx)\sin(mx) = \cos((m-n)x)/2 - \cos((m+n)x)/2$$

If $n = m$

$$\sin(mx)\sin(nx) = 1/2 - \tfrac{1}{2}\cos(2mx)$$

and for $m \neq n$

$$\int \sin(mx)\sin(nx)\,dx = (1/2)\int \cos((m-n)x)\,dx$$

$$-(1/2)\int \cos((m+n)x)\,dx \tag{30a}$$

Now if

$$\int \cos(x)\,dx = \sin(x)$$

then

$$\int \cos(ax)\,dx = (1/a)(\sin(ax)) \tag{31}$$

From (31), (30a) becomes

$$\int \sin(mx)\sin(nx)\,dx = (1/2(m-n))\sin((m-n)x)$$

$$-(1/2(m+n))\sin((m+n)x) \tag{30b}$$

For $m = n$

$$\int \sin(mx)\sin(nx)\,dx = 1/2x - (1/4n)\sin(2nx) \tag{30c}$$

If we now compute the definite integral between $-\pi$ and $+\pi$ we have

For $m \neq n$

$$= 0$$

$$\int_{-\pi}^{+\pi} \sin(mx)\sin(nx)\,dx = \tag{32}$$

For $m = n$

$$= \pi$$

This is so because $\sin(k\pi) = 0$ and so $\sin((m+n)\pi)$ and $\sin(2n\pi)$ are all zero.

Orthogonal relationships
By a similar procedure it is easy to show that

$$\int_{-\pi}^{+\pi} \sin(mx)\cos(nx)\,dx = 0 \tag{33}$$

and

$$= 0 \quad (m \neq n)$$

$$\int_{-\pi}^{+\pi} \cos(mx)\cos(nx)\,dx$$

$$= \pi \quad (m = n)$$

Expressions (32), (33), (34) also mean that

$$\int_{-\pi}^{+\pi} \sin(x)\cos(x)\,dx = 0$$

while

$$\int_{-\pi}^{+\pi} \sin^2(x)\,dx \neq 0$$

and

$$\int_{-\pi}^{+\pi} \cos^2(x)\,dx \neq 0$$

Relationships (32), (33) and (34) are called the *orthogonal relationships* of the trigonometric functions.

APPENDIX 4. The Taylor series

It is sometimes convenient to expand a function in a power series, and this is particularly convenient in the case of transcendental functions. The power series that is more frequently used is the Taylor series which describes a function in the neighbourhood of a point in terms of its derivatives. We will apply this method first to the case of a polynomial. If we take a general polynomial

$$P(x) = a_0 + a_1 x + a_2 x^2 + \cdots + a_n x^n$$

where $a_0, a_1, a_2, \ldots, a_n$ are the coefficients of the polynomial, then derivative of $P(x)$ is $P'(x)$:

$$P'(x) = (d/dx)(a_0 + a_1 x + a_2 x^2 + \cdots + a_n x^n) = (d/dx)(a_0) +$$
$$a_1(d/dx)(x) + a_2(d/dx)(x^2) + \cdots + a_n(d/dx)(x^n)$$
$$= a_1 + 2a_2 x + 3a_3 x^2 + \cdots + na_n x^{n-1}$$

If we make $x = 0$, then

$$P'(0) = a'$$

We now obtain the second derivative $P''(x)$:

$$P''(x) = (d/dx)(P'(x)) = 2a_2 + 3\cdot 2a_3 x + \cdots + n(n-1)a_n x^{n-2}$$

and we again make $x = 0$. So

$$P''(0) = 2a_2 \quad \text{or} \quad a_2 = P''(0)/2$$

The third derivative is $P'''(x)$:

$$P'''(x) = (d/dx)(P''(x)) = 3\cdot 2a_3 + \cdots$$

and for $x = 0$

$$P'''(0) = 3\cdot 2a_3 \quad \text{or} \quad a_3 = P'''(0)/3!$$

since $3 \cdot 2 \cdot 1 = 3!$.

If we continue with this procedure we find for the nth derivative that a_n is

$$a_n = P^{n'}(0)/n!$$

where $P^{n'}(0)$ means the nth derivative. Finally, if we compute the value of the function for $x = 0$

$$P(0) = a_0$$

We can now rewrite the polynomial as

$$P(x) = P(0) + P'(0)x + (P''(0)/2!)x^2 + \cdots + (P^{n'}(0)/n!)x^n$$

and this is the *Taylor series*. Near $P(0)$ we can describe the function $P(x)$ in terms of the first, second . . . nth derivative at that point. Each nth derivative is multiplied by x^n and divided by $n!$ (for $n = 0, 1, 2, \ldots$).

Let us now apply the same method to the exponential function $\exp(x)$. So

$$f(x) = e^x$$

But for this function (see Appendix 2)

$$f(x) = f'(x) = f''(x) = \cdots = f^n(x)$$

so

$$f(0) = f'(0) = f''(0) = \cdots = f^n(0) = 1$$

Thus

$$f(x) = 1 + x + x^2/2! + x^3/3! + \cdots + x^n/n!$$

an expression already derived earlier.

If, instead of $x = 0$, we want $x = a$, this is equivalent to shifting the function along the x axis by a. To do this we just substitute $(x - a)$ for x. So the Taylor series becomes

$$f(x - a) = f(a) + f'(a)(x - a) + (f''(a)/2!)(x - a)^2 + \cdots$$
$$+ (f^{n'}(a)/n!)(x - a)^n$$

APPENDIX 5. Stirling's formula

Stirling's formula states that

$$n! \rightarrow \sqrt{(2\pi)}n^{n+1/2}\exp(-n) + \text{error} \tag{1}$$

when $n \rightarrow \infty$, where the error term is defined as

$$\text{error} = |n! - \sqrt{(2\pi)}n^{n+1/2}\exp(-n)| \tag{2}$$

The error term increases with n. It can be shown that the *absolute* error increases with n; however, the relative error ($\text{error}/n!$) decreases with n. Stirling's formula has many applications and is particularly important in probability theory.

The formula is obtained by calculating the area under the curve $\ln(x)$. The exact area (S) (see Appendix 2) is defined from the integral

$$S = \int_1^x \ln(x)\,dx$$

If we rewrite S as

$$S = \int_1^x \underbrace{\ln(x)}_{u}\,\underbrace{(dx/dx)\,dx}_{dv}$$

This integral may be obtained by integration by parts. So

$$S = [uv]_1^x - \int_1^x v\,du$$

but

$$\ln(x) = u$$

and

$$du = (d/dx)\ln(x)\,dx = (1/x)\,dx$$
$$dv = (d/dx)(x)\,dx$$

or

$$dv = dx$$

then

$$v = x$$

so

$$S = \int_1^x \ln(x)\,dx = [x\ln(x)]_1^x - \int_1^x dx$$
$$= [x\ln(x) - x]_1^x$$

or

$$S = x\ln(x) - x + 1 \tag{3a}$$

The *approximate* area (Sa) under the curve $\ln(x)$ can be seen from Figure A5.1 to be

$$Sa = (\ln(1) + \ln(2))/2 + (\ln(2) + \ln(3))/2$$
$$+ (\ln(3) + \ln(4))/2 + \cdots + (\ln(n-2) + \ln(n-1))/2$$
$$+ (\ln(n-1) + \ln(n))/2$$

Each of the terms on the right-hand side is obtained by approximating the area between J and $J+1$ (2 and 3, for example) by a trapezium of base 1 and vertical sides in (J) and $\ln(J+1)$.

After simplifying, Sa becomes

$$Sa = \ln(2) + \ln(3) + \ln(4) + \cdots + \ln(n-1) + \tfrac{1}{2}\ln(n)$$
$$= \ln(2) + \ln(3) + \ln(4) + \cdots + \ln(n-1) + \ln(n) - \tfrac{1}{2}\ln(n)$$

or

$$Sa = \ln(n!) - \tfrac{1}{2}\ln(n) \tag{3}$$

But *Sa* can also be seen as a sum of *n* strips of base 1 under $f(x)$. The area under one of such strips is (see Figure A5.1b) from the definition of a definite integral

$$S_J = [x \ln(x) - x]_{J-1}^{J}$$

While the area of each trapezium (Sa_J) is

$$Sa_J = (\ln(J) + \ln(J+1))/2$$

Fig.A5.1

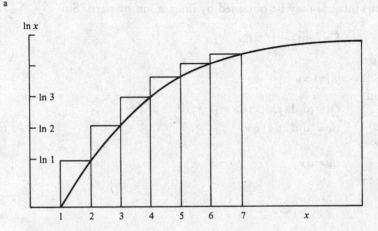

a

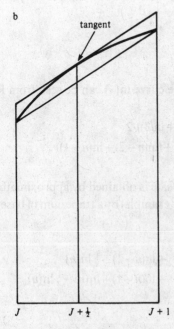

b

The difference $S_J - Sa_J$ is smaller than the difference $S_{TJ} - Sa_J$ where S_{TJ} is the area under the tangent to the curve at the point

$$(J + J + 1)/2 = J + \tfrac{1}{2}$$

so

$$S_J - Sa_J < S_{TJ} - Sa_J$$

Since the triangles a and b in Figure A5.1c are identical, the area under the tangent is simply $\ln(J + \tfrac{1}{2})$. Then

$$S_{TJ} - Sa_J = \ln(J + \tfrac{1}{2}) - \tfrac{1}{2}\ln(J) - \tfrac{1}{2}\ln(J + 1)$$

so

$$S_J - Sa_J < \ln(J + \tfrac{1}{2}) - \tfrac{1}{2}\ln(J) - \tfrac{1}{2}\ln(J + 1)$$

But

$$\ln(J + \tfrac{1}{2}) - \tfrac{1}{2}\ln(J) - \tfrac{1}{2}\ln(J + 1)$$

$$= \tfrac{1}{2}\ln(J + \tfrac{1}{2}) + \tfrac{1}{2}\ln(J + \tfrac{1}{2}) - \tfrac{1}{2}\ln(J) - \tfrac{1}{2}\ln(J + 1)$$

$$= \tfrac{1}{2}\ln\left(J\left(1 + \frac{1}{2J}\right)\right) + \tfrac{1}{2}\ln\left(J\left(1 + \frac{1}{2J}\right)\right) - \tfrac{1}{2}\ln(J) - \tfrac{1}{2}\ln\left(J\left(1 + \frac{1}{J}\right)\right)$$

$$= \tfrac{1}{2}\ln(J) + \tfrac{1}{2}\ln\left(1 + \frac{1}{2J}\right) + \tfrac{1}{2}\ln J + \tfrac{1}{2}\ln\left(1 + \frac{1}{2J}\right) - \tfrac{1}{2}\ln(J)$$

$$- \tfrac{1}{2}\ln(J) - \tfrac{1}{2}\ln\left(1 + \frac{1}{J}\right)$$

$$= \tfrac{1}{2}\ln\left(1 + \frac{1}{2J}\right) - \tfrac{1}{2}\ln\frac{1 + \dfrac{1}{J}}{1 + \dfrac{1}{2J}}$$

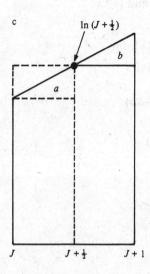

So

$$S_{TJ} - Sa_J = \tfrac{1}{2} \ln\left(1 + \frac{1}{2J}\right) - \tfrac{1}{2} \ln\left(\left(1 + \frac{1}{J}\right)\Big/\left(1 + \frac{1}{2J}\right)\right)$$

On the right-hand side the second term inside the parentheses can be rearranged, so that

$$\left(1 + \frac{1}{J}\right)\Big/\left(1 + \frac{1}{2J}\right) = (2J + 2)/(2J + 1) = 1 + \frac{1}{(2J+1)} > 1 + \frac{1}{2(J+1)}$$

so

$$S_{TJ} - Sa_J < \frac{1}{2}\left[\ln\left(1 + \frac{1}{2J}\right) - \ln\left(1 + \frac{1}{2(J+1)}\right)\right]$$

But since

$$S_J - Sa_J < S_{TJ} - Sa_J < \frac{1}{2}\left[\ln\left(1 + \frac{1}{2J}\right) - \ln\left(1 + \frac{1}{2(J+1)}\right)\right]$$

then

$$\sum_{J=1}^{J=n} (S_J - Sa_J) < \sum_{J=1}^{J=n} (S_{TJ} - Sa_J) < \frac{1}{2}\sum_{J=1}^{J=n}\left[\ln\left(1 + \frac{1}{2J}\right) - \ln\left(1 + \frac{1}{2(J+1)}\right)\right]$$

But the third summation is

$$\ln(1 + \tfrac{1}{2}) - \ln(1 + \tfrac{1}{4}) + \ln(1 + \tfrac{1}{4}) - \ln(1 + \tfrac{1}{6}) + \cdots$$

So all the terms cancel, except the first and last. Then

$$\sum_{J=1}^{J=n} (S_J - Sa_J) < \tfrac{1}{2}\ln(3/2) - \tfrac{1}{2}\ln\left(1 + \frac{1}{2n}\right) < \tfrac{1}{2}\ln(3/2)$$

This means that the difference between the two areas can never be larger than $\tfrac{1}{2}\ln(3/2)$. Also

$$\sum_{J=1}^{J=n} (S_J - Sa_J) S - Sa \quad \text{(from (3a) and (3))}$$

so

$$S - Sa = n\ln(n) - n + 1 - \ln(n!) + \tfrac{1}{2}\ln(n)$$
$$= (n + \tfrac{1}{2})\ln(n) - n + 1 - \ln(n!)$$

or

$$\ln(n!) = (n + \tfrac{1}{2})\ln(n) - n + 1 - (S - Sa)$$

Let us call $(S - Sa)$ the variable a_n, so

$$\ln(n!) = (n + \tfrac{1}{2})\ln(n) - n + (1 - a_n)$$

or

$$n! = n^{n+1/2}\exp(-n)\exp(1 - a_n)$$

If we define b_n as

$$b_n = \exp(1 - a_n) \tag{4}$$

then

$$n! = n^{n+1/2}\exp(-n)b_n \tag{5}$$

In this expression we have to find the value (limit) b_n.

In Appendix 6 it is shown that

$$\sqrt{\pi} = \lim_{n \to \infty} [(n!)^2 2^{2n}/((2n)! \sqrt{n})]$$

Since equation (5) is valid for any value of n it is valid when we substitute $2n$ for n. So

$$(2n!) = (2n)^{2n+1/2} \exp(-2n)b_{2n}$$
$$= 2^{2n+1/2}n^{2n+1/2} \exp(-2n)b_{2n} \tag{5a}$$

and

$$(n!)^2 = n^{2n+1} \exp(-2n)b_n^2$$

so

$$\sqrt{\pi} = \lim_{n \to \infty} [(n^{2n+1} \exp(-2n)b_n^2 2^{2n})/(n^{2n+1/2} \exp(-2n)b_{2n}2^{2n+1/2}n^{1/2})]$$

$$= \lim_{n \to \infty} (b_n^2/b_{2n}\sqrt{2})$$

We saw already that a_n can never be larger than $\frac{1}{2}\ln(3/2)$, but it can be shown (empirically or analytically) that as n increases a_n also increases. An implication of this is that as $n \to \infty$, a_n tends to a finite limit (a, for example), so

$$\lim_{n \to \infty} (a_n) = a \quad \text{and} \quad \lim_{n \to \infty} (b_n) = \exp(1-a) = b$$

Also

$$\lim_{n \to \infty} (b_{2n}) = b$$

so

$$\sqrt{\pi} = b^2/(b\sqrt{2}) \quad \text{or} \quad b = \sqrt{(2\pi)}$$

so

$$n! \approx \sqrt{(2\pi)}n^{n+1/2} \exp(-n)$$

which is the result we wanted to demonstrate.

APPENDIX 6. The Wallis formula – the recurrence formula for integration

This formula, discovered by Wallis in the middle seventeenth century, can be used to compute π and is

$$\sqrt{\pi} = \lim_{n \to \infty} [(n!)^2 2^{2n}/(2n)! \sqrt{n}] \tag{1}$$

Wallis's formula is used in the derivation of Stirling's formula (see

Appendix 5) and is obtained by integrating

$$\int \sin^n(x)\,dx \tag{2}$$

This integration can be written as

$$\int \sin^{n-1}(x) \sin(x)\,dx$$

and is carried out by the technique of integration by parts (see Appendix 2).
  If we define

$$u = \sin^{n-1}(x) \quad \text{and} \quad dv = \sin(x)\,dx$$

then

$$du = (n-1)\sin^{n-2}(x)\cos(x)\,dx$$

and

$$v = -\cos(x)$$

so

$$v\,du = -(n-1)\sin^{n-2}(x)\cos^2(x)\,dx$$

But

$$\cos^2(x) = 1 - \sin^2(x)$$
$$v\,du = -(n-1)\sin^{n-2}(x) + (n-1)\sin^n(x)$$

or

$$\int \sin^n(x)\,dx = -\sin^{(n-1)}(x)\cos(x)$$

$$+ (n-1)\int \sin^{n-2}(x)\,dx - (n-1)\int \sin^n(x)\,dx$$

so

$$\int \sin^n(x)\,dx = -\left(\frac{1}{n}\right)\sin^{n-1}(x)\cos(x) + ((n-1)/n)\int \sin^{n-2}(x)\,dx$$

If we integrate (2) between 0 and $\pi/2$

$$\int_0^{\pi/2} \sin^n(x)\,dx = (1/n)[0-0] + ((n-1)/n)\int_0^{\pi/2} \sin^{n-2}(x)\,dx$$

or

$$\int_0^{\pi/2} \sin^n(x)\,dx = ((n-1)/n)\int_0^{\pi/2} \sin^{n-2}(x)\,dx$$

we can also write

$$\int_0^{\pi/2} \sin^{n-2}(x)\,dx = ((n-3)/(n-2))\int_0^{\pi/2} \sin^{n-4}(x)\,dx$$

and so on. Or, in general,

$$\int_0^{\pi/2} \sin^{2n}(x)\,dx = ((2n-1)/2n)\int_0^{\pi/2} \sin^{2(n-1)}(x)\,dx \tag{3}$$

If we expand the right-hand side of (3) we obtain

$$\int_0^{\pi/2} \sin^{2n}(x)\,dx = ((2n-1)(2n-3)(2n-5)\cdots 1)/$$

$$((2n)(2n-2)(2n-4)\cdots 2) \int_0^{\pi/2} dx$$

or

$$\int_0^{\pi/2} \sin^{2n}(x)\,dx = [((2n-1)(2n-3)(2n-5)\cdots 1)/$$

$$((2n)(2n-2)(2n-4)\cdots 2)]\pi/2 \quad (4)$$

Similarly

$$\int_0^{\pi/2} \sin^{2n+1}(x)\,dx = [((2n)(2n-2)(2n-4)\cdots 2)/$$

$$((2n+1)(2n-1)(2n-3)\cdots 3)](\pi/2) \quad (5)$$

where the last term is

$$\int_0^{\pi/2} \sin(x)\,dx = 1 - 0 = 1$$

If we divide (4) by (5) we obtain

$$\int_0^{\pi/2} \sin^{2n}(x)\,dx \Big/ \int_0^{\pi/2} \sin^{2n+1}(x)\,dx$$

$$= [((2n+1)(2n-1)\cdots 9\cdot 9\cdot 7\cdot 7\cdot 5\cdot 5\cdot 3\cdot 3\cdot 1\cdot 1)/$$

$$((2n)(2n)\cdots 10\cdot 10\cdot 8\cdot 8\cdot 6\cdot 6\cdot 4\cdot 4\cdot 2\cdot 2)]\pi/2 \quad (6)$$

From (6) the value of 2 is

$$\pi/2 = ((2n)(2n)\cdots 4\cdot 4\cdot 2\cdot 2)/((2n+1)(2n+1)\cdots 3\cdot 3\cdot 1\cdot 1)$$

$$\times \left[\int_0^{\pi/2} \sin^{2n}(x)\,dx \Big/ \int_0^{\pi/2} \sin^{2n+1}(x)\,dx \right] \quad (7)$$

Since $|\sin(x)| \leqslant 1$ and $\sin(x)$ is positive between 0 and $\pi/2$ then

$$\sin^{2n-1}(x) \geqslant \sin^{2n}(x) \geqslant \sin^{2n-1}(x) > 0$$

If we integrate the three terms we obtain

$$\int_0^{\pi/2} \sin^{2n-1}(x)\,dx \geqslant \int_0^{\pi/2} \sin^{2n}(x)\,dx \geqslant \int_0^{\pi/2} \sin^{2n+1}(x)\,dx > 0$$

But

$$\int_0^{\pi/2} \sin^{2n+1}(x)\,dx = (2n)/(2n+1) \int_0^{\pi/2} \sin^{2n-1}(x)\,dx$$

If we divide the three terms by

$$\int_0^{\pi} \sin^{2n+1}(x)\,dx$$

We obtain

$$(2n+1)/2n \geqslant \int_0^{\pi/2} \sin^{2n}(x)\,dx \bigg/ \int_0^{\pi/2} \sin^{2n+1}(x)\,dx \geqslant 1 > 0$$

or

$$1 + 1/2n \geqslant \int_0^{\pi/2} \sin^{2n}(x)\,dx \bigg/ \int_0^{\pi/2} \sin^{2n+1}(x)\,dx \geqslant 1$$

So

$$\lim_{n \to \infty} \left(\int_0^{\pi/2} \sin^{2n}(x)\,dx \right) \bigg/ \left(\int_0^{\pi/2} \sin^{2n+1}(x)\,dx \right) = 1 \qquad (8)$$

From (7) and (8)

$$\pi/2 = \lim_{n \to \infty} ((2n)(2n) \cdots 4 \cdot 4 \cdot 2 \cdot 2 / ((2n+1)(2n-1) \cdots 3 \cdot 3 \cdot 1 \cdot 1)) \qquad (9)$$

But

$$\lim_{n \to \infty} 2n/(2n+1) = \lim_{n \to \infty} 1/(1+1/2n) = 1$$

So

$$\lim_{n \to \infty} [(2n \cdot 2n \cdots 4 \cdot 4 \cdot 2 \cdot 2) / ((2n+1)(2n-1) \cdots 3 \cdot 3 \cdot 1 \cdot 1)]$$

$$= \lim_{n \to \infty} [(2/3)^2 (4/5)^2 (6/7)^2 \cdots ((2n-2)/(2n-1))^2 2n] \qquad (10)$$

From (9) and (10) and taking the square root

$$\sqrt{(\pi/2)} = \lim_{n \to \infty} [((2 \cdot 4 \cdot 6 \cdots (2n-2))/(3 \cdot 5 \cdot 7 \cdots (2n-1)))\sqrt{(2n)}]$$

Multiplying top and bottom of the right-hand side by $[2 \cdot 4 \cdot 6 \cdots (2n-2)]$

$$= \lim_{n \to \infty} [((2 \cdot 2 \cdot 4 \cdot 4 \cdot 6 \cdot 6 \cdots)/(2 \cdot 3 \cdot 4 \cdot 5 \cdot 6 \cdot 7 \cdots))\sqrt{(2n)}] \text{ that is}$$

$$= \lim_{n \to \infty} [((2^2 \cdot 4^2 \cdots (2n-2)^2)/(2n-1)!)\sqrt{(2n)}]$$

Multiplying top and bottom by $(2n)^2$ and rearranging:

$$= \lim_{n \to \infty} [(2^2 \cdot 4^2 \cdots (2n)^2/(2n)!)(\sqrt{(2n)}/2n)]$$

But

$$2^2 \cdot 4^2 \cdot 6^2 \cdot 8^2 \cdots = 2^2 \cdot 2^2 \cdot 2^2 \cdot 2^2 \cdot 3^2 \cdot 2^2 \cdot 4^2 \cdots$$

$$= 2^2 \cdot 2^2 \cdot 2^2 \cdot 2^2 \cdot \underbrace{2^2 \cdot 3^2 \cdot 4^2 \cdots}_{(n!)^2}$$

so

$$\sqrt{(\pi/2)} = \lim_{n \to \infty} [(n!)^2 2^{2n} \sqrt{2} \sqrt{n}/(2n)!\, 2n]$$

or

$$\sqrt{\pi} = \lim_{n \to \infty} [(n!)^2 2^{2n}/(2n)! \sqrt{n}]$$

which is Wallis's formula.

It is possible to derive in a similar way the following *recurrence formulae*:

$$\int \cos^n(x)\,dx = (1/n)\cos^{n-1}(x)\sin(x) + ((n-1)/n)\int \cos^{n-2}(x)\,dx$$

and

$$\int \sin^p(x)\cos^q(x)\,dx = ((\sin^{p+1}(x)\cos^{q-1}(x))/(p+q))$$

$$+ ((q-1)/(p+q))\int \sin^p(x)\cos^{q-2}(x)\,dx$$

APPENDIX 7. Introduction to probability theory

Frequency and probability

When we throw a die we can obtain six possible results: 1, 2, 3, 4, 5, 6. If we throw the die a large number of times we will obtain 1 in about 1/6 of the times, 2 in about 1/6 of the times, etc. However, the result will never be *exactly* 1/6 and this difference may be the result of at least three things. Firstly because we did not throw the die a sufficient number of times. Secondly because we threw the die in such a way that some numbers are more likely to appear than others. Thirdly because the die is not a perfect cube of homogeneous density. None of these hypotheses can be completely tested, so we can never be sure that the frequency with which 1 appears will be a fixed number. That is, if we throw the die N times and 1 appears n times we cannot, for sure, say that

$$f = n/N \to P = 1/6$$

when

$$N \to \infty$$

where P (the probability of throwing a 1) is exactly one sixth.

Definition of probability

We cannot use the frequency (f) of an event measured in a physical experiment to define the *mathematical* probability of the event. The approach used by mathematicians to define P is to use conceptual *random* experiments (or *thought* experiments). In other words, we define a perfect die and postulate that it is *equally likely* that from any throw the numbers 1, or 2, or 3, or 4, or 5, or 6 will be obtained. We then say that in a *conceptual random experiment* where, by definition, all the conditions are defined, the probability that A takes place is given by the ratio n/N, provided that

    (i) there are N possible outcomes,

    (ii) that all the outcomes are mutually exclusive,

    (iii) that all the outcomes are equally likely, and

    (iv) that n of these outcomes result in event A.

In the case of a *thought* die there are

    (i) six possible outcomes ($N=6$),

    (ii) these outcomes are mutually exclusive (that is, the numbers 1 and 6 cannot appear at the same time), and

    (iii) all the outcomes are equally likely.

We can thus write that the probability of throwing a 1 ($n=1$) is

$$P_{(1)} = n/N = 1/6$$

Simple and compound events

In this case A is a *simple event*, but we might think of A being a *compound event*. For example, what is the probability of throwing a die twice and obtaining a sum of 4. The N possible outcomes are 36 and this is shown in Table 1 where all possible permutations of the die throwing are shown. With this table we can derive some of the rules of probability.

The addition rule

If, as a result of a random conceptual experiment, event A occurs only in the mutually exclusive forms $A_1, A_2, \ldots, A_n$ then the probability of event A is the sum of the probabilities of $A_1, A_2, \ldots, A_n$ (rule of addition).

Table 1. *Permutations of die throwing*

1, 1	1, 2	1, 3	1, 4	1, 5	1, 6
2, 1	2, 2	2, 3	2, 4	2, 5	2, 6
3, 1	3, 2	3, 3	3, 4	3, 5	3, 6
4, 1	4, 2	4, 3	4, 4	4, 5	4, 6
5, 1	5, 2	5, 3	5, 4	5, 5	5, 6
6, 1	6, 2	6, 3	6, 4	6, 5	6, 6

and $n=3$ so

$$P = 3/36 = 1/12$$

In the experiment described above

Event	Outcome	Probability
A_1	1, 3	1/36
A_2	2, 2	1/36
A_3	3, 1	1/36
$A = A_1 + A_2 + A_3$		3/36

Also, if as a result of a conceptual random experiment the probability of occurrence of two mutually exclusive events A_1 and A_2 is respectively $P(A_1)$ and $P(A_2)$, the probability of the joint occurrence of A_1 and A_2 is the product $P(A_1)$ times $P(A_2) = P(A_1, A_2)$ (rule of multiplication).

The multiplication rule

In Table 1 the probability of the first die showing a 1 ($P(A_1)$) is $6/36 = 1/6$. The probability of the second die showing a 1 ($P(A_2)$) is also $6/36 = 1/6$. The probability of both dies showing a 1 ($P(A_1, A_2)$) is then

$$P(A_1, A_2) = P(A_1)P(A_2) = 1/6 \times 1/6 = 1/36 \tag{1}$$

which agrees with the result that can be obtained by inspection of the table.

To find the probability of the following compound event:

(a) that one of the throws shows 1 (A_1), and

(b) that the sum of the values of the two throws is 4 (A_2),

we first compute the probability of obtaining one with the first throw (event B_1) – it is 1/6. Then we compute the probability of obtaining one with the second throw (event B_2); it is again 1/6.

We then apply the addition rule

$$P(B_1) + P(B_2) = 1/6 + 1/6 = 2/6 = 12/36 \tag{2}$$

Then we subtract the probability of both dies being one (1/36) since it is not a favourable outcome.

So

$$P(A_1) = 11/36$$

Conditional probabilities

Yet the correct result, which can be obtained from the table, is 10/36. The reason why the application of the addition rule leads to the *wrong* result is because B_1 and B_2 are *not* independent events. We should compute the joint probability of getting one in the first throw ($P(B_1)$), and of *not* getting one in the second throw ($P(\bar{B}_2)$) and then we should compute the joint probability of getting 1 in the second throw $(P(B_2))$ and not getting 1 in the first throw $(P(\bar{B}_1))$.

So the probability of obtaining only one in the two throws is

$$P(A_1) = P(\bar{B}_2/B_1) + P(\bar{B}_1/B_2)$$

$P(\bar{B}_2/B_1)$ is the *conditional probability* of throwing 1 in the first throw and not 1 in the second. $P(\bar{B}_1/B_2)$ is the probability of getting 1 in the second throw and of not throwing 1 in the first throw.

But

$$P(\bar{B}_2/B_1) = P(\bar{B}_2) \cdot P(B_1) = 30/36 \cdot 6/36$$

and

$$P(\bar{B}_1/B_2) = 30/36 \cdot 6/36$$

so

$$P(A_1) = (10 \cdot 30)/(36 \cdot 36) = (2 \cdot 5 \cdot 6 \cdot 6)/6^2 \cdot 6^2 = 10/36$$

Let us now compute the probability $(P(A_2))$ of obtaining the sum of 4 (A_2) with the two throws. From the table

$$P(A_2) = 3/36$$

If we apply the multiplication rule

$$P(A_1, A_2) = P(A_1)P(A_2)$$
$$= (10/36)(3/36) = 30/36^2$$

But the actual value obtained from the table is 2/36.

The multiplication rule produced the wrong result because A_1 and A_2 are *not* independent events. We should not compute the absolute probability of getting a sum of 4 but the *conditional* probability of getting a sum of 4 when one of the throws shows 1 $(P(A_1/A_2))$, so

$$P(A_1/A_2) = 2/10$$

and

$$P(A_1, A_2) = P(A_1)P(A_1/A_2)$$
$$= (10/36)(2/10) = 20/360 = 2/36 \tag{3}$$

which is the correct result (from Table 1).

The average or expected value

In order to find the *average* sum that is obtained when we throw two dice we first define the average $(\bar{x})$ of a set of n values $(x_1, x_2, \ldots, x_n)$ by

$$\bar{x} = (x_1 + x_2 + x_3 + \cdots + x_n)/n$$
$$= \sum_{i=1}^{n} x_i/n \tag{4}$$

the values of the sums are given in the following table.

Table 2. *Average sums in throwing two dies*

2	3	4	5	6	7
3	4	5	6	7	8
4	5	6	7	8	9
5	6	7	8	9	10
6	7	8	9	10	11
7	8	9	10	11	12

From the table it can be computed (with equation (4)) that

$$\bar{x} = 7$$

Let us now construct a table where we write the number of times (n_i) each value (x_i) is observed, and its corresponding probability.

Table 3. *The numbers of times individual values are observed*

x_i	n_i	$P(x_i)$	$P(x_i)$	$x_i - x$	$(x_i - x)^2$
2	1	1/36	1/36	−5	25
3	2	2/36	3/36	−4	16
4	3	3/36	6/36	−3	9
5	4	4/36	10/36	−2	4
6	5	5/36	15/36	−1	1
7	6	6/36	21/36	+0	0
8	5	5/36	26/36	+1	1
9	4	4/36	30/36	+2	4
10	3	3/36	33/36	+3	9
11	2	2/36	35/36	+4	16
12	1	1/36	36/36	+5	25

From this table it can be seen that $\bar{x}$ (7) occurs most frequently ($n_i = 6$). Although in empirical measurements this might not be the case, in conceptual random experiments it always is. For this reason the *mean* (or average) is also known as the *expected value* ($E[x_i]$). So

$$E[\bar{x}_i] = \bar{x} = \text{mean or average}$$

From Table 3 it can also be seen that

$$n_i = P(x_i)N$$

The number of times a given value is observed is given by the product of its probability of occurrence ($P(x_i)$) and the number of observations (N). For $x_i = 5$

$$P(x_i) = 4/36$$
$$N = 36$$
$$n_5 = 4/36 \times 36 = 4$$

The mean ($\bar{x}$) can also be obtained from the individual probabilities by the relationship

$$\bar{x} = \sum_{i=1}^{n} P(x_i)x_i \tag{5}$$

$$= (1/36) \times 2 + (2/36) \times 3 + (3/36) \times 4 \cdots$$

$$= (1 \times 2 + 2 \times 3 + 3 \times 4 \cdots)/36$$

$$= (2 + 3 + 3 + 4 + 4 + 4 + \cdots)/36$$

Probability distribution function

There is a one-to-one correspondence between the first and the third column of Table 3; that is, for every x_i there is a corresponding $P(x_i)$. We can thus say that $P(x_i)$ is a function of x_i (see Appendix 2) and $P(x_i)$ is called the *probability distribution function*.

Cumulative distribution function

In column four of Table 3 we have computed the probability that x_i is equal to, or smaller than, a given value ($P(x_i)$). For example, the probability that x_i is equal to or smaller than 5 is 10/36. $P(x_i)$ is called the *cumulative distribution function*.

The variance

Although the average gives some information about the possible outcome of an event (its expected value) it does not provide a measure of the uncertainty of such an outcome. For example, we might have an experiment in which the outcomes, instead of ranging between 1 and 12, range between 6 and 8. The average is seven but the spread of the observations would be much less. In characterizing this spread we are not able to use the average values of the differences between individual observations (x_i) and the average value ($\bar{x}_i$). This is because this average is zero, since the total sum of the differences is zero:

$$\sum_{i=1}^{n} (x_i - x)P(x_i) = -5/36 - 8/36 - 9/36 - 5/36 + 0$$

$$+ 5/36 + 8/36 + 9/36 + 8/36 + 5/36$$

$$= 0$$

If we compute instead the *square* of the differences, every difference will make a positive contribution to the total and now the result will be non-zero.

$$\sum_{i=1}^{n} (x-x_i)^2 P(x_i) = 25/36 + 32/36 + 27/36 + 16/36 + 5/36 + 0$$
$$+ 5/36 + 16/36 + 27/36 + 32/36 + 25/36$$
$$= 210/36$$

In this calculation we have summed all the squares of the differences and divided by their number (36). However, this is not correct because we started with 36 observations, computed a new value $(\bar{x})$, and then computed 36 differences. But only 35 of the differences are independent, since $\bar{x}$ is obtained from the 36 values. This means that once we know 35 differences the last one is not independent so we should divide the sum of the square by 35. The value obtained is called the *variance* (s^2), so

$$s^2 = \sum_{i=1}^{n} (x_i - \bar{x})^2 / (n-1) \tag{6}$$

Standard deviation and standard error of the mean

The square root of the variance is called the *standard deviation* (s or σ) and the ratio between s (or σ) and $\sqrt{n}$ is called the *standard error of the mean*.

Although tables such as Table 1 or 3 may be very useful if we want to make predictions about random events, rather than construct tables every time it is easier to obtain analytical expressions from which we can derive the probability of a given event.

In order to obtain such expressions we first set up a mathematical model of the conceptual random experiment. When we do this we obtain a limited number of analytical expressions which can be used for a wide range of situations.

Probability of a certain event and of an impossible event

But before we obtain these expressions we need to introduce other basic concepts of probability theory. The first is that the probability of a *certain* event is *one* and the second is that the probability of an *impossible* event is *zero*. The third is that in conceptual random experiments where the only possible events of the experiment are $A_1, A_2, \ldots, A_n$, then

$$P(A_1) + P(A_2) + P(A_3) + \cdots + P(A_n) = 1 \tag{7}$$

If the conceptual random experiment can produce N independent outcomes and if event A_1 corresponds to n_1 of these outcomes, event A_2 to

n_2 of these outcomes, and so on, then

$$P(A_1) = n_1/N$$
$$P(A_2) = n_2/N$$
$$\vdots$$
$$P(A_K) = n_K/N$$

and

$$P(A_1) + P(A_2) + \cdots + P(A_n) = n_1/N + n_2/N + \cdots + n_K/N$$
$$= (n_1 + n_2 + n_3 + \cdots + n_K)/N$$
$$= N/N = 1$$

Equation (7) implies that the probability of any one event is then

$$P(A_1) = 1 - (P(A_2) + P(A_3) + \cdots + P(A_n))$$

Another useful concept is the probability of an event *not* taking place. If the probability of the event A_1 is $P(A_1)$, then the probability of event A_1 not taking place ($P(\bar{A}_1)$) is given by

$$P(\bar{A}_1) = 1 - P(A_1) \tag{8}$$

The binomial distribution

With these basic concepts and our introductory remarks we should now be able to derive a number of mathematical models, the first of which leads to the *binomial distribution*. In order to do this we assume that we are performing a conceptual random experiment with only two possible outcomes. For example, when we throw a die and we consider only two possible outcomes, such as obtaining the number 1 (one) or of not obtaining a 1 (one). If the probability of getting a favourable outcome is θ (1/6), then if we throw the die twice the probability of a favourable outcome (getting 1 twice) will be θ^2 (by the multiplication rule). The probability of an unfavourable outcome on both throws (not getting 1 twice) is then $(1 - \theta)^2$. The third possibility is that we get only one favourable outcome out of the two throws. This result can occur in two different ways, that is, if 1 occurs in the first throw and does not occur in the second throw, and if 1 does not occur in the first throw but does occur in the second throw. The probability of the first event is (multiplication rule) $\theta(1 - \theta)$ while the probability of the second event is $(1 - \theta)\theta$. By the addition rule the probability ($P(1)$) of getting only a one in both throws is $2\theta(1 - \theta)$.

So we can write

$$P(0) = (1 - \theta)^2$$
$$P(1) = 2\theta(1 - \theta)$$
$$P(2) = \theta^2$$

We can check that these probabilities are right by seeing whether the sum of all the probabilities is equal to one:

$$P(0) + P(1) + P(2) = (1 - \theta)^2 + 2\theta(1 - \theta) + \theta^2$$
$$= 1 - 2\theta + \theta^2 - 2\theta - 2\theta^2 + \theta^2$$
$$= 1$$

The possible outcomes from throwing the die three times are

$$\theta\theta\theta = \theta^3$$
$$\theta\theta(1 - \theta) = \theta^2(1 - \theta)$$
$$\theta(1 - \theta)\theta = \theta^2(1 - \theta)$$
$$(1 - \theta)\theta\theta = \theta^2(1 - \theta)$$
$$\theta(1 - \theta)(1 - \theta) = \theta(1 - \theta)^2$$
$$(1 - \theta)(1 - \theta)\theta = \theta(1 - \theta)^2$$
$$(1 - \theta)\theta(1 - \theta) = \theta(1 - \theta)^2$$
$$(1 - \theta)(1 - \theta)(1 - \theta) = (1 - \theta)^3$$

so

$$P(0) = (1 - \theta)^3$$
$$P(1) = 3\theta(1 - \theta)^2$$
$$P(2) = 3\theta^2(1 - \theta)$$
$$P(3) = \theta^3$$

If we follow a similar procedure to compute the outcome of throwing the die four times we obtain

$$P(0) = (1 - \theta)^4$$
$$P(1) = 4\theta(1 - \theta)^3$$
$$P(2) = 6\theta^2(1 - \theta)^2$$
$$P(3) = 4\theta^3(1 - \theta)^2$$
$$P(4) = \theta^4$$

Table 4 shows the results obtained so far. This table shows that the

Table 4. *Die-throwing forecasts*

1 throw	2 throws	3 throws	4 throws
			$P(0) = 1\ (1 - \theta)^4$
		$P(0) = 1\ (1 - \theta)^3$	
	$P(0) = 1\ (1 - \theta)^2$		$P(1) = 4\ (1 - \theta)^3\theta$
$P(0) = 1\ (1 - \theta)$		$P(1) = 3\ (1 - \theta)^2\theta$	
	$P(1) = 2\ \theta(1 - \theta)$		$P(2) = 6\ (1 - \theta)^2\theta^2$
$P(1) = 1\ \theta$		$P(2) = 3\ (1 - \theta)\theta^2$	
	$P(2) = 1\ \theta^2$		$P(3) = 4\ (1 - \theta)\theta^3$
			$P(4) = 1\ \theta^4$

probability of any outcome $(P(0), P(1), \ldots, P(n))$ depends upon the number of times the die is thrown. If we examine the numerical coefficients in this table they can be seen to give the following pattern:

1 throw	2 throws	3 throws	4 throws
			1
		1	
	1		4
1		3	
	2		6
1		3	
	1		4
		1	
			1

This pattern is Pascal's triangle (see Appendix 2) and represents the coefficients of the expansion of the binomial series $(a+x)^n$. The terms in the binomial expansion are the same as the terms in Table 4 if $0 = a$ and $(1-\theta) = x$. So, we can write

$$P_n(x) = (n!/x!\,(n-x)!)\theta^x(1-\theta)^{n-x} \tag{9}$$

Equation (9) gives the probability $(P_n(x))$ of obtaining outcome x in a conceptual random experiment performed n times. If, for example, $\theta = 1/6$ then $(1-\theta) = 5/6$. The probability of obtaining a 1 three times $(x=3)$ when we throw the die 5 times $(n=5)$, is

$$P_5(3) = 5!/(3!\,2!) \times (1/6)^3 \times (1-1/6)^2$$
$$= 5 \times 2 \times 0.00463 \times 0.694$$
$$= 0.032$$

Expression (9) is called the *binomial distribution*, and the binomial distribution is completely defined once we know θ and n. We can also compute the mean (expected value) and the variance of this distribution.

The mean of a binomial distribution
By definition

$$\bar{x} = \sum_{x=0}^{n} xP(x) = \sum_{x=0}^{n} [x(n!/x!\,(n-x)!)\theta^x(1-\theta)^{n-x}]$$

$$= \sum_{x=0}^{n} n[(x(n-1)!/(x-1)!\,x(n-x)!)\theta^x(1-\theta)^{n-x}]$$

$$= n\theta \sum_{x=1}^{n} [((n-1)!/(x-1)!\,(n-x)!)\theta^{x-1}(1-\theta)^{n-x}]$$

If $a = x - 1$, then $n - x = n - a - 1$, and

$$\bar{x} = n\theta \sum_{a=0}^{n} ((n-1)!/a!\,(n-a-1)!)\theta^a(1-\theta)^{n-a-1}$$

But the sum of the expression under the summation sign is equal to 1, since it is the sum of all possible outcomes where value a is obtained from $n-1$ trials, so

$$\bar{x} = n\theta \tag{10}$$

The variance of a binomial distribution

The variance is, by definition,

$$s^2 = \sum_{1}^{n} (x - \bar{x})^2/n$$

(Note that for large n we can use n instead of $n-1$.) But

$$\sum_{1}^{n} (x - \bar{x})^2 = \sum_{1}^{n} (\bar{x}^2 - 2\bar{x}x + x^2)$$

$$= \sum_{1}^{n} \bar{x}^2 - 2\bar{x} \sum_{1}^{n} x + \sum_{1}^{n} x^2$$

$$= n\bar{x}^2 - 2n\bar{x}^2 + \sum_{1}^{n} x^2 \quad \left(\text{since } n\bar{x} = \sum_{1}^{n} x\right)$$

$$= \sum_{1}^{n} x^2 - n\bar{x}^2 = \left(\left(\sum_{1}^{n} x(x-1)/n\right) - \bar{x}(\bar{x}-1)\right)n$$

Since

$$s^2 = \sum_{1}^{n} (x - \bar{x})^2/n$$

then

$$s^2 = n\left(\sum_{1}^{n} (x(x-1)/n) - \bar{x}(\bar{x}-1)\right)\Big/n$$

$$s^2 = \sum_{1}^{n} (x(x-1)/n) - \bar{x}(\bar{x}-1)$$

Also

$$\sum_{1}^{n} x(x-1)/n = \sum_{0}^{n} x(x-1)P_n(x)$$

$$= \sum_{0}^{n} x(x-1)(n!/(n-x)!\,x!)\theta^x(1-\theta)^{n-x}$$

$$= n(n-1)\theta^2 \sum_{2}^{n} ((n-2)!/(x-2)!\,(n-x)!)\theta^{x-2}(1-\theta)^{n-x}$$

If $x - 2 = a$, then $x = a + 2$, and

$$\sum_{1}^{n} x(x-1)/n = n(n-1)\theta^2 \underbrace{\sum_{0}^{n-2} ((n-2)!/a!\,(n-a-2)!)\theta^a(1-\theta)^{n-a-2}}_{=1}$$

But the value of the sum is 1, so

$$\sum_1^n x(x-1)/n = n(n-1)\theta^2$$

so

$$s^2 = \overbrace{n(n-1)\theta^2}^{\bar{x}} - \overbrace{n\theta\,(n\theta-1)}^{(\bar{x}-1)} = n\theta(1-\theta)$$

So, for a binomial distribution the mean and variance are:

$$\bar{x} = n\theta$$
$$s^2 = n\theta(1-\theta) \tag{11}$$

The Poisson distribution

The binomial distribution tends to two other distributions under some special conditions. These are the Poisson distribution or the normal distribution. Let us first deal with the Poisson distribution.

If θ decreases as n increases, that is,

$$\theta = \varepsilon/n$$

where ε is a constant, so that when $n \to \infty$ it tends to zero and the binomial distribution tends to the Poisson distribution. If we substitute θ by ε/n

$$P(x) = (n!/x!\,(n-x)!)(\varepsilon/n)^x(1-\varepsilon/n)^{n-x}$$
$$= (n(n-1)(n-2)\cdots(n-x+1)/x!)\varepsilon^x/n^x(1-\varepsilon/n)^{n-x}$$
$$= [(1-1/n)(1-2/n)\cdots(1-(x-1)/n)(1-\varepsilon/n)^{-x}](\varepsilon^x/x!)(1-\varepsilon/n)^n$$

When $n \to \infty$ every term in the denominator tends to zero. Thus the product inside the brackets tends to 1. Also

$$\lim_{n \to \infty}(1-\varepsilon/n)^n = \exp(-\varepsilon) \quad \text{(see Appendix 2)}$$

So

$$P(x) \underset{n \to \infty}{=} (\varepsilon^x/x!)\exp(-\varepsilon) \tag{12}$$

which is the expression for the Poisson distribution. Thus equation (12) was derived from the binomial distribution, with the assumption that the number of trials is infinite and that the probability of a favourable outcome (θ) is very small ($\to 0$).

The mean of the Poisson distribution

By definition the mean of the Poisson distribution is given by

$$\bar{x} = \sum_{x=0}^{x=n} xP(x) = \sum_{x=0}^{x=n} x(\varepsilon^x/x!)\exp(-\varepsilon)$$
$$= 0 + \varepsilon\exp(-\varepsilon) + \varepsilon^2\exp(-\varepsilon) + (\varepsilon^3/2!)\exp(-\varepsilon) + (\varepsilon^4/3!)\exp(-\varepsilon) + \cdots$$
$$= \varepsilon\exp(-\varepsilon)(1 + \varepsilon + \varepsilon^2/2! + \varepsilon^3/3! + \cdots)$$

But the term inside the brackets is the power series expansion of $\exp(\varepsilon)$ (see Appendix 2) so

$$\bar{x} = \varepsilon \exp(-\varepsilon)\exp(\varepsilon) = \varepsilon$$

or

$$\bar{x} = \varepsilon \tag{13}$$

So ε is the mean of the Poisson distribution.

The variance of the Poisson distributions

The variance can also be found from our original definition of s^2

$$s^2 = \sum_{x=0}^{\infty} (\bar{x}-x)^2 P(x)$$

$$= \sum_{x=0}^{\infty} (\bar{x}^2 P(x) - 2xP(x))\bar{x} + x^2 P(x)$$

$$= \sum_{x=0}^{\infty} \bar{x}^2 P(x) - \sum_{0}^{\infty} 2xP(x)\bar{x} + \sum_{0}^{\infty} x^2 P(x)$$

$$= \bar{x}^2 \sum_{0}^{\infty} P(x) - 2\bar{x}\sum_{0}^{\infty} xP(x) + \sum_{0}^{\infty} x^2 P(x)$$

But

$$\sum_{0}^{\infty} P(x) = 1$$

and

$$\sum_{0}^{\infty} xP(x) = \bar{x} = \varepsilon$$

so

$$s^2 = \varepsilon^2 - 2\varepsilon^2 + \sum_{0}^{\infty} x^2 P(x)$$

$$= \sum_{0}^{\infty} x^2 P(x) - \varepsilon^2$$

But

$$\sum_{0}^{\infty} x^2 P(x) = \sum_{0}^{\infty} x^2 (\varepsilon^x/x!)\exp(-\varepsilon)$$

$$= 0 + \varepsilon\exp(-\varepsilon) + 2\varepsilon^2\exp(-\varepsilon) + \frac{3\varepsilon^3\exp(-\varepsilon)}{2!} + \frac{4\varepsilon^4\exp(-\varepsilon)}{3!}$$

$$= \varepsilon\exp(-\varepsilon)(1 + 2\varepsilon + 3\varepsilon^2/2! + 4\varepsilon^3/3! + \cdots)$$

But the term inside the brackets is $(\varepsilon+1)\exp(\varepsilon)$ because

$$\exp(\varepsilon) = 1 + \varepsilon + \varepsilon^2/2! + \varepsilon^3/3! + \varepsilon^4/4! + \cdots$$

and

$$\varepsilon\exp(\varepsilon) = \varepsilon + \varepsilon^2 + \varepsilon^3/2! + \varepsilon^4/3! + \varepsilon^5/4! + \cdots$$

so

$$\exp(\varepsilon) + \varepsilon \exp(\varepsilon) = \exp(\varepsilon)(\varepsilon + 1) = 1 + 2\varepsilon + (3/2!)\varepsilon^2 + (4/3!)\varepsilon^3 + \cdots$$

since the term inside the bracket is $(\varepsilon + 1)\exp(\varepsilon)$, then

$$\sum_0^\infty x^2 P(x) = \varepsilon \exp(-\varepsilon)(\varepsilon + 1)(\exp(\varepsilon))$$

$$s^2 = (\varepsilon + 1)\exp(\varepsilon)\exp(-\varepsilon)\varepsilon - \varepsilon^2 = \varepsilon^2 + \varepsilon - \varepsilon^2 = \varepsilon$$

so

$$s^2 = \varepsilon \tag{14}$$

We thus see that in the Poisson distribution the mean and the variance are the same.

The normal distribution

Another distribution that can be derived from the binomial distribution is the *normal distribution*. The normal distribution has even wider applications than the binomial or the Poisson distribution. It can be shown that the following mathematical relationship holds (see Hald).

$$\lim(n!/x! \, (n-n)!)\theta^x(1-\theta)^{n-x}$$

$$\approx (1/\sqrt{(2\pi n\theta(1-\theta))}) \exp(-(x-n\theta)^2/2n\theta(1-\theta))$$

if we define

$$\varepsilon = n\theta \tag{15}$$

and

$$s^2 = n\theta(1-\theta)$$

then the right-hand side becomes

$$P(x) = (1/\sqrt{(2\pi s^2)}) \exp(-[(x-\varepsilon)/\sqrt{2s}]^2) \tag{16}$$

Equation (16) is the probability distribution function of the *normal distribution*. In this distribution the random variable can take any real value and $n \to \infty$. If there are an *infinite number* of different possible outcomes, then the probability associated with any value of x becomes infinitesimal. This means that (16) is not a probability distribution function in the same sense as the binomial, or the Poisson distribution, functions. It is called a *probability density function*. However, we can associate a finite probability to finding x, between x_1 and $x_1 + \Delta x$, and this probability will be

$$\Delta P(x) \approx p(x)\Delta x \tag{17}$$

For small Δx, (17) becomes

$$dP(x) = p(x)\,dx$$

the probability of x being between 0 (zero) and x will then be

$$P(x) = \int_0^x p(x)\,dx = 1/\sqrt{(2\pi s^2)} \int_0^x \exp(-[(x-\varepsilon)/\sqrt{2s}]^2)\,dx \tag{18}$$

From (18) one can see that

$$(d/dx)P(x) = p(x)$$

dP/dx is the rate of change of the cumulative probability with x, so $p(x)$ is a probability per unit of x. It can be directly compared with *density* defined as

$$dM/dv$$

where M is mass and v is volume, hence the term *density* in probability density function. $P(x)$ is called the *cumulative distribution function* for the case where the random variable (x) is continuous. It is cumulative because we are integrating (summing) over x.

If we define u as

$$u = (x - \varepsilon)/\sqrt{2s} \tag{19}$$

then

$$du = dx/\sqrt{2s} \quad \text{or} \quad dx = \sqrt{2s}\, du \tag{20}$$

and

$$x = \sqrt{2su} + \varepsilon = a \tag{21}$$

The error function

If we substitute (19), (20) and (21) into (18) we obtain

$$P(x) = \frac{1}{\sqrt{\pi}} \int_0^a e^{-u^2}\, du \tag{22}$$

which is half the *error function*; it is divided by 2 because we only considered the occurrence of x between zero and x in equation (18). Since the normal distribution is symmetrical around $u = 0$, the probability of finding a value of x between 0 and x is half that of finding it between $-x$ and x. The error function is used in Chapters 3 and (8).

We shall now generalize the definitions of *mean* and *average* to the case of a continuous random variable. (In a discrete distribution the random variable x can only have values (x_i). In a continuous distribution x may be *any* real value.) The definition of an average was given in (5).

The mean of the normal distribution

Returning to equation (5)

$$\bar{x} \ (\text{or } \varepsilon) = \sum_{i=1}^{n} P(x_i) x_i \tag{5}$$

For the case of a continuous variable $P(x_i)$ becomes

$$P(x_i) \rightarrow p(x)\, \Delta x$$

discontinuous x continuous x

also $n \to \infty$. So (5) becomes

$$\bar{x} = \lim_{\substack{n \to \infty \\ \Delta x \to 0}} \sum_1^n xp(x)\Delta x = \int_0^\infty xp(x)\,dx \tag{23}$$

The variance of the normal distribution

Similarly while for a discontinuous random variable the variance s^2 is given by

$$s^2 = \sum_1^n P(x)(\bar{x} - x_i)^2$$

for a continuous variable

$$s^2 = \lim_{\substack{n \to \infty \\ x \to 0}} \sum_1^n (\bar{x} - x)^2 P(x)\Delta x$$
$$= \int_0^\infty (\bar{x} - x)^2 p(x)\,dx \tag{24}$$

APPENDIX 8. Partial fractions

The solution of linear differential equations by the Laplace transform method leads to solutions in the p domain (see Appendix 14) of the type

$$Y(p) = R(p)/Q(p) \tag{1}$$

where $R(p)$ and $Q(p)$ are polynomials in p of order $n-1$ or smaller, and n respectively. In order to obtain the inverse Laplace transform of (1) it is often convenient to expand the fraction into a sum of simpler fractions of the type

$$A/(p+a) \tag{2}$$

or

$$(Ap + B)/(p^2 + ap + b) \tag{3}$$

The inverse transforms of these simpler fractions can then be obtained directly from tables of Laplace transforms.

Expressing equation (1) as a sum of fractions of types (2) and (3) is known as the expansion into *partial fractions*, a method that is also used to integrate rational functions (a rational function is defined as a ratio between any two polynomials). The first step in the expansion is to express $Q(p)$ as products of factors of the type

$$(p+\alpha)^m \quad \text{or} \quad (p^2 + ap + b)^n$$

where m and n can be 1, 2, ... and α, a and b can be any real numbers including zero. If the factor is of the form

$$(p+\alpha)$$

then the partial fraction is of the form

$$A/(p+\alpha)$$

where A is a real number or a constant to be determined. If the factor is of the form

$$(p+\alpha)^2 \quad \text{or} \quad (p^2+ap+b)$$

then the partial fraction is of the form

$$(Ap+B)/(p+\alpha)^2 \quad \text{or} \quad (Ap+B)/(p^2+ap+b)$$

where A and B are real numbers to be determined. For factors of the form $(p+\alpha)^3$ the partial fraction is of the form

$$(Ap^2+Bp+C)/(p+\alpha)^3$$

where A, B and C are real numbers or constants to be determined. In order to show how A, B and C can be determined we will work through the following example. If $Y(p)$ is of the form

$$Y(p)=(a_2 p^2+a_1 p+a_0)/(b_3 p^3+b_2 p^2+b_1 p+b_0) \tag{4}$$

then $Y(p)$ can be rearranged as

$$Y(p)=(a_2/b_3)(p^2+(a_1/a_2)p+(a_0/a_2))/$$
$$(p^3+(b_2/b_3)p^2+(b_1/b_3)p+b_0/b_3)$$
$$=(a_2/b_3)(p^2+a_1'p+a_0')/(p^3+(b_2/b_3)p^2+(b_1/b_3)p+(b_0/b_3))$$

Let us assume that the denominator can be expanded as the product

$$(p+\alpha)(p^2+B_1 p+B_0)$$

so

$$Y(p)=(a_2/b_3)(p^2+a_1'p+a_0')/(p+\alpha)(p^2+B_1 p+B_0) \tag{5}$$

We can now expand (5) in partial fractions, so

$$Y(p)=(a_2/b_3)[A/(p+\alpha)+(B_1 p+C)/(p^2+B_1 p+B_0)] \tag{6}$$

where A is given by the value of

$$A=(p^2+a_1'p+a_0')/(p^2+B_1 p+B_0)$$

for $p=-\alpha$.

We then add the fractions inside the brackets of the right-hand side of (6) to obtain

$$((A+B_1)p^2+(AB_1+\alpha B_1+C)p+(\alpha C+AB_0))/(p+\alpha)(p^2+B_1 p+B_0) \tag{7}$$

If we compare (7) with the fractions on the right-hand side of (5) the two fractions have the same denominator so their numerators must be equal, since (5) is assumed to be equal to (6) so

$$A+B_1=1 \quad \text{coefficient of } p^2 \tag{8}$$

$$AB_1 + \alpha B_1 + C = a_1' \quad \text{coefficient of } p$$
$$\alpha C + AB_0 = a_0' \quad \text{independent term} \tag{9}$$

Since we know A we can obtain B_1 from (8) and C from (9).

APPENDIX 9. Integration of differential equations: the separation of variables technique

Differential equations arise naturally in the description of physical systems as it is often possible to relate rates of change (with time or with distance) with the value of a function.

Analysis of an RC circuit: first-order differential equation

Let us take for an example the simple electrical circuit shown in Figure A9.1. This consists of a battery (E), a switch (s), a resistor (R) and a capacitor (C). We shall write the equation of the circuit and then compute V_C, the voltage across the capacitor. By Kirchhoff's law for the voltage when the switch is closed

$$E = V_R + V_C \tag{1}$$

where V_R is the voltage across R and V_C is the voltage across C. By Ohm's Law

$$V_R = IR \tag{2}$$

where I is the current flowing in the circuit. The relationship between V_C and $I_c \, (= I)$ is

$$I_c = I = C(\mathrm{d}/\mathrm{d}t)(V_C)$$

Fig.A9.1

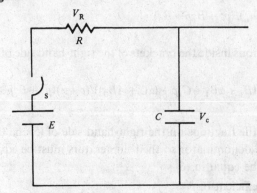

as

$$V_C = V \quad \text{then} \quad I = C \, dV/dt \tag{3}$$

From (2) and (3)

$$V_R/R = C \, dV/dt$$

But from (1)

$$V_R = E - V_c = E - V$$

so

$$(E - V)/R = C \, dV/dt \tag{4}$$

We can rearrange equation (4) as

$$dV/dt + V/RC = E/RC$$

If we define

$$RC = T$$

then

$$dV/dt + V/T = E/T \tag{5}$$

Equation (5) is a differential equation since it relates V, dV/dt and t. This equation can be solved in at least two ways. One way is by the technique known as separation of variables and another is by the integrating factor method described in Appendix 10.

To solve by separation of variables we first rearrange (5) as

$$dV/dt = -(V/T - E/T) = -(1/T)(V - E)$$

or

$$dV/(V - E) = -(1/T) \, dt \tag{6}$$

In equation (6) we have terms in V on the left-hand side and terms in t on the right-hand side. We now integrate each of the two sides since we want to obtain V as a function of t.

$$\int (1/(V - E)) \, dV = \phi V + C$$

where

$$(d/dx)\phi(V) = 1/(V - E)$$

Let us make the substitution (see Appendix 2)

$$x = V - E$$

then

$$dx = dV$$

so

$$\int dx/x = \ln(x) + C$$

$$= \ln(V - E) + C_1$$

Let us now integrate the right-hand side

$$\int -(1/T)\,dt = -(1/T)\int dt = -t/T + C_2$$

so

$$\ln(V-E) + C_1 = -t/T + C_2$$

If we now define c as

$$c = C_2 - C_1$$

In order to find c we have to go back to the physical system. If at $t = 0$ there was no charge $(q_0 = 0)$ across the capacitor then

$$V_0 = q_0/c = 0$$

so

$$\ln(-E) = c$$

or

$$\ln(V-E) = -t/T + \ln(-E)$$

or

$$\ln(V-E) - \ln(-E) = -t/T$$

thus

$$\ln((V-E)/(-E)) = -t/T$$

and

$$(V-E)/(-E) = \exp(-t/T) \tag{7}$$

or

$$V = E(1 - \exp(-t/T))$$

Solution (7) could have been obtained in a slightly different way: if we had used the definition of the definite integral (see Appendix 2)

$$\int_{V(0)}^{V(t)} dV/(V-E) = -(1/T)\int_0^t dt$$

The left-hand side means the definite integral between V for $t = 0$ and V for $t = t$, the right-hand side means the definite integral between time zero and time t. Since we said that

$$V(0) = 0$$

then

$$\int_0^V dV/(V-E) = -(1/T)\int_0^t dt$$

so

$$[\ln(V-E)]_0^V = -(1/T)[t]_0^t$$

or

$$\ln(V-E) - \ln(-E) = -t/T - 0$$

or

$$V = E(1 - \exp(-t/T))$$

APPENDIX 10. Integration of differential equations by the integrating factor

Let us consider a differential equation of the form

$$d(Y)/dx + a(x)y = b(x) \tag{1}$$

Where both $a(x)$ and $b(x)$ are functions of x. We now define function u as

$$u = \int a(x)\, dx \tag{2}$$

then

$$d(u)/dx = a(x) \tag{3}$$

by the fundamental rule of calculus.

If we define a function z by the relationship

$$z = \exp(u) \tag{4}$$

then

$$d(z)/dx = (d(z)/du)(d(u)/dx) \tag{5}$$

But

$$d(z)/du = \exp(u) \tag{6}$$

so

$$d(z)/dx = \exp(u)a(x) = \exp\left(\int a(x)\, dx\right)a(x) \tag{7}$$

If we now obtain the derivative of the product yz

$$d(yz)/dx = z(d(y)/dx) + y(d(z)/dx) \tag{8}$$

From (4), (7) and (8)

$$(d/dx)\left(y\exp\left(\int a(x)\, dx\right)\right)$$

$$= \exp\left(\int a(x)\, dx\right)(d(y)/dx) + a(x)y\exp\left(\int a(x)\, dx\right)$$

$$= \exp\left(\int a(x)\, dx\right)(d(y)/dx + a(x)y)$$

and

$$\exp\left(-\int a(x)\, dx\right)(d/dx)\left(y\exp\left(\int a(x)\, dx\right)\right) = d(y)/dx + a(x)y = b(x)$$

or

$$\exp\left(-\int a(x)\, dx\right)(d/dx)\left(y\exp\left(\int a(x)\, dx\right)\right) = b(x) \tag{9}$$

If we multiply both sides of (9) by $\exp\left(\int a(x)\, dx\right)$ we obtain

$$(d/dx)\left(y\exp\left(\int a(x)\, dx\right)\right) = \exp\left(+\int a(x)\, dx\right)b(x)$$

or

$$\int (d/dx)\left(y \exp\left(\int a(x)\,dx \right)\right) dx = \int \exp\left(+ \int a(x)\,dx \right) b(x)\,dx + C$$

so

$$y \exp\left(\int a(x)\,dx \right) = \int \exp\left(+ \int a(x)\,dx \right) b(x)\,dx + C$$

then

$$y = \exp\left(- \int a(x)\,dx \right)\left[\int \left(\exp\left(\int a(x)\,dx \right) b(x) \right) dx + C \right] \qquad (10)$$

Equation (10) is the solution of equation (1) where C is the integration constant and the function $\exp(u)$ is called the *integrating factor*.

APPENDIX 11. The Fourier expansion

Expansion of a periodic function in a series of trigonometric functions

It can be shown that most periodic functions observed in nature can be adequately represented by a Fourier series of the type

$$f(x) = a_0 + \sum_{n=1}^{n=\infty} (a_n \cos(nx) + b_n \sin(nx)) \qquad (1)$$

(In fact, only periodic functions that have a finite number of discontinuities within a period can be expanded in a Fourier series, but the proof of this is beyond the scope of this book.)

Since we are interested mainly in *time functions* we shall use sinusoids of the type

$$a_n \cos(n\omega t) \quad \text{and} \quad b_n \sin(n\omega t)$$

So in the Fourier series expression (1) becomes

$$f(t) = a_0 + \sum_{n=1}^{n=\infty} (a_n \cos(n\omega t) + b_n \sin(n\omega t)) \qquad (2)$$

Radians, radians per second and cycles per second

Since the argument (x) of $\sin(x)$ or $\cos(x)$ is either degrees or radians the arguments of the sinusoids in expression (2), $n\omega t$, must have the dimensions of degrees or radians (usually radians are used). Since n is a dimensionless integer, the dimensions of ω must be radians $\cdot$ s^{-1}. So

$$\omega = \text{radians} \cdot \text{s}^{-1}$$

and ω is thus an angular velocity. The function $\cos(n\omega t)$ or $\sin(n\omega t)$ repeats itself every T seconds and this is known as the *time period* of the function.

When $t = T$, T is then the time period of the function,

$$n\omega T = n2\pi \quad \text{or} \quad \omega T = 2\pi$$

so

$$\omega = 2\pi/T$$

If the function repeats itself f times in a second, we call f the frequency. The unit of frequency is the Hertz, and one Hertz is one cycle per second. So

$$f = 1/T = T^{-1} \quad \text{(no. of cycles per second)}$$

and

$$\omega = 2\pi f$$

The two sinusoidal functions within the brackets under the summation sign can be added to give a sinusoid. In Appendix 3 we saw that

$$\cos(x - \theta_n) = \cos(\theta_n)\cos(x) + \sin(\theta_n)\sin(x)$$

or, more generally, multiplying both sides by A_n,

$$A_n \cos(x - \theta_n) = A_n \cos(\theta_n)\cos(x) + A_n \sin(\theta_n)\sin(x) \tag{3}$$

If we make

$$x = n\omega t$$

and compare (3) with the sum

$$a_n \cos(n\omega t) + b_n \sin(n\omega t)$$

then

$$a_n = A_n \cos(\theta_n) \quad \text{and} \quad b_n = A_n \sin(\theta n)$$

so

$$a_n^2 + b_n^2 = A_n^2 (\cos^2(\theta_n) + \sin^2(\theta_n))$$

but

$$\cos^2(\theta_n) + \sin^2(\theta_n) = 1 \quad \text{(see Appendix 3)}$$

so

$$A_n = \sqrt{(a_n^2 + b_n^2)} \tag{4}$$

Also

$$b_n/a_n = +\sin(\theta_n)/\cos(\theta_n) = +\tan(\theta_n) \text{or}$$

or

$$\theta_n = \tan^{-1}(-b_n/a_n)$$
$$= -\tan^{-1}(b_n/a_n) \tag{5}$$

From (3), (4) and (5)

$$a_n \cos(n\omega t) + b_n \sin(n\omega t) = A_n \cos(n\omega t - \theta_n) \tag{6}$$

We can think of the term a_n as the projection in the x axis of a line of length A_n making an angle (θ_n) with the x axis. The arc θ_n is called a *phase* (or *phase angle* or *phase arc*).

The parameters of a sinusoid

A sinusoid is thus characterized by three constants, which are

(i) the angular frequency ($n\omega$) or the linear frequency (nf),

(ii) the amplitude (A_n), and

(iii) the phase (θ_n).

Expressions (2) and (6) mean that the expansion of the periodic function $f(t)$ contains a constant term (a_0) and a series of sinusoid harmonics (a_n and b_n or A_n). The series of sinusoids consists of the *fundamental* (a_1, b_1 or A_1) with the same period T of $f(t)$ given by the expression

$$T = 2\pi/\omega \tag{7}$$

and the remaining components with double the frequency (2ω), three times the frequency (3ω) and so on.

In order to expand $f(t)$ we need to compute $a_0, a_1, \ldots, a_n, b_1, b_2, \ldots, b_n$ from $f(t)$.

The constant value a_0 is the average value of $f(t)$ and is given by

$$a_0 = (1/T') \lim_{T' \to \infty} \int_{-T'/2}^{+T'/2} f(t)\, dt = (1/T) \int_{-T/2}^{+T/2} f(t)\, dt \tag{8}$$

The average value of a periodic function

Equation (8) states that the average value of a periodic function for $T' \to \infty$ is equal to the average value calculated over a period.

Let us assume that $T' = nT + \tau$, where $\tau < T$, then

$$(1/T') \int_{-T'/2}^{+T'/2} f(t)\, dt = \lim_{n \to \infty}(1/(nT+\tau)) \int_{-(nT+\tau)/2}^{+(nT+\tau)/2} f(t)\, dt$$

The right-hand side is the integration between $-T/2$ and $+T/2$, $T/2$ and $3T/2$, $-T/2$ and $-3T$ and so on. So

$$(1/T') \lim_{T' \to \infty} \int_{-T'/2}^{+T'/2} f(t)\, dt = \lim_{n \to \infty} n(1/(nT+\tau)) \int_{-T/2}^{+T/2} f(t)\, dt$$

$$+ \lim_{n \to \infty}(1/(nT+\tau)) \int_{-(nT+\tau)/2}^{-nT/2} f(t)\, dt$$

$$+ \lim_{n \to \infty}(1/(nT+\tau)) \int_{nT/2}^{(nT+\tau)/2} f(t)\, dt$$

When $n \to \infty$

$$\lim[n/(nT+\tau)] \to 1/T$$

for if we divide top and bottom by n

$$n/(nT+\tau) = 1/(T+\tau/n)$$

then, when $n \to \infty$, $\tau/n \to 0$. Furthermore,

$$\lim_{n \to \infty}(1/(nT+\tau)) \to 0$$

so

$$(1/T') \lim_{T' \to \infty} \int_{-T'/2}^{+T'/2} f(t)\, dt = (1/T) \int_{-T/2}^{+T/2} f(t)\, dt \tag{9}$$

The value of a_0 is very easy to compute since the average value of a sinusoid is zero (see Appendix 2). Furthermore, integrating over the period 0 to T is the same as integrating over the period $-T/2$ to $+T/2$; the period's position along the time axis is just shifted. So

$$(1/T) \int_0^T f(t) \, dt = (1/T) \int_{-T/2}^{+T/2} a_0 \, dt$$

$$+ (1/T) \int_{-T/2}^{+T/2} \sum_{n=1}^{n} (a_n \cos(n\omega t) + b_n \sin(n\omega t)) \, dt$$

$$= (1/T) \int_{-T/2}^{+T/2} a_0 \, dt \to (1/T)(a_0)[T/2 + T/2] = a$$

$$+ (1/T) \sum a_n \int_{-T/2}^{+T/2} \cos(n\omega t) \, dt \to \text{zero}$$

(see Appendix 3)

$$+ (1/T) \sum b_n \int_{-T/2}^{+T/2} \sin(n\omega t) \, dt \to \text{zero}$$

(see Appendix 3)

We can now use the *orthogonality* relationships to compute $a_n b_n$ (see Appendix 3).

If we multiply $f(t)$ by $\cos(m\omega t)$ and compute, we obtain

$$\int_{-T/2}^{+T/2} f(t) \cos(m\omega t) \, dt$$

$$= a_0 \int_{-T/2}^{T/2} \cos(m\omega t) \, dt + \sum a_n \int_{-T/2}^{+T/2} \cos(n\omega t) \cos(m\omega t) \, dt$$

$$+ \sum b_n \int_{-T/2}^{+T/2} \sin(n\omega t) \cos(m\omega t) \, dt \tag{10}$$

The parameters of the periodic (sinusoid) components of a periodic function

The first term on the right-hand side is the *average value* of a sinusoid which is zero. We can obtain the integration of the second term from Appendix 3. It is zero when $m \neq n$. When $m = n$ it becomes

$$a_n \int_{-T/2}^{+T/2} \cos^2(n\omega t) \, dt = a_n T/2$$

Finally the third term can also be obtained from Appendix 3 and it is zero. So

$$a_n = (2/T) \int_{-T/2}^{+T/2} f(t) \cos(n\omega t) \, dt$$

If we multiply $f(t)$ by $\sin(m\omega t)$ we again obtain a first term

$$a_0 \int_{-T/2}^{+T/2} \sin(m\omega t)\, dt = 0$$

a second group of terms of the type

$$a_n \int_{-T/2}^{+T/2} \cos(n\omega t) \sin(m\omega t)\, dt = 0$$

and a third group of terms of the type

$$b_n \int_{-T/2}^{+T/2} \sin(n\omega t) \sin(m\omega t)\, dt$$

which is zero when $m \neq n$ (Appendix 3), and for $m = n$ it is

$$b_n \int_{-T/2}^{+T/2} \sin^2(n\omega t)\, dt = b_n \int_{-T/2}^{+T/2} dt/2 - \frac{1}{2} \int_{-T/2}^{+T/2} \cos(2m\omega t)\, dt$$

$$\downarrow \qquad\qquad\qquad\qquad\qquad \downarrow$$

$$= b_n T/2 \qquad\qquad\qquad\qquad \text{zero}$$

so

$$b_n = (2/T) \int_{-T/2}^{+T/2} f(t) \sin(n\omega t)\, dt \qquad\qquad (11)$$

So with (9), (10), and (11) we are able to determine a_0, a_n, and b_n.

An example of the Fourier expansion of a periodic signal

If we now apply these relationships to the case of a pulse of amplitude A, and duration τ, which repeats itself every T seconds (see Figure A11.1), then

$$a_0 = (1/T) \int_{-T/2}^{+T/2} f(t)\, dt$$

As the pulse exists only between 0 and τ, and has a constant amplitude A

Fig.A11.1

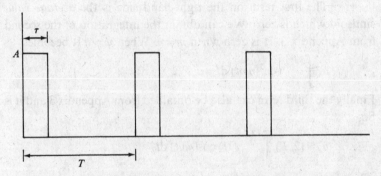

during that time, then

$$a_0 = (1/T) \int_0^\tau A \, dt = (A/T)[t]_0^\tau = A\tau/T$$

so the *average value* is just the area of the pulse $(A\tau)$ *divided by T*. Also

$$a_n = (2/T) \int_0^\tau A \cos(n\omega t) \, dt$$

$$= (2A/T)[\sin(n\omega t)]_0^\tau / n\omega$$

or

$$a_n = (2A\tau/T) \sin(n\omega \tau)/(n\omega \tau)$$

So a_n is a periodic function in which the amplitude $((2A\tau/n\omega\tau))$ decreases as n increases.

Finally, following a similar approach

$$b_n = -(2A/n\omega T)[\cos(n\omega t)]_0^\tau$$

or

$$b_n = -((2A\tau/T)/n\omega\tau)[\cos(n\omega\tau) - 1]$$

so

$$f(t) = (A\tau/T)\left[1 + \sum_{n=1}^{\infty} (2/n\omega\tau)\sin(n\omega\tau)\cos(n\omega t) \right.$$

$$\left. - \sum_{n=1}^{\infty} (2/n\omega\tau)[\cos(n\omega\tau) - 1]\sin(n\omega t) \right]$$

Since $\omega T = 2\pi$ we can also write

$$f(t) = (A/\pi)\left[(\omega\tau)/2 + \sum_{n=1}^{n=\infty} (1/n)(\sin(n\omega\tau)\cos(n\omega t)) \right.$$

$$\left. - \sum_{n=1}^{n=\infty} (1/n)((\cos(n\omega\tau) - 1)\sin(n\omega t)) \right]$$

The constant term (a_0) and the periodic components $(a_n \cos(n\omega t)$ and $b_n \sin(n\omega t))$ are called the *Fourier components* or the frequency components of $f(t)$.

Power spectrum of a signal

At this point we need to introduce the concept of the power spectrum of a periodic signal. Later we shall use the power spectrum concept in the description of non-periodic signals.

If we expand the square of equation (2) $(f(t))$ we obtain terms of the following types:

(i) $a_n a_m \cos(n\omega t) \sin(n\omega t)$ $(n \neq m)$

(ii) $a_0 a_n \cos(n\omega t)$

(iii) $a_0 b_n \sin(n\omega t)$

(iv) a_0^2

(v) $a_n^2 \cos^2(n\omega t)$

(vi) $b_n^2 \sin^2(n\omega t)$

(vii) $a_n \cos(n\omega t)b_n \sin(n\omega t)$

(viii) $a_n \cos(n\omega t)b_m \sin(n\omega t)$

(ix) $b_n \sin(n\omega t)b_m \sin(n\omega t)$

Terms of the type (i), (ii), (iii), (vii), (viii) and (ix) (see Appendix 3) will result in null integrals. So if we then compute the average value of $f(t)$ and $f(t)$ squared $(f^2(t))$ we obtain:

$$(1/T) \int_{-T/2}^{+T/2} f^2(t)\, dt$$

$$= (1/T)\left[\int_{-T/2}^{+T/2} a_0^2\, dt + \sum_{n=1}^{n=\infty} \int_{-T/2}^{+T/2} a_n^2 \cos(n\omega t)\, dt \right.$$

$$\left. + \sum_{n=1}^{n=\infty} \int_{-T/2}^{+T/2} b_n^2 \sin(n\omega t)\, dt \right]$$

If we represent this function

$$(1/T) \int_{-T/2}^{+T/2} f^2(t)\, dt \quad \text{by} \quad \bar{f}^2(n)$$

then we say that

$$\bar{f}^2(n) = a_0^2 + \sum_{n=1}^{n=\infty} (1/2)a_n^2 + \sum_{n=1}^{n=\infty} (1/2)b_n^2 \qquad (12)$$

is the *power spectrum* of $f(t)$, which is the time average of the squared function.

Exponential form of the Fourier series

In addition to (2) and (7) there is a third way of representing a Fourier series; this is the exponential form, and is introduced below. Consider the pair of terms

$$a_n \cos(n\omega t) + b_n \sin(n\omega t)$$

In order to simplify the notation let us define θ_n as

$$n\omega t$$

and $f(n)$ as

$$a_n \cos(\theta_n) + b_n \sin(\theta_n)$$

Now compare the Taylor expansion (see Appendix 4) of $\sin(\theta_n)$ and $\cos(\theta_n)$. So

$$\sin(\theta_n) = \theta_n - \theta_n^3/3! + \theta_n^5/5! - \theta_n^7/7! + \cdots$$

and

$$\cos(\theta_n) = 1 - \theta_n^2/2! + \theta_n^4/4! - \theta_n^6/6! + \cdots$$

If we add
$$\sin(\theta_n)+\cos(\theta_n)=1+\theta_n-\theta_n^2/2!-\theta_n^3/3!+\theta_n^4/4!+\cdots \tag{13}$$
If we compare (13) with the series expansion (see Appendix 2) given by
$$e^\theta=1+\theta+\theta^2/2!+\theta^3/3!+\theta^4/4!+\cdots \tag{14}$$
We see that the two series have exactly the same terms and differ only by the signs ($\pm$) in front of each term. If we now substitute $j\theta_n$ for θ in (14) and change the left-hand side of (13) into
$$\cos(\theta_n)+j\sin\theta_n$$
The expansion of this sum now becomes
$$\cos(\theta_n)+j\sin(\theta_n)=1+j\theta_n-\theta_n^2/2!-j\theta_n^3/3!+\theta_n^4/4!+\cdots \tag{15}$$
while
$$e^{j\theta_n}=1+j\theta_n+(j)^2\theta_n^2/2!+(j)^3\theta_n^3/3!+(j)^4\theta_n^4/4!+\cdots$$

The complex exponential
In Appendix 1 we saw that
$$j^2=-1$$
$$j^3=-j$$
$$j^4=1$$
$$j^5=j$$
$$j^6=-1$$
where
$$j=\sqrt{-1}$$

De Moivre's theorem
Equation (15) is identical to the following expression
$$\cos(\theta_n)+j\sin(\theta_n)=1+j\theta_n+(j)^2\theta_n^2/2!$$
$$+(j)^3\theta_n^3/3!+(j)^4\theta_n^4/4!+\cdots$$
So
$$\cos(\theta_n)+j\sin(\theta_n)=e^{j\theta_n}=\exp(j\theta_n) \tag{16}$$
where $\exp(j\theta_n)$ is an exponential with a complex exponent (complex exponential). Equation (16) is geometrically described in Figure A11.2, in which we represent $\cos(\theta_n)$ as the projection of a rotating radius in the R axis and $j\sin(\theta_n)$ as the projection of the same radius in the j axis. The vector $\exp(j\theta_n)$ is the *vectorial sum* of $\cos(\theta_n)$ and $j\sin(\theta_n)$.

Equation (16) is known as De Moivre's theorem and can be used to relate the exponential function to the sinusoidal function. Thus
$$\exp(j\theta_n)=\cos(\theta_n)+j\sin(\theta_n) \tag{16}$$
$$\exp(-j\theta_n)=\cos(\theta_n)-j\sin(\theta_n) \tag{17}$$

If we add (16) to (17) we obtain

$$\exp(j\theta_n) + \exp(-j\theta_n) = 2\cos(\theta_n)$$

or

$$\cos(\theta_n) = (\exp(j\theta_n) + \exp(-j\theta_n))/2 \qquad (18)$$

If we subtract (17) from (16) and rearrange, we obtain

$$\sin(\theta_n) = (\exp(j\theta_n) - \exp(-j\theta_n))/2j \qquad (19)$$

Equations (18) and (19) express the sine and cosine of an angle θ_n in terms of two exponentials. If we now substitute (18) and (19) in (2) with $\theta_n = n\omega t$ we obtain

$$f(t) = a_0 + \sum_{n=1}^{n=\infty} [(a_n/2)(\exp(j\theta_n) + \exp(-j\theta_n))$$
$$- (jb_n/2)(\exp(j\theta_n) - \exp(-j\theta_n))] \qquad (20)$$

Let us expand the terms inside the summation sign

$$(a_n/2)\exp(j\theta_n) + (a_n/2)\exp(-j\theta_n) - (jb_n/2)\exp(j\theta_n)$$
$$+ (jb_n/2)\exp(-j\theta_n)$$

Collecting terms and substituting $n\omega t$ for θ_n we obtain

$$[(a_n - jb_n)/2]\exp(jn\omega t) + [(a_n + jb_n)/2]\exp(-jn\omega t)$$

Let us define C_n and C_{n-} by

$$C_n = (a_n - jb_n)/2$$
$$C_{n-} = (a_n + jb_n)/2$$

Fig.A11.2

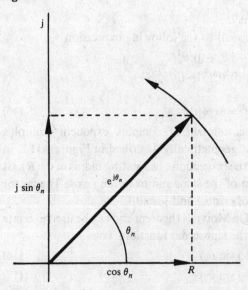

Thus C_{n-} is the complex conjugate of C_n (see Appendix 1). If we define C_0 as

$$C_0 = a_0$$

then (20) can be rewritten as

$$f(t) = C_0 + \sum_{n=1}^{n=\infty} C_n \exp(jn\omega t) + \sum_{n=1}^{n=\infty} C_{n-} \exp(-jn\omega t)$$

If we now redefine C_{n-} as the value of C_n for negative values of n, then

$$f(t) = C_0 + \sum_{n=1}^{n=\infty} C_n \exp(jn\omega t) + \sum_{n=-1}^{n=-\infty} C_m \exp(jn\omega t) \tag{21}$$

The three terms on the right-hand side of (21) can now be put together as follows

$$f(t) = \sum_{n=-\infty}^{n=\infty} C_n \exp(jn\omega t) \tag{22}$$

since for $n = 0$, $C_0 \exp(0) = C_0$. The right-hand side of (22) is the exponential form of the Fourier series of the periodic function $f(t)$. This form of the Fourier series involves a slight difficulty since we now have components with *negative frequencies*, that is, the terms:

$$n\omega \quad \text{for} \quad n \text{ negative}$$

These negative frequencies are mathematical entities as are a_n and b_n. In (7) we showed that the trigonometric form of the Fourier series contains only a component of each frequency of amplitude A_n and we also showed that

$$A_n^2 = a_n^2 + b_n^2$$

Now if we make the product $C_n C_{n-}$ we obtain

$$C_n C_{n-} = (a_n - jb_n)(a_n + jb_n)/4 = (a_n^2 + b_n^2)/4 = A_n^2/4$$

So the amplitude A_n of any component of frequency now is given by

$$A_n = 2\sqrt{(C_n C_{n-})}$$

Finally we can relate a_n and b_n to C_n and C_{n-}.

By definition

$$C_n = (a_n - jb_n)/2$$

and

$$C_{n-} = (a_n + jb_n)/2$$

Adding and subtracting these two equations and rearranging we obtain

$$a_n = 2(C_n + C_{n-})$$

and

$$b_n = (2/j)(C_{n-} - C_n) = 2j(C_n - C_{n-}) \tag{23}$$

We can now obtain expressions for the value of C_n (and C_{n-}) once we know $f(t)$.

We use (22) to perform the following integration

$$(1/T) \int_{-T/2}^{+T/2} f(t) \exp(-jm\omega t)\, dt \qquad (24)$$

If we substitute (22) into (24) we obtain

$$(1/T) \int_{-T/2}^{+T/2} \sum_{n=-\infty}^{n=+\infty} C_n \exp(jn\omega t)\exp(-jm\omega t)\, dt$$

$$= \sum_{n=-\infty}^{n=+\infty} (C_n/T) \int_{-T/2}^{+T/2} \exp(j(n-m)\omega t)\, dt$$

$$= \sum_{n=-\infty}^{n=+\infty} (C_n/T)(1/j(n-m)\omega)[\exp(j(n-m)\omega t)]_{-T/2}^{+T/2} \qquad (25)$$

In order to understand this integration let us use Figure A11.3. According to whether $n\omega t$ is 0, $\pi/2$, π, $(3/2)\pi$ or 2π the vector $\exp(jn\omega t)$ will have the values $1, j, -1, -j$. These values will be repeated after every 2π rotation. So

$$\exp((2k+1)\pi j) = -1 \quad \text{and} \quad \exp((2k+3/2)\pi j) = -j$$

In expression (25) when $n \neq m$ or $n-m=k$ the term inside the square brackets will be

$$\exp(j(\omega T)k/2) - \exp(-j(\omega T)k/2)$$

but

$$\omega T = 2\pi$$

so

$$j\omega Tk/2 = jk\pi \quad \text{and} \quad -j\omega Tk/2 = -jk\pi$$

Fig.A11.3

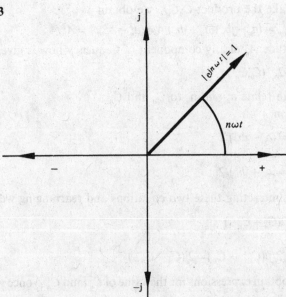

so
$$\exp(jk\pi) - \exp(-jk\pi) = -1 - (-1) = 0$$

Expression (25) also shows that when $n = m$ the integral becomes indeterminate because the term $n - m = 0$ in the denominator of the second fraction in the expression. This indetermination can be removed if we go one step back. The expression

$$(C_n/T) \int_{-T/2}^{+T/2} \exp(j\omega t(n-m)) \, dt$$

For $n = m$, becomes

$$(C_n/T) \int_{-T/2}^{T/2} dt = (C_n/T)[t]_{-T/2}^{+T/2} = C_n$$

so

$$C_n = (1/T) \int_{-T/2}^{+T/2} f(t) \exp(-jn\omega t) \, dt \tag{26}$$

Description of a signal in the time and in the frequency domain

Expressions (22) and (26) describe the interconversion between the *time domain* ($f(t)$) and the *frequency domain* (C_n). (See Figure A11.4.)

Fig.A11.4

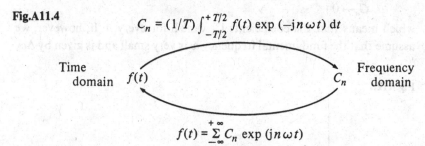

$$C_n = (1/T) \int_{-T/2}^{+T/2} f(t) \exp(-jn\omega t) \, dt$$

Time
domain $f(t)$ C_n Frequency
                                                                  domain

$$f(t) = \sum_{-\infty}^{+\infty} C_n \exp(jn\omega t)$$

We say that C_n gives a description in the *frequency domain* because C_n gives the amplitude ($A_n = 2\sqrt{(C_n C_{n-})}$) and phase ($-\tan^{-1} b_n/a_n = \tan^{-1}((C_n + C_{n-})/j(C_n - C_{n-}))$) of the frequency components of the time function $f(t)$. While, on the other hand, $f(t)$ gives the value of the function at every instant in time.

APPENDIX 12. The Fourier integral

The method described in the previous Appendix of expanding a function $f(t)$ into a series of sinusoidal (or complex exponential) functions can also be applied to non-period functions. We shall consider here the case of *pulse* functions.

Pulse functions

A pulse function is defined as a function that has a non-zero value during a certain interval, τ, and is zero outside this interval (see Figure A12.1a). If we wish to calculate the Fourier coefficients (C_n) for a pulse function the integration has to be performed between $-\infty$ and $+\infty$, since it is not a periodic function. So

$$C_n = (1/T) \int_{-T/2}^{+T/2} f(t) \exp(-jn\omega t)\, dt \qquad \qquad (1)$$

$$T \rightarrow \infty$$

If $f(t)$ is a rectangular pulse of amplitude A and duration τ (Figure 12.1b), then

$$C_n = (1/T) \int_0^\tau A \exp(-jn\omega t)\, dt$$

$$T \rightarrow \infty$$

$$= A[(\exp(-jn\omega\tau) - 1)/(jn\omega T)] \quad T \rightarrow \infty \qquad (2)$$

For any value of n the numerator of (2) is constant while, in the denominator, $T \rightarrow \infty$. That is

$$C_n \rightarrow 0$$

which means that the coefficients C_n vanish for every n. If, however, we assume that the fundamental frequency ω is very small and is given by $\Delta\omega$,

Fig.A12.1

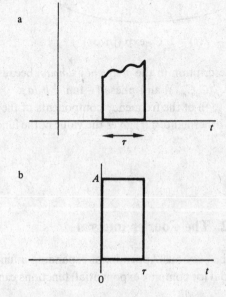

a

b

A

τ

0

t

then (1) becomes:

$$C_n = (1/T) \lim_{T \to \infty} \int_{-T/2}^{+T/2} f(t) \exp(-jn \, \Delta\omega t) \, dt \tag{3}$$

We can think of a pulse function as the limiting case of a periodic function when the period (T) becomes infinitely long. Since

$$\omega = 2\pi/T$$

when T becomes very large ω becomes very small, so $\Delta\omega = 2\pi/T$ when $T \to \infty$ or

$$T = 2\pi/\Delta\omega \tag{4}$$

(We note that $\Delta\omega \to 0$ as $T \to \infty$.)

If we now substitute (4) into (3) we obtain

$$C_n = (\Delta\omega/2\pi) \int_{-\pi/\Delta\omega}^{+\pi/\Delta\omega} f(t) \exp(-jn \, \Delta\omega t) \, dt \tag{5}$$

Substitution of (5) into the formula for the Fourier series of a periodic signal (see Appendix 11),

$$f(t) = \sum_{-\infty}^{+\infty} C_n \exp(jn\omega t)$$

gives

$$f(t) = \sum_{-\infty}^{+\infty} (\Delta\omega/2\pi) \left[\int_{-\pi/\Delta\omega}^{+\pi/\Delta\omega} f(t) \exp(-jn \, \Delta\omega t) \, dt \right] \exp(jn \, \Delta\omega t)$$

on rearranging

$$f(t) = (1/2\pi) \sum_{-\infty}^{+\infty} \exp(jn \, \Delta\omega t) \left[\Delta\omega \int_{-\pi/\Delta\omega}^{+\pi/\Delta\omega} f(t) \exp(-jn \, \Delta\omega t) \, dt \right]$$

Since ω has to take a finite value, it follows that if $\Delta\omega \to 0$ as $\omega = n \, \Delta\omega$ then n must $\to \infty$. When $\Delta\omega$ approaches zero then $\pi/\Delta\omega \to \infty$ and so the summation sign becomes an integral. So

$$f(t) = (1/2\pi) \int_{-\infty}^{+\infty} \exp(j\omega t) \, d\omega \int_{-\infty}^{+\infty} f(t) \exp(-j\omega t) \, dt \tag{6}$$

To calculate the second integral for an impulse function of amplitude A, interval τ,

$$\int_0^\tau A \exp(-j\omega t) \, dt = (A/(-j\omega))[\exp(-j\omega t)]_0^\tau$$

$$= A[1 - \exp(j\omega\tau)]/(j\omega)$$

The Fourier integral

This integral does not vanish any more and is now a *continuous function of* ω, which we shall call $F(\omega)$, so (6) becomes

$$f(t) = (1/2\pi) \int_{-\infty}^{+\infty} F(\omega) \exp(j\omega t)\, d\omega \qquad (7)$$

where

$$F(\omega) = \int_{-\infty}^{+\infty} f(t) \exp(-j\omega t)\, dt \qquad (8)$$

We can now compare the pair of equations derived in the previous Appendix for a periodic signal

$$f(t) = \sum_{n=-\infty}^{+\infty} C_n \exp(jn\omega t) \qquad \text{(A11 (22))}$$

$$C_n = (1/T) \int_{-T/2}^{+T/2} f(t) \exp(-jn\omega t)\, dt \qquad \text{(A11 (26))}$$

with the pair (7) and (8).

Spectral density

In the case of a periodic function, the function is transformed into a *discrete* sum (series) of sinusoidal (complex exponential) terms. In the case of equation (7) a pulse signal is transformed into a *continuous* function $(F(\omega))$ of angular frequency (ω). $F(\omega)$ (like C_n) is a weighting function for the amplitudes of the frequency components. We should not speak of amplitudes, but of *spectral density* or, more precisely, of the spectral content $(F(\omega)\, d(\omega))$ that occurs within a given range of frequencies $d(\omega)$. (We shall recall we defined $\Delta\omega$ as $=\omega/n$, where n is the number of harmonics and $n \to \infty$, that is, $d\omega = \omega/n$, for very large n; this then gives us a *range* of frequencies.) $F(\omega)$ is called the *Fourier transform* of $f(t)$.

Digital data processing

Until digital computers and instrumental methods for analysing time functions (signals) were developed, Fourier techniques were essentially mathematical tools used by physicists and engineers in the description of signals or systems.

However, we are now able to record time signals in such a way that it is possible to analyse those signals directly with a computer. The signals can be recorded directly onto magnetic tape and then 'replayed' and analysed as many times as required. Alternatively the signals can be 'sampled' and recorded as numbers on magnetic tapes or magnetic discs and then fed to a computer. This sampling consists of taking periodic measurements of the signal. These measurements are represented in Figure A12.2a by the dots.

In order to obtain a measurement, an elementary unit of measurement is defined. The computer then counts how many of these units are contained in the measured value. For example, in Figure A12.2b we represent a signal being measured at t_1. The value of the signal falls between 7 and 8 units of measurement. Since we cannot use a precision greater than one unit of measurement the value of the signal is 7. In practice, we might divide 1 volt into at least 2^{10} levels, that is, 1024 levels. The precision with which we would measure the signal would then be $\frac{1}{1024}$ volts or 0.9766 mV. If we require greater precision we use smaller steps. The value of the signal will then be represented by an *integer* number of these steps and it is with these steps that computers operate.

The effect of time sampling: sampling frequency

The next problem is that even though we are measuring the signal with sufficient precision we might be distorting the signal $(t_0, t_1, t_2, \ldots, t_n)$ by sampling at discrete intervals in time. Although the sampled signal is now no longer continuous we can still recover the original signal provided we sample at an appropriate rate. This rate is defined precisely by Shannon's theorem. In order to introduce this theorem, and for the sake of simplicity, we shall consider the simplest case. Let us then sample a sinusoid $A \cos(\omega_0 t)$ with *adequate accuracy* (that is, sufficiently small steps) over τ seconds and assume that the sampling time is infinitely short. The sinusoidal function (Figure A12.3a) will then be represented by T/τ values

Fig.A12.2

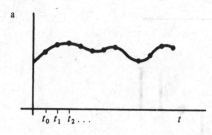

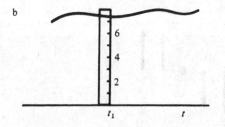

where T is the period of the sinusoid. If we Fourier-transform the function

$$f(t) = A \cos(\omega_0 t) = (A/2)(\exp(j\omega_0 t) + \exp(-j\omega_0 t))$$

the Fourier series of $f(t)$ is then

$$C_n = (A/2T) \int_{-T/2}^{+T/2} (\exp(j\omega_0 t) + \exp(-j\omega_0 t)) \exp(-jn\omega t) \, dt$$

$$= (A/2T) \int_{-T/2}^{+T/2} \exp(j(\omega_0 - n\omega)t) \, dt$$

$$+ (A/2T) \int_{-T/2}^{+T/2} \exp(-j(\omega_0 + n\omega)t) \, dt$$

Only when $n\omega = \omega_0$ is the first integral on the right-hand side not zero for $n > 1$, while the second integral is always zero. So

$$C_n = (A/2T) \int_{-T/2}^{+T/2} dt = A/2$$

Fig.A12.3

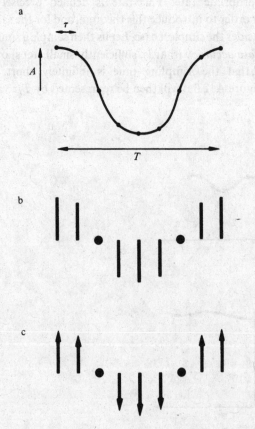

For $n<0$ the first integral is zero and the second becomes $A/2$. The amplitude of ω_0 is thus

$$C_n + C_{n-} = A$$

or

$$A = 2C_n$$

If we Fourier-transform the function represented in Figure A12.3b, which we shall call $fs(t)$ (the sampled function of t), we obtain

$$C_n(s) = (1/T) \int_{-T/2}^{+T/2} fs(t) \exp(-jn\omega t)\, dt$$

$$= (1/T) \int_{0}^{+T} fs(t) \exp(-jn\omega t)\, dt$$

$$= (1/T)\left[\int_{0-}^{0+} A \cos(\omega_0 t) \exp(-jn\omega t)\, dt \right.$$

$$+ \int_{\tau-}^{\tau+} A \cos(\omega_0 t) \exp(-jn\omega t)\, dt + \cdots$$

$$\left. + \int_{m\tau-}^{m\tau+} A \cos(\omega_0 t) \exp(-jn\omega t)\, dt \right] \tag{9}$$

where $m = T/\tau$. The limits $0-$ and $0+$ mean that the value of the function is non-zero during a short Δt around $t=0$. Similarly $\tau-$, $\tau+$, etc.

Let us deal with the first integral (see Appendix 3)

$$(1/T) \int_{-\Delta t/2}^{+\Delta t/2} A \cos(\omega_0 t) \exp(-jn\omega t)\, dt$$

$$= (A/2T) \int_{-\Delta t/2}^{+\Delta t/2} (\exp(j\omega_0 t) + \exp(-j\omega_0 t) \exp(-jn\omega t))\, dt$$

$$= (A/2T)[(1/j(\omega_0 - n\omega)) \exp(j(\omega_0 - n\omega)t)$$

$$- (1/j(\omega_0 + n\omega)) \exp(-j(\omega_0 - n\omega)t)]_{-\Delta t/2}^{+\Delta t/2}$$

As $\Delta t \to 0$ this integral tends to zero. This is not unexpected as the Fourier-transform of a pulse (see Appendix 11) when $\tau \to 0$ is zero. So this means that (9) is not the correct mathematical procedure with which to deal with sampled functions.

The numerical computation of Fourier spectra from sampled functions must involve a different mathematical approach. The sampled function is represented by a series of infinitely short pulses of infinite amplitude but of finite area (strength) (see Figure A12.3c). The sampling procedure is as if the function to be sampled signal ($A \cos(\omega_0 t)$) is multiplied by a periodic function, which consists of a train of pulses of infinitely short duration, infinite amplitude and of area equal to one. Such pulses are called *delta functions* (for example, a rectangular pulse of width Δt and amplitude $1/\Delta t$

will behave as a delta function as $\Delta t \rightarrow 0$) and are represented by the symbol

$$\delta(t) \quad \text{or in general} \quad \delta(t-T)$$

and by definition

$$\int_{-\infty}^{\infty} \delta(t)\,dt = \int_{0-}^{0+} \delta(t)\,dt = 1 = \int_{-T}^{+T} \delta(t-T)\,dt = 1$$

The Fourier series of a train of impulse functions $(\delta_T(t))$ can be easily found,

$$C_n = (1/T) \int_{-T/2}^{+T/2} f(t) \exp(-jn\omega t)\,dt$$

$$= (1/T) \int_0^{\delta} \delta_T(t) \exp(-jn\omega t)\,dt$$

where $\omega = 2\pi/T$ and T is the period of sampling.

In the interval of time between 0 and δ the function $\delta_T(t)$ has a non-zero value only at $t=0$ so the product $\delta_T(t)\exp(-jn\omega t)$ only has a non-zero value $(\delta_T(T)\exp(0)=\delta_T(T))$ at $t=0$. So

$$(1/T) \int_0^{\delta} \delta_T(t) \exp(-jn\omega t)\,dt = (1/T) \int_0^{\delta} \delta_T(t)\,dt = 1/T$$

and thus $C_n = 1/T$. If we expand $\delta_T(t)$ in a Fourier series we obtain

$$\delta_T(t) = \sum_{n=-\infty}^{n=+\infty} C_n \exp(-jn\omega t) = (1/T) \sum_{n=-\infty}^{n=+\infty} \exp(jn\omega t)$$

If we assume that the sampled function $fs(t)$ is the product of $f(t)$ by $\delta_T(t)$

$$fs(t) = f(t)\,\delta_T(t) = (f(t)/T) \sum_{n=-\infty}^{n=+\infty} \exp(jn\omega t)$$

If $f(t)$ is a simple sinusoid of the form

$$f(t) = A\cos(\omega_0 t) = (A/2)(\exp(j\omega_0 t) + \exp(-j\omega_0 t))$$

then

$$fs(t) = (A/2T)(\exp(j\omega_0 t) + (-j\omega_0 t)) \sum_{n=-\infty}^{n=+\infty} (jn\omega t)$$

It helps to understand the product of exponentials in this expression if we expand the sum of exponentials and then multiply out:

$$(\exp(j\omega_0 t) + \exp(-j\omega_0 t))(+\cdots + \exp(-jn\omega t) + \cdots$$
$$+1+\cdots+\exp(jn\omega t)+\cdots)$$
$$=(+\cdots+\exp(j(\omega_0 - n\cdot\omega)t)) + \cdots + \exp(-j\omega t)$$
$$+\exp(j\omega t)+\cdots+\exp((\omega_0 + n\cdot\omega)jt)+\cdots)$$

If we now collect terms we obtain

$$= +\cdots+(\exp(j(\omega_0 - n\omega)t)+\exp(-j(\omega_0 - n\omega)t))+\cdots$$
$$+(\exp(j\omega t)+\exp(-j\omega t))+\cdots$$
$$+(\exp(j(\omega_0 + n\omega)t)+\exp(-j(\omega_0 + n\omega)t))+\cdots$$

So

$$+ \cdots + 2\cos[(\omega_0 - n\omega)t] + \cdots + 2\cos(\omega_0 t) + 2\cos[(\omega_0 + n\omega)t] + \cdots$$

The effect of the sampling procedure is thus

$$A\cos(\omega_0 t) \xrightarrow{\text{sampling at frequency } \omega} \frac{A}{T} \sum_{n=-\infty}^{n=\infty} \cos[(\omega_0 + n\omega)t] \qquad (10)$$

The mathematical operation in (10) describes the effect of sampling a simple sinusoid at a frequency ω. That (10) is an accurate representative of the sampling procedure, and that our analysis is correct, can be verified experimentally by sampling a sinusoid and then computing by numerical methods the Fourier series of this function. It turns out that such a series

Fig.A12.4

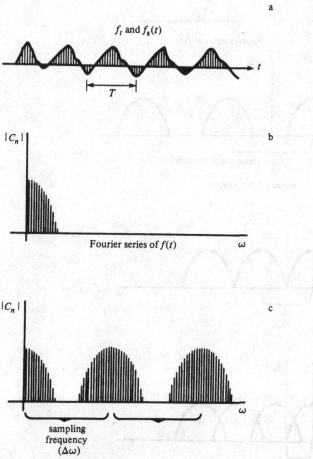

a

f_t and $f_s(t)$

T

$|C_n|$

b

Fourier series of $f(t)$ ω

$|C_n|$

c

sampling
frequency
$(\Delta\omega)$

Fourier series of $f_s(t)$

does correspond to the right-hand side of (10) so that the mathematical representation of the sampling procedure as the multiplication of the function ($f(t)$) by the sampling function $\delta_T(t)$ is correct. A rigorous non-experimental mathematical verification of (10) is beyond the scope of this book.

The sampled signal, in addition to containing a scaled down A/T (or attenuated version of the original signal (for $n = 0$)), also contains an infinite

Fig.A12.5

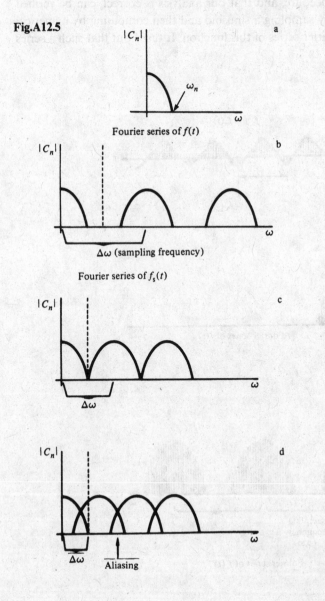

Fourier series of $f(t)$

Fourier series of $f_s(t)$

number of components of the same amplitude (A/T) but of frequencies $\omega_0 \pm \omega$, $\omega_0 \pm 2\omega$, $\omega_0 \pm 3\omega$, etc.

The spectrum of the original signal is repeated in the frequency domain with a periodicity of ω_0, the sampling frequency. This means that if we have a method of eliminating the newly generated frequencies (by filtering) we can recover an attenuated version $(A/T)\cos(\omega_0 t)$ of the original signal from the sampled signal.

Sampling non-sinusoidal functions

The effect of sampling more complex signals is similar to our description of the simple sinusoid. In Figure A12.4a we represent a periodic non-sinusoidal signal which was sampled. In A12.4b we have plotted the modulus $(|C_n|)$ of the Fourier components of the signal, that is $(a_n^2 + b_n^2)/2$ and in A12.4c the spectrum of the sampled signal. It can be seen that the effect of the sampling is to generate a periodic repetition of the spectrum in the frequency domain such that for each frequency component, ω_0, of the original signal there are frequency components of frequency $\omega_0 \pm \Delta\omega$, $\omega_0 \pm 2\Delta\omega$, $\omega_0 \pm 3\Delta\omega$, and so on, where $\Delta\omega$ is the frequency of sampling. In Figure A12.5a we have again represented the spectrum of the periodic signal $f(t)$. In this figure, ω_n is the highest frequency component of $f(t)$. In Figure A12.5b, c and d we represent the spectrum of $f(t)$ when sampled at three different sampling frequencies $(\Delta\omega)$.

Shannon's sampling theorem

We can see that when $\Delta\omega < 2\omega_n$ the additional frequency components generated by the sampling procedure are superimposed upon the original spectrum. This superposition is known as *aliasing*. When there is *aliasing* we cannot recover the original signal, because if we removed all the frequency components above ω_n (see A12.5d) we would be left with the spectrum of the original signal plus other components of the next spectrum. This means that in order to sample a signal without distortion we have to sample at a frequency that is at least *twice* the highest frequency component of the original signal. This rule is known as the *sampling theorem* and was discovered by Shannon.

APPENDIX 13. Harmonic analysis of non-periodic signals

Most of the signals that we have to deal with are neither periodic nor pulse signal. If, for example, we record (with sufficient sensitivity) the current flowing across a resistor, after applying a constant voltage across it, we observe that the current fluctuates continuously around a mean value. Or, if we were able to record the pressure of a gas against the wall of the container with sufficient sensitivity, we would also record fluctuations of the pressure around a mean level. Those fluctuations reflect the fact that current is not a continuous 'fluid' in movement, but involves the movement of discrete currents of charge (electrons), and that the pressure exerted by a gas is due to the collision of molecules with the walls of the container. Neither the current fluctuations nor the pressure fluctuations can be described by an analytical function which will give us the current or pressure precisely at time t (in contrast to this, a sinusoidal function is completely defined from $-\infty$ to $+\infty$ in time). However, if we know enough about the molecular mechanisms responsible for the fluctuations one should be able to make predictions about, for example, the size of the fluctuations. Thus, for example, we should be able to say that the fluctuations of current might be of the order of microamps and not of amps. In order to make these predictions we need to use probability theory.

Stationary signals

The first assumption we have to make, in order to apply probability theory to the description of a random signal, is that if we observe the signal one day for a sufficient length of time and if we observe the signal at any other time we should still get the same *average* results. We then say that the random signal is a *stationary* signal.

Let us now imagine that a random signal and the value of the signal, at any time t, is the result of the random choice between n possible levels and that *all levels* are *equally likely* to be chosen. Or, more formally, the probability of choosing any one level is the same as the probability of choosing any other level. (With this assumption we are performing a *conceptual random experiment* (see Appendix 7) and, as shown in Appendix 7, we need *conceptual random experiments* in order to define probabilities.)

Statistical description of non-periodic signals

In this experiment we shall also assume that we have an infinite number of identical sources (I_i), each producing a random signal (Figure A13.1). We can now make a number of measurements on the signals of these sources. For example, at time t_1 we can measure the values of the signals produced by the sources ($x_1, x_2, \ldots, x_n$) and with these values we can obtain the expected value or *mean*, that is,

$$\bar{x} = E[x_i] = \sum_{\substack{i=1 \\ n \to \infty}}^{n} x_i/n \tag{1}$$

or we can characterize the distribution of the values x_i and assign a probability (or probability density $P(x_i)$) to each value of x_i (see Appendix 7) so that

$$\bar{x} = E[x_i] = \sum_{\substack{i=1 \\ n \to \infty}}^{n} P(x_i)x_i \quad \text{or} \quad \int_0^\infty xP(x)\,dx \tag{2}$$

Ensembles

We call this average an ensemble average at t_1 ($\bar{x}(t_1)$). We say at t_1 because we call an *ensemble*, the *whole* collection of time signals.

We can also compute the ensemble average at t_2 ($\bar{x}(t_2)$).

The variance

If

$$\bar{x}(t_1) = \bar{x}(t_2) = \cdots = \bar{x}(t_n) = \cdots \bar{x}(t_{-n}) \tag{3}$$

from $t \to -\infty$ to $t \to +\infty$ we say that we have a stationary ensemble. We can also compute the *variance* of the ensemble at time t_1 or $t_2 \ldots$

Fig.A13.1

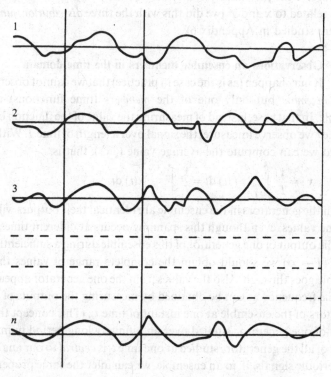

$$s^2 = E[(\bar{x} - x_i)^2] = \sum_{\substack{i=1 \\ n \to \infty}}^{n} (\bar{x} - x_i)^2/n$$

(4)

$$= \sum_{\substack{i=1 \\ n \to \infty}}^{n} (\bar{x} - x_i)^2 P(x_i)$$

or

$$s^2 = \int_0^\infty (\bar{x} - x)^2 P(x)\,\mathrm{d}x$$

for a stationary ensemble

$$s^2(t_1) = s^2(t_2) = \cdots = s^2(t_n) = s^2(t_{n-1})$$

(5)

Distribution functions

If, besides being able to observe the output signals of the generators that produce the signals, we also know how the generators are made and how they work, then we are able to produce a *probabilistic model*. If our generator is a dice or a roulette wheel thrown or spun at known time intervals, we can derive full, time-dependent, probabilistic models of, for example, the chance of throwing or obtaining certain numbers. In this way we can derive the probability distribution (or density) function which can then be related to $\bar{x}$ and s^2 (we did this with the three *distribution functions* that were studied in Appendix 6).

Observations on ensemble members in the time domain

It may happen (as is the case in practice) that we cannot observe the whole *ensemble* but only one of the *members* (time functions) of the ensemble. In that case, instead of measuring the value of the function only at one time t we observe (measure) the signal over a length of time T. With such a record we can compute the average value ($\langle x \rangle$), that is,

$$\langle x \rangle = \frac{1}{T} \int_{-T/2}^{+T/2} f(t)\,\mathrm{d}t = \frac{1}{T} \int_{-T/2}^{+T/2} x(t)\,\mathrm{d}t$$

(6)

Since all the generators in the ensemble are identical their outputs will span the same values, even though this spanning occurs at different times. If we study the output of one generator of this ensemble during a sufficiently long period ($T \to \infty$) we should obtain the complete range of values that the ensemble goes through. Also the values from the one generator appear with the same frequency as can be obtained by measuring the outputs of all the generators of the ensemble at one instant of time t_i. (This concept that the output of one generator studied over an infinitely long period mimics the output of all the generators studied at one time t_i is *central* to our analysis of non-periodic signals. If, in an ensemble, we can infer the same properties of the signal from either studying them *all* at a fixed time, or any *one* of the members of the ensemble for a long time, we say that the ensemble is *ergodic*.) This means that

$$\bar{x} = \frac{1}{T} \int\limits_{\substack{-T/2 \\ (T\to\infty)}}^{+T/2} x_j(t)\, dt = \langle x_j \rangle = E[x_i] \tag{7}$$

where i goes from 1 to ∞, and x_i is the output of the generator i at time t, while j means an individual member of the ensemble.

Thus for this type of ensemble the *ensemble average* is equal to the time average of *one* ensemble member. We can follow a similar procedure to compute variance. We have already shown that

$$s^2 = E[(\bar{x} - x_i)^2] = \sum_{i=1}^{n} (\bar{x} - x_i)^2/n = \sum_{i=1}^{n} x_i^2/n - \bar{x}^2$$
$$= E[x_i^2] - E[x_i]^2 \tag{7a}$$

By the same reasoning used to derive equation (7)

$$E[x_i^2] = \frac{1}{T} \int\limits_{\substack{-T/2 \\ T\to\infty}}^{+T/2} x_j^2(t)\, dt \tag{8}$$

Equations (7) and (8) have been written on an intuitive basis and those interested in a more complete mathematical description should consult Lee. Expression (8) means that if we multiply the signal by itself and then compute the time average of the resulting signal we obtain the average (*or expected*) square of the ensemble.

In order to understand (7) and (8) we may think of a random signal as a sequence of bars of variable amplitude in time. Figure A13.2 shows such a random signal, which is also one of the members of an ensemble. We can think that the other members of the ensemble are generated by changing, in a random way, the orders of the bars. For example, another function would have the following sequence of bars

4, 11, 8, 14, 1, 6, 2, 13, 15, 5, 10, 3, 8, 9, 11

We can then assume that we can have at least as many bars as ensemble members.

This is an over-simplification as in a *physical* generator the output current (or voltage) will not jump *instantaneously* from one value to a much larger or much smaller value. This means that the values of $x(t)$ at time t are not necessarily independent of the values of $x(t)$ for, say, $t - \tau$. And, in fact, as τ gets smaller they become less and less independent.

The autocorrelation function

There is a function which *reflects* this dependence, which is called the *autocorrelation* function, and it is defined by

$$\phi_{tt}(\tau) = \frac{1}{T} \int_{-T/2}^{+T/2} f(t)f(t-\tau)\,dt = \frac{1}{T} \int_{-T/2}^{+T/2} f(t)f(t+\tau)\,dt \qquad (9)$$

In Figure A13.2b we show the shifted time function $(f(t-\tau))$. In order to compute $\phi_{tt}(\tau)$ we first multiply $f(t-\tau)$ by $f(t)$, that is,

$x(1)x(-1)$

$x(2)x(0)$

$x(3)x(1)$

etc.

Then we multiply each product by Δt, add them all up to compute the integral and divide by T. $\phi_{tt}(\tau)$ is a kind of time average but is a function of τ.

Fig.A13.2

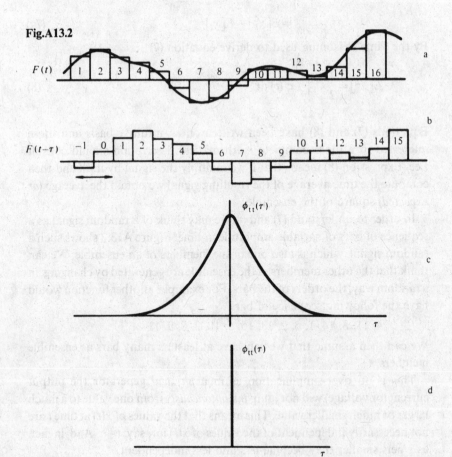

Since the values of $x(t)$ become unrelated to the values of $x(t-\tau)$ it will be equally likely that we obtain both positive and negative products and, furthermore, *all* values are equally likely. We expect that for very large τ the sum of the products will cancel, that is,

$$\phi_{tt}(\tau) \to 0 \quad \text{for} \quad \tau \to \infty$$

$\phi_{tt}(\tau)$ is an even function (see Appendix 3), so if

$$\phi_{tt}(\tau) = (1/T) \int_{\substack{-T/2 \\ T \to \infty}}^{T/2} f(t)f(t+\tau)\,dt$$

and we define

$$y = t + \tau$$

then

$$t = y - \tau \quad \text{and} \quad dt = dy$$

so

$$\phi_{tt}(\tau) = \frac{1}{T} \int_{-T/2}^{+T/2} f(y-\tau)f(y)\,dy$$

For a random signal we expect the autocorrelation function to be as represented in Figure A13.2c. If $x_i(t)$ was totally uncorrelated (independent) of $x_i(t-\tau)$ we should expect the autocorrelation function to be as represented in A13.2d. To recapitulate, up to this point we have obtained the autocorrelation function by recording the signal $f(t)$ over a sufficient length of time $(T \to \infty)$ and applying to the recorded values the operation defined by equation (9). This operation creates a replica of $f(t)$ displaced in time $(f(t-\tau))$, then for each value of τ (where τ goes from $-T/2$ to $+T/2$ $(T \to \infty)$) the two functions are multiplied together, and the resulting function integrated between $-T/2$ and $+T/2$. In this way a value $\phi_{tt}(\tau)$ is obtained.

We shall now assume (a similar assumption was made on page 378) that the autocorrelation function of an ensemble can be obtained *either* by studying (over a sufficient period of time) one of its members *or* by studying all the members of an ensemble at the two instants of time, t_i and $t_i + \tau$. In order to do this, for each member of the ensemble, we multiply its value at time t ($x_i(t)$) by its value at $t+\tau$ ($x_i(t+\tau)$). And then we compute the expected value (or average) of these products, that is,

$$E[x_i(t)x_i(t+\tau)]$$

or

$$E[x_i(t)x_i(t+\tau)] \tag{10}$$

Since we have assumed that the set of values $x_i(t_i)$ of an ensemble of functions at time t_i is equivalent, neglecting the order, to a set of values obtained from one member of the ensemble over a particularly long period of time $(-\infty < t < +\infty)$, we can write

$$\phi_{tt}(\tau) = \frac{1}{T} \int\limits_{\substack{-T/2 \\ T \to \infty}}^{+T/2} f(t)f(t-\tau)\,dt = E[x_i(t)x_i(t-\tau)] \tag{11}$$

But for large ensembles and for long periods of observation

$$E[x_i(t)x_i(t-\tau)] = \bar{x}_i(t)\bar{x}_i(t-\tau)$$

so

$$\phi_{tt}(\tau) = \bar{x}_i(t)\bar{x}_i(t-\tau) \tag{12}$$

where $\bar{x}_i(t)$ and $\bar{x}_i(t-\tau)$ are the expected values of x_i at t and $t-\tau$. Equation (11) is the basis of most methods used in the analysis of membrane noise (see Chapter 10). The mathematical analysis of a noise signal is model dependent and one obtains $x_i(t)$ and $x_i(t-\tau)$. Substituting these in equation (12) we obtain an analytical expression for the autocorrelation function. This analytical expression can then be fitted to a set of values obtained by computer processing a record of the noise from expression (9). In this way a model of the process is *fitted* to experimental data.

Harmonic analysis of the autocorrelation function

The autocorrelation function $\phi_{tt}(\tau)$ has some interesting properties. These can be demonstrated by applying the autocorrelation function to periodic signals. As shown in Appendix 11, we can expand a periodic time function $f(t)$ in a Fourier series. So

$$f(t) = \sum_{n=-\infty}^{n=+\infty} C_n \exp(jn\omega_0 t) \tag{13}$$

and

$$f(t-\tau) = \sum_{n=-\infty}^{n=+\infty} C_n \exp(jn\omega_0(t-\tau)) \tag{14}$$

so

$$f(t)f(t-\tau) = \sum_{n=-\infty}^{n=+\infty} C_n \exp(jn\omega_0 t) \sum_{n=-\infty}^{n=+\infty} C_n \exp(jn\omega_0(t-\tau)) \tag{15}$$

Equation (15) generates the following types of products

(a) C_0^2

(b) $C_n C_m \exp(-jn\omega_0\tau) \exp(j\omega_0 t(n+m))$

(c) $C_n C_m \exp(jn\omega_0\tau) \exp(j\omega_0 t(n-m))$

(d) $C_{n-} C_m \exp(-jn\omega_0\tau) \exp(-j\omega_0 t(n-m))$

(e) $C_0 C_n \exp(jn\omega_0 t)$

(f) $C_m C_0 \exp(-jn\omega_0\tau) \exp(-jm\omega_0 t)$

$$(16)$$

If we want to compute the autocorrelation function ($\phi_{tt}(\tau)$), that is,

$$\phi_{tt}(\tau) = \frac{1}{T} \int\limits_{\substack{-T/2 \\ T \to \infty}}^{+T/2} f(t) f(t-\tau) \, dt$$

we will have to integrate functions (16). So

(a) $\dfrac{1}{T} \int\limits_{\substack{-T/2 \\ T \to \infty}}^{+T/2} C_0^2 \, dt = C_0^2$

(b) $\dfrac{1}{T} \int\limits_{-T/2}^{+T/2} C_n C_m \exp(-jn\omega_0\tau) \exp(j\omega_0 t(m+n)) = 0$

(c) $Z = \dfrac{1}{T} \int\limits_{-T/2}^{+T/2} C_n C_m \exp(-jn\omega_0\tau) \exp(j\omega_0 t(n-m))$

$= C_n C_m \exp(jn\omega_0 t)$

for $n \neq m = 0 \Rightarrow z = 0 \quad n = m \Rightarrow z = C_n^2 \exp(jn\omega_0\tau) \, dt$

(d) is identical to (c), so for $m = n$

integral $= C_{n-} C_m \exp(-jn\omega_0\tau)$

(e) is zero

(f) is zero

We are thus left with

$$\phi_{tt}(\tau) = C_0^2 + \sum (C_n C_{n-} \exp(jn\omega_0 t) + C_{n-} C_n \exp(-jn\omega_0\tau))$$

but

$$C_n C_n = C_{n-} C_n$$

So

$$\phi_{tt}(\tau) = C_0^2 + \sum_{n=1}^{n=\infty} A_n^2 \cos(n\omega_0\tau) \tag{17}$$

where

$$A_n^2 = 2C_n C_{n-} = (a_n^2 + b_n^2)/2$$

Power spectrum of a non-periodic signal

If we now Fourier transform (15) we obtain $\phi(\omega)$ which is known as the *power spectrum* of the original signal.

Using the same procedure it is easy to show that the Fourier transform of the autocorrelation function ($\phi_{tt}(\tau)$) of a pulse signal ($f(t)$) gives the *power density spectrum* of the signal ($F(\omega)$).

The Fourier transform can also be applied to random signals. That is, we can also think of a random signal as resulting from the summation of an infinite number of frequency components in which the phase and amplitude is randomly distributed among the components. If there was a fixed relation between the phases or amplitudes of the different frequency components their addition would not produce a random signal.

In order to Fourier transform a random signal we first assume that the signal exists for a limited period of time T. We then compute the Fourier series for such a signal. So

$$f(t) = \sum_{n=-\infty}^{n=+\infty} \exp(jn\omega_0 t)(1/T) \int_{-T/2}^{+T/2} f(t) \exp(-jn\omega_0 t)\,dt$$

But

$$T = 2\pi/\omega_0$$

so

$$f(t) = (1/2\pi) \sum_{n=-\infty}^{n=+\infty} \omega_0 \exp(jn\omega_0 t) \int_{-T/2}^{+T/2} f(t)\exp(-jn\omega_0 t)\,dt$$

$$= (1/2\pi) \sum_{n=-\infty}^{n=+\infty} \exp(jn\omega_0 t)\omega_0 \int_{-T/2}^{+T/2} f(t)\exp(-jn\omega_0 t)\,dt$$

$$(18)$$

If we now allow T to become large, $T \to \infty$, $\omega_0 \to d\omega$ and $n\,d\omega = \omega$, so the integral in the right-hand side of (18) becomes

$$F(\omega) = (1/2\pi) \int_{-\infty}^{+\infty} f(t)\exp(-j\omega t)\,dt$$

$$f(t) = \int_{-\infty}^{+\infty} F(\omega)\exp(j\omega t)\,d\omega \qquad (19)$$

Thus $F(\omega)$ becomes an *amplitude density spectrum* since the spectrum is now continuous.

As in the case of the Fourier transform of a pulse signal, $F(\omega)$ is a function of a complex variable with a real part $(R(\omega))$ and an imaginary part $(I(\omega))$, that is,

$$F(\omega) = R(\omega) + jI(\omega) \qquad (20)$$

the amplitude density of component ω is the modulus of $F(\omega)$

$$|F(\omega)| = \sqrt{(R^2(\omega) + I^2(\omega))} \qquad (21)$$

and the phase angle of each component $(\theta(\omega))$ is given by

$$\theta(\omega) = \tan^{-1} I(\omega)/R(\omega) \qquad (22)$$

Power density spectrum of a non-periodic signal

In Figure A13.3 we see that the autocorrelation function of a random signal is a pulse function of τ, symmetrical around zero. This means that we cannot compute the Fourier series of the autocorrelation function of a random signal. However, if we can compute its Fourier transform the result will be the *power density spectrum.*

$$|F(\omega)|^2 = R^2(\omega) + I^2(\omega) \tag{23}$$

In general, there will be a frequency-independent term equivalent to the C_0^2 obtained from the Fourier series of the autocorrelation function of a periodic signal. This term is the square of the average value of the signal given by

$$\bar{f} = (1/T) \int_{-\infty}^{+\infty} f(t)\, dt \tag{24}$$

Since we do not obtain, separately, $R(\omega)$ and $I(\omega)$, but only $|F(\omega)|^2$, we cannot obtain the phase of the components from the Fourier transform of the autocorrelation function.

In neurophysiology most studies of membrane random signals (noise) start with the autocorrelation of the recorded signal. The autocorrelation function is then Fourier transformed and the constant component $\bar{f}^2$ is subtracted. In (12) we showed that

$$\phi_{tt}(\tau) = \bar{x}_i(t)\bar{x}_i(t-\tau) \tag{25}$$

But A_n^2 is the value of the autocorrelation function for $\tau = 0$. In this case

$$\phi_{tt}(0) = (1/T) \int_{-T/2 \atop T \to \infty}^{+T/2} f(t)f(t)\, dt = (1/T) \int_{-T/2 \atop T \to \infty}^{+T/2} f(t)^2\, dt = \bar{f}^2 \tag{26}$$

Fig.A13.3

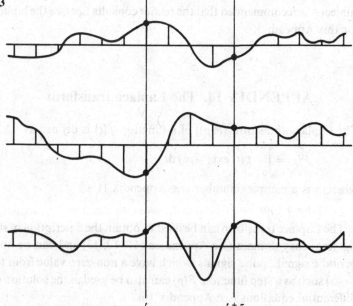

so from (12) and (14)

$$\phi_{tt}(0) = \bar{x}_i(0)\bar{x}_i(0) \tag{27}$$

But for large values of τ, $x_i(t)$ becomes independent of $x_i(t+\tau)$, that is,

$$\bar{x}_i(t) = x_i(t+\tau) \tag{28}$$

for very large τ.

Equation (28) means that the signal is *stationary*, the assumption we made at the start of this Appendix. So

$$\bar{x}_i(\infty) = \bar{x}_i(0) \tag{29}$$

If we substitute (29) into (27) we obtain

$$\phi_{tt}(0) = \bar{x}_i(\infty)\bar{x}_i(\infty) \tag{30}$$

Autocovariance

If we subtract (30) from (12) we obtain the *autocovariance* function C. This is frequently used by electrophysiologists when they study membrane noise.

$$C = \phi_{tt}(\tau) - \phi_{tt}(0) = \bar{x}_i(t)\bar{x}_i(t-\tau) - \bar{x}_i(\infty)\bar{x}_i(\infty)$$

Power-density spectrum

If we Fourier transform the autocovariance function we obtain the *power-density spectrum* of the signal with the square of the average component removed. That is, we obtain the power-density spectrum of the fluctuations around a mean value. For a more-detailed analysis of this subject it is recommended that the reader consults Lee (see the bibliography for this Appendix).

APPENDIX 14. The Laplace transform

The Laplace transform $(F(p))$ of a function $f(t)$ is defined as

$$F(p) = \int_0^\infty f(t) \exp(-pt)\, dt$$

where p is a complex number (see Appendix 1), so

$$p = \alpha + j\omega$$

The Laplace transform can be used to obtain the description of signals in the frequency domain (see Appendices 11, 12, 13) and can be applied to periodic signals, pulse signals (which have a non-zero value from $t = 0$ to $t \rightarrow \infty$) such as a step function. $F(p)$ can also be used in the solution of linear differential equations (see Appendix 16).

For convenience we shall first derive some of the most important properties of the Laplace transform.

The Laplace transform of a constant
If $f(t) = A = $ constant, then

$$\int_0^\infty A \exp(-pt)\,dt = A \int_0^\infty \exp(-pt)\,dt = (A/p)(-1)[\exp(-pt)]$$

$\exp(-pt)$ when $t \to \infty$ is zero, so

$$\int_0^\infty A \exp(-pt)\,dt = A/p \tag{1}$$

The Laplace transform of a delta function $(\delta(t))$
A delta function is introduced in Chapter 10 and its Laplace transform is

$$\int_0^\infty \delta(t) \exp(-pt)\,dt$$

since $\delta(t)$ only exists for $t = 0$ and $\exp(0) = 1$

$$\int_0^\infty \delta(t) \exp(-pt)\,dt = \int_{0-}^{0+} \delta(t)\,dt = 1 \quad \text{(by definition)} \tag{2}$$

The Laplace transform of the derivative of a function
Let

$$f'(t) = (d/dt)(f(t))$$

so

$$F(p) \int_0^\infty f'(-t) \exp(-pt)\,dt = \int_0^\infty \exp(-pt)(d/dt)(f(t))\,dt$$

if we integrate by parts (see Appendix 2)

$$u = \exp(-pt) \quad du = -p \exp(-pt) \quad dV = (d/dt)(f(t))\,dt$$

so

$$v = f(t)$$

Since

$$\int u\,dv = uv - \int v\,du$$

then

$$\int f'(-t) \exp(-pt)\,dt = [f(t) \exp(-pt)]_0^{-\infty}$$

$$+ p \int_0^\infty f(t) \exp(-pt)\,dt$$

The first term on the right-hand side is zero for $t \to \infty$ since $\exp(-\infty) = 0$ and is $f(0)$ at $t = 0$ since $\exp(0) = 1$. The second term on the right-hand side is $pF(p)$, so

$$\int_0^\infty (f'(t)) \exp(-pt)\, dt = -f(0) + p \int_0^\infty f(t) \exp(-pt)\, dt \qquad (3)$$

The Laplace transform of a second-order derivative
From (3) we have

$$\int_0^\infty f''(t) \exp(-pt)\, dt = -f'(0) + p \int_0^\infty f'(t) \exp(-pt)\, dt$$

Also from (3)

$$\int_0^\infty f''(t) \exp(-pt)\, dt = -f'(0) - pf(0) + p^2 \int f(t) \exp(-pt)\, dt$$

$$= -f'(0) - pf(0) + p^2 F(p)$$

so for an nth derivative

$$\int_0^\infty f^{n}(t) \exp(-pt)\, dt = -f^{(n-1)'}(0) - pf^{(n-2)'}(0) - \cdots$$

$$- p^{n-1} f(0) + p^n F(p)$$

The Laplace transform of a function delayed by τ $(f(t-\tau))$
(See Chapter 9 for delayed function.)

$$\int_0^\infty f(t-\tau) \exp(-pt)\, dt$$

Let us define u as

$$u = t - \tau$$

so

$$t = u + \tau \quad \text{and} \quad dt = du$$

Thus

$$\int_0^\infty f(u) \exp(-p(u+\tau))\, du = \int_0^\infty f(u) \exp(-pu) \exp(-p\tau)\, du$$

$$= \exp(-p\tau) \int_0^\infty f(u) \exp(-pu)\, du$$

Integral $\int_0^\infty f(u) \exp(-pu)\, du$ is the Laplace transform of $f(t)$ since it is independent of u, so

$$\int_0^\infty f(t-\tau) \exp(-pt)\, dt = \exp(-p\tau) F(p)$$

The Laplace transform of an exponential $(\exp(-at))$

$$\int_0^\infty \exp(-at)\exp(-pt) = \int_0^\infty \exp(-(a+p)t)\, dt$$

$$= -\frac{1}{a+p}[\exp(-(a+p)t)]_0^\infty$$

$$= \frac{1}{a+p}$$

or

$$\int_0^\infty \exp(-at)\exp(-pt)\, dt = \frac{1}{a+p}$$

The Laplace transform of $\cos(\omega t)$

If we use the expansion $\cos(\omega t) = \frac{1}{2}\exp(+j\omega t) + \frac{1}{2}\exp(-j\omega t)$ (see Appendix 3), then

$$\cos(\omega t)\exp(-pt)\, dt = \frac{1}{2}\int_0^\infty \exp(-(p-j\omega)t)\, dt$$

$$+ \frac{1}{2}\int_0^\infty \exp(-(p+j\omega)t)\, dt$$

From the transform of an exponential, and if we define $a = j\omega$ and $-a = -j\omega$, then

$$\int_0^\infty \cos(\omega t)\exp(-pt)\, dt = \frac{1}{2(p-j\omega)} + \frac{1}{2(p+j\omega)} = \frac{p}{p^2+\omega^2}$$

Using a similar procedure we obtain

$$\int_0^\infty \sin(\omega t)\exp(-pt)\, dt = \frac{\omega}{p^2+\omega^2}$$

The Laplace transform of a sum $(H(t))$ **of functions** $(f(t)$ and $g(t))$

$$\int_0^\infty H(t)\exp(-pt)\, dt = \int_0^\infty f(t)\exp(-pt)\, dt$$

$$+ \int_0^\infty g(t)\exp(-pt)\, dt$$

$$= F(p) + G(p)$$

or

$$H(p) = F(p) + G(p)$$

With these results we can make the following table:

t domain ($f(t)$)	p domain ($F(p)$)
A	A/p
$\delta(t)$	1
$f'(t)$	$-f(0)+\beta F(\beta)$
$f(t-\tau)$	$\exp(-p\tau)F(p)$
$\cos(\omega t)$	$p/(\omega^2+p^2)$
$\sin(\omega t)$	$\omega/(\omega^2+p^2)$
$f(t)+g(t)$	$F(p)+G(p)$

In order to obtain an *inverse transform* of any function $G(p)$ we first decompose it into a sum of Laplace transforms which are tabulated and then look up the corresponding inverse transforms. These tables are produced in two ways.

One way is by calculating the Laplace transform of a known function and constructing tables (as was carried out above). The other is to start with an $F(p)$ function and obtain the corresponding $f(t)$ function by integrating the function

$$f(t)=\frac{1}{2\pi}\int_{\alpha-j\omega}^{\alpha+j\omega} F(p)\exp(pt)\,\mathrm{d}t$$

This integration is often complicated.

APPENDIX 15. Fundamental circuit equations

Section I: general considerations
In Appendix 23 we derive Coulomb's law which states that

$$F=(kqq')/a^2$$

where q and q' are two point charges, a the distance that separates them and k is a constant. The value of k depends on the medium that surrounds the charges and on the system of units adopted.

When F is given in newtons, q and q' in coulombs, a in metres and the system is in a vacuum,

$$k=9\times10^9\ \mathrm{N\cdot m^{-2}\cdot C^2}$$

where a newton is the *force* that when applied to a mass of one kilogram causes the mass to accelerate 1 metre per second per second. It is usual to define a quantity ε_0 such that

$$\varepsilon_0=1/4\pi k$$

in which case

$$\varepsilon_0 = 8.85 \times 10^{-12} \, C^2 \cdot N^{-1} \cdot m^{-2}$$

ε_0 is called the *permittivity* of free space. When the surrounding medium is other than vacuum, then Coulomb's law becomes

$$F = (1/(4\pi\varepsilon))(qq'/a^2)$$

where

$$\varepsilon = k\varepsilon_0$$

so

$$k = \varepsilon/\varepsilon_0$$

k is a dimensionless quantity called the *dielectric constant*, or coefficient of the medium. (In the c.g.s. system the dielectric constant of a vacuum is 1.) Then

$$F = (1/k)(1/4\pi\varepsilon_0)(qq'/a^2)$$

We shall now consider some basic definitions used frequently in circuit equations.

The coulomb (*C*) is defined as the quantity of charge which repels an identical charge, 1 metre away, with a force of 9×10^9 newtons. The elementary charge (*e*), that is, the charge of a proton ($+e$) or an electron ($-e$), is

$$e = 1.602\,06 \times 10^{-19} \, \text{coulomb}$$

Since the Faraday (*F*)

$$F = N_A e$$

where N_A is the Avogadro number, and the Faraday (F) = 96 495 coulomb (approximately). The unit of charge in the c.g.s. system is the electrostatic unit of charge (esu).

The potential difference (*V*) between two points (*A*, *B*) is the work required to transfer a unit charge from *A* to *B*. In the MKS system *V* is measured in volts and its units are

$$V = \text{joule} \cdot \text{coul}^{-1}$$

The joule (*J*) is the work performed by a force of 1 newton when the force displaces its point of application along its direction by 1 metre.

The current (*I*) in the MKS system current is measured in amperes and a flow of charge of 1 coulomb per second is called a current of 1 ampere. So

$$\text{ampere} = \text{coulomb} \cdot s^{-1} = C \cdot s^{-1}$$

or

$$\text{ampere} = dq/dt$$

The second definition is more general since it applies when the current (I) is not steady. If I is a current flowing through an area S, then the current density $(\bar{I}) = I/S$.

When the current flows across a conductor the potential difference across the conductor is given by

$$V = RI$$

or   (Ohm's law)

$$I = GV$$

so

$$G = 1/R$$

where R is the resistance and G the conductance.

The resistance (R) is measured in ohms (Ω) and so

$$\Omega = \text{volt} \cdot \text{amp}^{-1} = \text{V} \cdot \text{amp}^{-1}$$

The conductance (G) is measured in siemens (S) and so

$$S = \text{amp} \cdot \text{V}^{-1}$$

The resistance of a conductor is related to its intrinsic properties and to its geometry by the expression

$$R = \rho l/s$$

where l is the length and s the cross-sectional area of the conductor. ρ is called the resistivity or specific resistance and is usually given by

$$\rho = Rs/l = \Omega \cdot \text{cm}^2 \cdot \text{cm}^{-1} = \Omega \cdot \text{cm}$$

so the *specific conductance* (λ) *is defined by*

$$\lambda = 1/\rho = 1/\Omega \cdot cm^{-1} = S \cdot cm^{-1}$$

When a capacitor is charging (or discharging), charge is accumulating in (or moving away from) one of its plates and moving away from (or accumulating in) the other plate. This is equivalent to a current flowing through the capacitor (the displacement current). This current can be derived from the relationship

$$V_c = q/C$$

or

$$q = CV_c$$

so

$$dq/dt = C \, dV_c/dt$$

But dq/dt is a current (I_c), so

$$I_c = C \, dV_c/dt$$

Alternatively

$$V_c = (1/C) \int I \, dt$$

The capacitance (C) is measured in *Farads* and

$$Farads = coul./volt = C \cdot V^{-1}$$

The capacitance of a capacitor depends on the material between the plates (dielectric material), the geometry of the plates, and the distance that separates them

$$C = (k\varepsilon_0 A)/l$$

where k = dielectric constant of the dielectric material, ε_0 = permittivity of vacuum, A = area of the plates, and l = distance between the plates.

For a square centimetre of a plasma membrane (where $A = 1$) we can calculate the membrane capacitance (C_m) as follows:

$$k = 2\text{--}5 \text{ (dielectric constant of lipid core)}$$
$$\varepsilon_0 = 8.35 \times 10^{-12} \text{ C} \cdot \text{N}^{-1} \cdot \text{m}^{-2}$$
$$l = 50\text{--}100 \times 10^{-10} \text{ m} \quad (50\text{--}100 \text{ Å})$$

Then

$$C_m = 5 \times 5.85 \times 10^{-12}(\text{coul.}^2/(\text{N} \cdot \text{m}^2)) \times 10^{-4} \text{ m}^2/50 \times 10^{-10} \text{ m}$$
$$= 0.89 \times 10^{-6} \text{ C} \cdot \text{V}^{-1}$$
$$= 1 \, \mu\text{F}$$

Section II: Kirchhoff's laws (see Figure A15.1a and b)

If currents I_1, I_2, I_3, ..., I_n flow on across electrical elements (resistors, capacitors, etc.) = 1, 2, 3, 4, ..., n, then (Figure A15.1a)

$$\sum_{i=1}^{n} I_i = 0 \quad \text{for each node}$$

This is known as the *Kirchhoff's law of the currents*.

If current (I) flows through elements 1, 2, 3, 4, ..., n and V_1, V_2, V_3, ..., V_n are the electrical potential differences (V_i) across respective elements 1, 2, 3, ..., n, V_i may be given by Ohm's law or by the expression for each loop

$$V_c = (1/c) \int I \, dt \quad \text{and} \quad \sum_{i=1}^{n} E_i = \sum_{i=1}^{n} V_i$$

This equation is *Kirchhoff's law of the voltages* where

$$V_i = R_i I \quad \text{or} \quad V_i = (1/c_i) \int I \, dt$$

and E_i are electromotive forces – batteries for example (by definition a pure electromotive force E has no internal resistance; see Figure A15.1b). Let us consider the circuit A15.1c where E is an electromotive force and elements

1, 2, 3 are resistors. Then, by Kirchhoff's law of the currents

$$I_T = I_1 + I_2 + \cdots + I_n$$
$$= E(1/R_1 + 1/R_2 + 1/R_3 + \cdots + 1/R_n)$$

so

$$I_T/E = 1/R_1 + 1/R_2 + \cdots + 1/R_n$$

But the left-hand side is the conductance of the parallel combination of resistors. So, for a parallel combination of resistances (conductances)

$$G_T = G_1 + G_2 + G_3 + \cdots + G_n$$

or

$$G_T = \sum_{i=1}^{n} G_i$$

where

$$G_i = 1/R_i$$

For $i = 2$

$$G_T = 1/R_1 + 1/R_2 = (R_1 + R_2)/R_1 R_2$$

Fig.A15.1

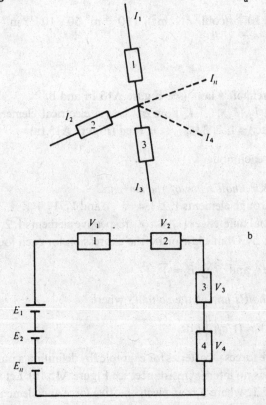

and
$$R_T = 1/G_T = R_1 R_2/(R_1 + R_2)$$

For the case where we have n equal conductance in series
$$1/R + 1/R + \cdots + 1/R = n/R = nG$$

where
$$G = 1/R$$

Let us consider a series combination of resistors $(R_1, R_2, \ldots, R_n)$ connected to an electromotive force (Figure A15.1d). From Kirchhoff's law of the voltages

$$
\begin{aligned}
E &= IR_1 + IR_2 + \cdots + IR_n \\
&= I(R_1 + R_2 + \cdots + R_n) \\
&= I \sum_{i=1}^{n} R_i
\end{aligned}
$$

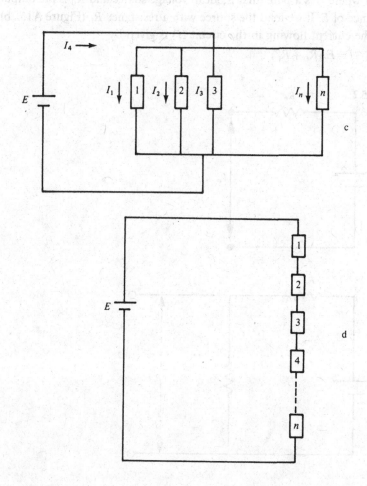

or

$$E/I = \sum_{i=1}^{n} R_i = R_T$$

so for resistors R_1, R_2, ... connected in series

$$R_T = \sum_{i=1}^{n} R_i$$

For $n=2$

$$R_T = R_1 + R_2$$

and

$$G_T = 1/R_T = 1/(1/G_1 + 1/G_2) = G_1 G_2/(G_1 + G_2)$$

Section III: voltage and current sources

Any voltage source (E) can be represented by the circuit of Figure A15.2a where E is a pure (that is, ideal) voltage source and R_0 is the output resistance of E. If we load the source with a resistance R_L (Figure A15.2b) then the current flowing in the circuit (I) is given by

$$I = E/(R_0 + R_L)$$

Fig.A15.2

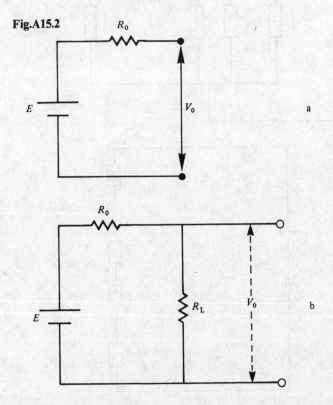

and the voltage (V_0) across the terminals of the source is given by

$$V_0 = IR_L = ER_L/(R_0 + R_L) = E(1/(1 + R_0/R_L))$$

when

$$R_L \gg R_0$$

then

$$V_0 = E$$

since for $I = 0$, V_0 is also E, E is the open circuit voltage of the voltage source.

Section IV: voltmeters and ammeters

An ideal *voltmeter* is a voltmeter with an *infinite* internal resistance R_i. Any real voltmeter can be represented by the circuit of Figure A15.3a. When we use a practical voltmeter to measure a voltage source (Figure A15.3b), the current flowing through the voltmeter (I) is given by

$$I = E/(R_i + R_0)$$

but

$$V = IR_i$$

Fig.A15.3

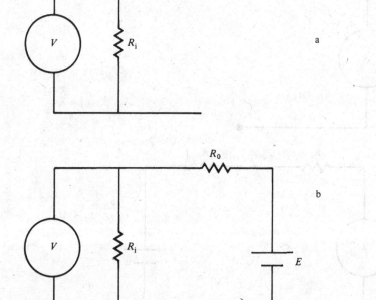

so
$$V = E(R_i/(R_i+R_0)) = E/(1 + R_0/R_i)$$
The volemeter will only measure E when
$$R_0 \ll R_i$$

An ideal current meter (ammeter) is a current meter with zero internal resistance. Any practical current meter can be represented by the circuit of Figure A15.4a. If we want to measure a current flowing through a resistor R_0 as a result of an electromotive force E (Figure A15.4b) the current flowing through A is given by
$$I = E/(R_0+R_i) \quad \text{Ohm's law}$$
The current we want to measure (I_0) is
$$I_0 = E/R_0$$
Substituting for E,
$$I_0 = \frac{I(R_0+R_i)}{R_0} = I(1/(1+R_i/R_0))$$
I will be equal to I_0 only when
$$R_i \ll R_0$$

Fig.A15.4

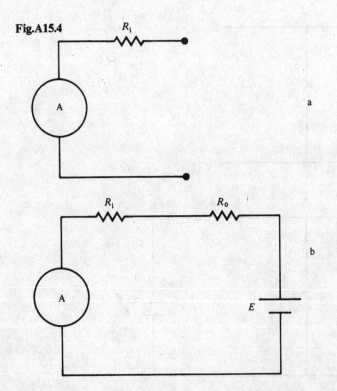

APPENDIX 16. Solution of linear differential equations by the Laplace transform

The Laplace transform can be used to solve differential equations of constant coefficients. These equations are known as linear differential equations.

Let us consider a second-order differential equation of the type

$$(d/dx)^2(Y) + a(d/dx)(Y) + bY = f(x) \tag{1}$$

For example

$$(d/dx)^2(Y) + 3(d/dx)(Y) + 2Y = \exp(-ax) \tag{1a}$$

If we Laplace transform both sides of equation (1a) we obtain

$$\int_0^\infty (d/dx)^2(Y)\exp(-px)\,dx$$

$$+3\int_0^\infty (d/dx)(Y)\exp(-px)\,dx + 2\int_0^\infty Y\exp(-px)\,dx$$

$$= \int_0^\infty \exp(-ax)\exp(-px)\,dx \tag{2}$$

From Appendix 17

$$\int_0^\infty (d/dx)^2(Y)\exp(-px)\,dx = -Y'(0) - pY(0) + p^2Y(p) \tag{3}$$

$$\int_0^\infty (d/dx)(Y)\exp(-px)\,dx = -Y(0) + pY(p) \tag{4}$$

$$\int_0^\infty Y\exp(-px)\,dx = Y(p) \tag{5}$$

and

$$\int_0^\infty \exp(-px)\exp(-ax)\,dx = 1/(p+a) \tag{6}$$

If we substitute (3), (4), (5) and (6) into (2) we obtain

$$-Y'(0) - pY(0) + p^2Y(p) - 3Y(0) + 3pY(p) + 2Y(p) = 1/(p+a) \tag{7}$$

If we collect terms in (7) and arrange

$$Y(p)[p^2 + 3p + 2] = 1/(p+a) + Y'(0) + Y(0)(p+3)$$

But

$$p^2 + 3p + 2 = (p+1)(p+2)$$

so

$$Y(p) = 1/(p+a)(p+1)(p+2) + (Y'(0) + Y(0)(p+3))/(p+1)(p+2) \tag{8}$$

The right-hand side can be expanded in partial fractions (see Appendix 8), so

$$1/(p+a)(p+1)(p+2) = A/(p+a) + B/(p+1) + C/(p+2) \tag{9}$$

and

$$(Y'(0) + (p+3)Y(0))/(p+1)(p+2) = D/(p+1) + E/(p+2) \qquad (10)$$

If we substitute (9) and (10) into (8) and rearrange we obtain

$$Y(p) = A/(p+a) + (D+B)/(p+1) + (C+E)/(p+2)$$

From a table of Laplace transforms we obtain that

$$Y(t) = A \exp(-at) + (D+B) \exp(-t) + (C+E) \exp(-2t) \qquad (11)$$

Equation (11) is the *general solution* for equation (1a). We have now to express A, $D+B$ and $C+E$ in terms of $Y'(0)$ and $Y(0)$, the *initial conditions*.

APPENDIX 17. The application of Laplace transforms to circuit theory: the concept of complex impedance

As shown in Chapter 4, the differential equation describing a circuit consisting of a resistor (R), a capacitor (C), a battery (E) and a switch (S) in series is

$$C \, dV/dt + V/R = E/R \qquad (1)$$

where V is the voltage across the capacitor. When the switch is closed the voltage across the capacitor (V_0) is zero. If we Laplace transform equation (1) we obtain

$$pCV(p) + V(p)/R = E(p)/R \qquad (2)$$

where $E(p)$ is given by $E(p) = E/p$ since E is a constant (see Appendix 14).

If we rearrange equation (2) to find $V(1)$ we obtain

$$V(p) = E(p)(1/R)/(pC + 1/R) \qquad (3)$$

If we multiply and divide top and bottom of (3) by R and pC respectively we obtain

$$V(p) = E(p)(1/pC)/((1/pC) + R) \qquad (4)$$

To understand the term $1/(pC)$ we need to analyse the relationship between the voltage and the current across a capacitor. In Appendix 15 we saw that

$$I_c = C \, dV/dt \qquad (5)$$

If we Laplace transform (5) with the assumption that the voltage across the capacitor (V_0) was zero when current I_c started to flow,

$$I_c(p) = pCV(p) \qquad (6)$$

where $I_c(p)$ and $pV(p)$ are the Laplace transforms of I_c and dV/dt. So

$$V(p)/I_c(p) = 1/pC \qquad (7)$$

If we now Laplace transform Ohm's law

$$V = I_R R$$

we obtain

$$V(p) = I_R(p)R$$

or

$$V(p)/I_R(p) = R \tag{8}$$

Equation (8) means that for the case of a resistor Ohm's law still applies in the p domain. Formally the right-hand sides of equations (7) and (8) are comparable. That is, the resistance term (R) in equation (8) is equivalent to the capacitance term $(1/pC)$ in equation (7). Both terms are the ratios of voltage to currents in the p domain and are known as impedances (Z). In the case of R the impedance (Z) is a real number, while in the case of $1/pC$ the impedance is a complex number, because p is itself a complex number. The reciprocal of an impedance (Z) is called an admittance (Y).

It is possible with Laplace-transformed voltages and currents to apply Kirchhoff's laws to circuits capacitors. If we apply this procedure to the circuit of Figure A17.1 we can see that, from Ohm's law,

$$I(p) = E(p)/(R + 1/pC) \tag{9}$$

and

$$V(p) = I(p)(1/pC)$$
$$V(p) = E(p)(1/pC)/(R + 1/pC) \tag{9}$$

When we are dealing with Laplace-transformed variables we say that we are in the p (or s) domain. We should note that equation (9) is identical to (4). By Laplace transforming differential equations that describe circuits that contain capacitors and resistors we are transforming differential equations into simpler algebraic equations. For example, the right-hand side of equations (3) or (9) can be expanded in partial fractions (see Appendix 8).

Fig.A17.1

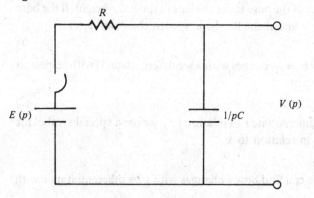

$E(p)$ R $V(p)$ $1/pC$

Since

$$E(p) = E/p$$

then equation (9) (or (3)) becomes (9a)

$$V(p) = (E/p)(1/pC)/(R + 1/pC) \tag{9a}$$

If we multiply top and bottom of the right-hand side by pC we obtain

$$V(p) = (E/p)/(pCR + 1) = (E/p)(1/(p\tau + 1))$$

or

$$V(p) = (E/\tau)(1/p(p + 1/\tau))$$

where τ is the time constant.

The right-hand side can be expanded in partial fractions

$$V(p) = E(1/p - 1/(p + 1/\tau))$$

or

$$V(t) = E(p - \exp(-t/\tau))$$

This solution was also obtained in Chapter 4 by solving equation (1) by other methods. Since this solution here was obtained by alternative means it is reasonable to assume that we can use complex impedances and apply Kirchhoff's laws.

The concept of complex impedance may be used when $V(t)$ and $I(t)$ are time functions of any type. They may be periodic signals, pulse signals, random signals or non-periodic signals with a non-zero average value such as a step function.

APPENDIX 18. Partial differentiation: the gradient and divergence

In a description of the physical world we frequently encounter functions of more than one variable. For example, the volume of a rectangular block is given as the product of the base times the length times the height. If the base is a square of side x and if the height is y, then the volume (v) is

$$v = x^2 y \tag{1}$$

If we want to know how v changes with x we differentiate (1) with respect to x and keep y constant:

$$(\partial v / \partial x)_y = 2xy \tag{2}$$

Since we can also differentiate v in relation to y we use a special symbol for the differentiation in relation to x

$$(\partial / \partial x)$$

In a similar way we can find how v changes with y by differentiating v with respect to y keeping x constant

$$(\partial v/\partial y)_x = \partial v/\partial y = x^2 \tag{3}$$

The differential of v with respect to x is then

$$dv_x = (\partial v/\partial x)\,dx \tag{4}$$

and the differential of v with respect to y is

$$dv_y = (\partial v/\partial y)\,dy \tag{5}$$

The differential of v in relation to both x and y (the total differential) is thus

$$dv = (\partial v/\partial x)\,dx + (\partial v/\partial y)\,dy$$

or

$$dv = 2xy\,dx + x^2\,dy \tag{6}$$

We can also calculate the second derivative of v in relation to both x and y, that is,

$$(\partial/\partial y)(\partial v/\partial x) \quad \text{or} \quad (\partial/\partial x)(\partial v/\partial x)$$

From (2)

$$(\partial/\partial y)(\partial v/\partial x) = (\partial/\partial y)(2xy) = 2x$$

or

$$(\partial/\partial x)(\partial v/\partial x) = (\partial/\partial x)(x^2) = 2x$$

Some functions are functions of x, y and z. For example, if the base of the rectangular cube is rectangular of sides x and y and its height is z the volume is given by

$$v = xyz$$

then

$$dv = yz(dx) + xz(dy) + xy(dz)$$

Gradient

We shall now define two functions, the gradient and the divergence, which have wide applications in physics. (For a more detailed and precise development of these two concepts the reader is referred to the Berkley Physics series on electricity and magnetism; see end of the Appendix.) If F is a function of x, y and z ($F(x, y, z)$), we call the *gradient* of F the following

$$\text{gradient of } F = \mathbf{i}(\partial/\partial x)(F(x, y, z)) + \mathbf{j}(\partial/\partial y)(F(x, y, z))$$
$$+ \mathbf{k}(\partial/\partial z)(F(x, y, z))$$

For the case of v we obtain

$$\text{grad } v = \mathbf{i}yz + \mathbf{j}xz + \mathbf{k}xy$$

The gradient tells us how the function varies along the three axes (x, y and z), and in order to specify this we write

$$\text{grad } F = \mathbf{i}(\partial/\partial x)(F) + \mathbf{j}(\partial/\partial y)(F) + \mathbf{k}(\partial/\partial z)(F) \tag{7}$$

The quantities **i, j, k** have a magnitude of 1 but are measured along x, y and z respectively. F is a quantity defined only by its magnitude. (Quantities defined by a magnitude and a direction are called *vectors* (**i, j, k**) while quantities that are defined only by a magnitude are called scalars.) Each term in (7) is a vector as we are multiplying a vector (**i, j** and **k**) by a quantity. So grad F is a vector. In order to compute the magnitude of grad F we use Pythagoras' theorem. First we compute the magnitude of g_1 in the xy plane (Figure A18.1),

$$g_1^2 = ((\partial/\partial x)F)^2 + ((\partial/\partial y)F)^2$$

then we compute the magnitude of grad v (g_2)

$$g_2^2 = g_1^2 + ((\partial/\partial z)F)^2$$

so

$$g_2^2((\partial/\partial x)F)^2 + ((\partial/\partial y)F)^2 + ((\partial/\partial z)F)^2$$
$$g_2 = |\text{grad } v| = \sqrt{(((\partial/\partial x)F)^2 + ((\partial/\partial y)F)^2 + ((\partial/\partial z)F)^2)}$$

(see Figure A18.1). By using trigonometrical relationships we can also define the angle of grad v with the xy, xz and yz planes.

Let us assume that a solute is dissolved in a solution and that the concentration of the solute is not uniform. That is, c is a function of x, y and z. Then

Fig.A18.1

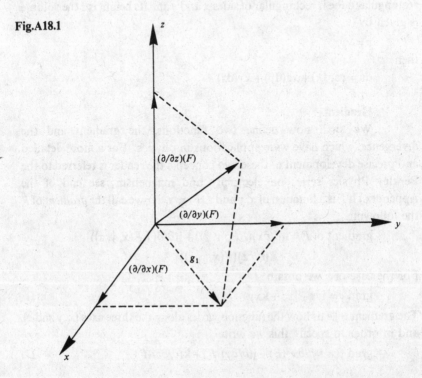

$$\text{grad } c(x, y, z) \equiv \mathbf{i}(\partial/\partial x)(c(x, y, z)) + \mathbf{j}(\partial/\partial y)(c(x, y, z))$$
$$+ \mathbf{k}(\partial/\partial z)(c(x, y, z))$$

since

$$|\text{grad } c| = \sqrt{(((\partial/\partial x)c)^2 + ((\partial/\partial y)c)^2 + ((\partial/\partial z)c)^2)}$$

and each term inside the square term is always positive. This means that the direction of grad c is the one along which there is the steepest rate of change of concentration.

The first law of Fick in three dimensions is thus

$$j = -D \text{ grad } c \tag{8}$$

and j, the flux (per unit area), is in the direction opposite to that of grad c. So

$$j = -D[\mathbf{i}(\partial/\partial x)(c) + \mathbf{j}(\partial/\partial y)(c) + \mathbf{k}(\partial/\partial z)(c)] \tag{9}$$

Divergence

The second function which we wish to introduce is the *divergence*. To understand the concept of divergence we need first to set up a physical model. Let us assume that a fixed amount of solute is produced per unit time in the centre of a cube of sides Δx, Δy, Δz and that the rate of production is

$$\rho \text{ mol} \cdot \text{s}^{-1}$$

(An example of such a system might be a mitochondrium at the centre of a cubic cell', producing ρ moles of ATP per second.) Let us also assume that the centre of the cube has coordinates

$$x + \Delta x/2, \quad y + \Delta y/2, \quad z + \Delta z/2$$

At steady-state the total flux will leave the box by the six faces. The components of these fluxes will be

$$j(x), j(y), j(z)$$

(fluxes per unit area in the x, y and z directions). The value of $j(x)$ varies along the y and z axis. Along the z axis the variation in $j(x)$ will be approximately

$$\Delta j(x) = (\partial/\partial z)(F(x)) \Delta z$$

For small Δz we may assume that $\partial/\partial z(F_x)$ is constant and that the average value of j_x along the z axis (see Figure A18.2) is

$$(\partial/\partial z)(j(x)) \Delta z/2$$

By using a similar reasoning for the other axis the net flux across the two faces parallel to the zy plane will be

$$\Delta z \, \Delta y \, [j(x)(x, y, z) + (\partial/\partial z)(j(x)) \Delta z/2 + (\partial/\partial y)(j(x)) \Delta y/2 + \Delta x(\partial/\partial x)(j(x))/2]$$

(i) area of   Flux per $\Delta z \times \Delta y$ area leaving the cube at $x + \Delta x$
       one of
       the faces

$$-\Delta z\,\Delta y\,[j(x)(x,y,z)+(\partial/\partial z)(j(x))\,\Delta z/2+(\partial/\partial y)j(x)\,\Delta y/2]$$

(ii) area of the   Flux per $\Delta z \times \Delta y$ area along the x axis, leaving the
opposite   cube at x
faces

The last term does not include $\Delta x(\partial/\partial x)x$ because the cube is placed between x and $x+\Delta x$, so one of the faces is at $x(\Delta x=0)$ and the other at $x+\Delta x$. This term is negative because the flux $j(x)$ is in the opposite direction to the $j(x)$ of the first term. The sum is simply

$$\Delta x\,\Delta y\,\Delta z(\partial/\partial x)(j(x))$$

By using a similar reasoning for the other components of the flux and adding all the components we obtain

$$j_{total}=\rho=\Delta x\,\Delta y\,\Delta z((\partial/\partial x)(j(x))+(\partial/\partial y)(j(y))+(\partial/\partial z)(j(z)))$$

or

$$j_{total}/(\Delta x\,\Delta y\,\Delta z)=\rho/\Delta x\,\Delta y\,\Delta z$$
$$=((\partial/\partial x)(j(x))+(\partial/\partial y)(j(y))+(\partial/\partial z)(j(z)))$$

The right-hand side is called the divergence of Y, that means that

$$\text{div}\,\mathbf{j}=\text{flux/volume}=\text{production/volume} \tag{10}$$

Divergence is thus a scalar quantity and is the sum of the derivatives of the three components $(j(x),j(y),j(z))$ of a vectorial quantity $(\mathbf{j})$ in relation to the corresponding directions (x,y,z).

Fig.A18.2

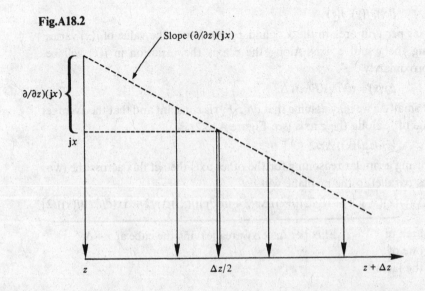

In (10) we showed the divergence to be a flux per unit volume; we should now examine this definition. If our system is a much larger cube (V) and if the solute is produced everywhere in the cube at a constant rate; we divide this cube into small elementary cubes of volume Δv and define Δv as $\Delta v = \Delta x\, \Delta y\, \Delta z$. Then there will be a flux of substance across the six elementary faces and the total flux across these elementary cubes will be the local flux j_i, times the local elementary area. Since the local flux is different at different points, in each elementary area ($\Delta x\, \Delta y$ or $\Delta y\, \Delta z$ or $\Delta x\, \Delta z$) we should divide each of these elementary areas into infinitesimal areas dA and multiply these infinitesimal areas by the local value of the flux j. For an elementary cube dv, the total flux will be then the sum of all these products, so

$$\text{total flux} = \sum_{i=1}^{n} j_i\, dA$$

As $n \to \infty$, $dA \to 0$, the sum tends to the integral and the total flux corresponding to elementary cube k (j_k) is then given by

$$j_k = \int_{\Delta S} j\, dA \qquad (11)$$

this integral is over the whole surface (ΔS) of the cube Δv. The total flux in the macroscopic cube (v) is thus

$$j_T = \sum_{i=1}^{k} \int_{\Delta S_i} j\, dA_i = \int_S j\, dA \qquad (12)$$

The integral $\int_S$ in (12) is known as a surface integral and is treated exactly like any other integral. We note that

$$S_i = 2(\Delta x\, \Delta y + \Delta z\, \Delta x + \Delta y\, \Delta z)$$

$$S = \sum_i S_i$$

In (11), as the fluxes across a face between adjacent cubes will cancel each other, the sum j_T is just the flux across the faces of cube v. This means that sum (12) does not tell us what is happening *inside* the cube v. As we keep adding adjacent elementary cubes we end up with the flux across the boundaries of the new volume. In order to examine what is happening inside the cube it is necessary to compute the ratio

$$\frac{j_k}{v_k}$$

that is, the ratio between the flux (j_k) across the boundaries of a volume element Δv_k and the volume. In the limit

$$\lim_{\Delta r_k \to 0} (1/\Delta v_k) \int_{\Delta S_k} j\, dA_k$$

we have now the flux per unit volume at each point and we call this limit the *divergence* of **j** (div). So

$$\text{div } j = \lim_{\Delta v_k \to 0} (1/\Delta v_k) \int_{\Delta S_k} j \, \mathrm{d}A_k \tag{13}$$

But from (12)

$$\int_S j \, \mathrm{d}A = \sum_{k=1}^{k=N} j \, \mathrm{d}A_k = \sum_{k=1}^{k=N} \Delta v_k \left[\int_{\Delta S_k} j \, \mathrm{d}A_k / \Delta v_k \right]$$

when $N \to \infty$

$$\Delta S_k \to 0$$

the term inside brackets tends to the div **j** and the summation tends to an integral over volume v. So

$$\int_S j \, \mathrm{d}A = \int_v \text{div } \mathbf{j} \, \mathrm{d}v \tag{14}$$

Gauss's theorem

Relationship (14) is known as *Gauss's theorem* as it relates the integral over an area of a vectorial quantity with the integral over the volume of its divergence. Let us consider now that we have a steady-state situation where our source of solute is in the middle of a sphere of radius a producing solute at a rate of q moles per unit time. The total flux across the boundary of the sphere (j_T) will be related to the flux per unit area (j) across such a boundary by the expression

$$j = j_T / 4\pi a^2$$

But since

$$j_T = q$$

(for we are at steady-state and there is no accumulation in the sphere so what is produced (q) must leave (j_T)), then

$$j = q / 4\pi a^2$$

Let us redefine the source ρ as being given by

$$\rho = q / 4\pi$$

then

$$j = \rho / a^2$$

and

$$j_T = 4\pi a^2 j = 4\pi a^2 \rho / a^2 = 4\pi \rho \tag{15}$$

We can see that j_T is totally independent of the radius. In fact, equation (15) applies to a surface of *any shape* because what is produced inside the surface must leave *through* the surface.

If instead of one source (q) we have a source for each element $\mathrm{d}v$, the total amount produced (q_T) will be given by

$$q_T = \int_v q \, dv$$

since

$$q = 4\pi\rho$$

then

$$j_T = 4\pi \int \rho \, dv \tag{16}$$

But j_T is just the flux per unit area (j) integrated over the whole area of the surface (S), so

$$j_T = \int_S j \, dA$$

so

$$\int j \, dA = 4\pi \int \rho \, dv \tag{17}$$

Equation (17) was derived by Gauss for the electrical field (E) (17) and it is often written in the form

$$\int E \, dA = 4\pi \int \rho \, dv \tag{18}$$

where E is the electrical field at the boundary (also called the flux of electrical field at the boundary) while $\int \rho \, dv$ is the total charge q enclosed by the boundary.

We can rewrite (14) for the electrical field as

$$\int_S E \, dA = \int_v \text{div } E \, dv \tag{19}$$

But we also know (see Appendix 22) that the electrical potential (ψ) is related to the electrical field by the expression

$$E = -(d/dx)(\psi) \tag{20}$$

This relation is for one dimension (x). For the three dimensions (x, y, z) it will be

$$E = -(i(\partial/\partial x)(\psi) + j(\partial/\partial y)(\psi) + k(\partial/\partial z)(\psi))$$

or from (7)

$$E = -\text{grad } \psi$$

so

$$\text{div } E = -\text{div grad } \psi$$
$$= -\text{div}(i(\partial/\partial x)(\psi) + j(\partial/\partial y)(\psi) + k(\partial/\partial z)(\psi))$$

$i(\partial/\partial x)(\psi)$, $j(\partial/\partial y)(\psi)$, $k(\partial/\partial z)(\psi)$ are the components of the vector grad along the x, y and z axes respectively. So

$$\text{div } \mathbf{E} = -[(\partial/\partial x)^2(\psi) + (\partial/\partial y)^2\psi + (\partial/\partial z)^2\psi] \tag{21}$$

But from (13), (14) and (18)

$$\text{div } \mathbf{E} = \lim_{\Delta r_k \to 0} 1/\Delta v_k \int_{\Delta S_k} j \, dA_k$$

$$= \lim_{\Delta r \to 0} (1/\Delta v)4\pi \int \rho \, dv$$

$$= (d/dv)\left(4\pi \int \rho \, dv\right) = 4\pi\rho$$

Poisson's equation

For the one-dimensional case

$$(\partial/\partial x)^2\psi = -4\pi\rho$$

This is the *Poisson equation* written in the c.g.s. system which relates the local electrical potential to the local charge density (charge per unit volume). In the MKS system the equation becomes

$$(\partial/\partial x)^2(\psi) = -4\pi\rho(1/\varepsilon)$$

This equation is used extensively in electrochemistry and can be applied to the calculation of the ionic concentrations and electrical potential in the solutions adjacent to membranes (Debye Layers). In Appendix 22 we analyse the Poisson equation in some detail.

APPENDIX 19. Partial differential equations: integration of the diffusion equation

Partial differential equations are differential equations that have derivatives of more than one variable. These equations arise from the description of physical systems when a variable is a function of more than one coordinate in space (x and y, for example), or is a function of both distance and time.

Fick's laws are examples of partial differential equations.

Integration of the diffusion equation

Integration of the diffusion equation depends upon the boundary or initial conditions. This thus means that a large number of different solutions may be obtained, but here we will consider only two of the possible solutions.

(I) Steady-state solution: the one-dimensional diffusion equation is

$$(\partial/\partial t)(c) = D(\partial/\partial x)^2 c \tag{1}$$

where c is a function of both distance and time $(c(x, t))$. In the steady-state the time derivative is zero, so

$$(\partial/\partial t)(c) = 0$$

and

$$D(d/dx)^2 c(x) = (d/dx)^2 c(x) = 0 \tag{2}$$

then

$$\int (d/dx)^2 c(x)\,dx = \int (d/dx)((d/dx)(c(x)))\,dx$$

$$= (d/dx)(c(x)) + a = 0$$

where a is the integration constant, and

$$\int (d/dx)(c(x))\,dx + \int a\,dx = c(x) + ax + b = 0$$

For $x = 0$

$$0 = c(0) + b \quad \text{or} \quad b = -c(0)$$

so

$$(d/dx)(c(x)) = -a \quad \text{and} \quad c(x) = c(0) - ax$$

But from the first law of Fick the flux (J) is given by

$$J = -D\,dc/dx$$
$$= Da \tag{3}$$

But

$$a = (c(0) - c(x))/x$$

so

$$J = D(c(0) - c(x))/x = (D/x)(c(0) - c(x))$$
$$= P(c(0) - c(x)) \tag{4}$$

where P is the permeability of a homogeneous slab through which the solute diffuses with a diffusion coefficient D.

(II) Non-steady-state solution: in equation (1) concentration is a function of both x and t. It can be integrated by several methods, but we shall use the Laplace transform technique (see Appendices 14, 16). Let us consider the cases where the concentration of the solute is both finite and infinite at $x = 0$.

(a) *Finite concentration at x = 0*
Let us assume that the solute is concentrated at time zero in a plane of cross-sectional area 1 cm^2, which is located at $x = 0$, and if the plane is bathed on both sides by semi-infinite baths of cross-sectional area 1. (The baths (1 and 2) are called semi-infinite because they extend from $x = 0$ to $x \rightarrow +\infty$ and x

$\rightarrow -\infty$, respectively.) Then the boundaries and initial conditions are at $t=0$ and $x>0$

$$c(0, x)=0$$

where the total amount of substance in the plane at time zero is Q_0. Since $c(x, t)$ is a function of both x and t we Laplace transform first in relation to one of the variables (t) and then in relation to the other (x). So

$$\int_0^\infty (\partial/\partial t)(c(x, t))\exp(-pt)\,\mathrm{d}t$$

$$=D\int_0^\infty (\partial/\partial x)^2 c(x, t)\exp(-pt)\,\mathrm{d}t \quad (5)$$

In order to integrate the left-hand side we use the method of integration by parts (see Appendix 2). Then

$$\int_0^\infty u\,\mathrm{d}v=[uv]_0^\infty-\int_0^\infty v\,\mathrm{d}u \qquad (5a)$$

where

$$u=\exp(-pt) \qquad (6)$$
$$\mathrm{d}v=(\partial/\partial t)(c(x, t)\,\mathrm{d}t) \qquad (7)$$

so

$$\mathrm{d}u=-p\exp(-pt)\,\mathrm{d}t \qquad (8)$$
$$v=c(x, t) \qquad (9)$$

If we substitute (6), (7), (8) and (9) into (5a) we obtain

$$\int_0^\infty \exp(-pt)(\partial/\partial t)(c(x, t))\,\mathrm{d}t$$

$$=[\exp(-pt)c(x, t)]_0^\infty+p\int_0^\infty c(x, t)\exp(-pt)\,\mathrm{d}t \quad (10)$$

The first term on the right-hand side of (10) is zero for $t\rightarrow\infty$. Because $\exp(-pt)$ is zero and is $c(x, 0)$ for $t=0$. But $c(x, 0)$ is zero. The second term on the right-hand side is the Laplace transform of $c(x, t)$. So

$$\int_0^\infty (\partial/\partial t)(c(x, t))\exp(-pt)\,\mathrm{d}t=pc(xp) \qquad (11)$$

The derivative on the right-hand side of (5) is with respect to x so it can be brought out of the integral. So

$$\int_0^\infty (\partial/\partial x)^2(c(x, t))\exp(-pt)\,\mathrm{d}t$$

$$=(\partial/\partial x)^2\int_0^\infty c(x, t)\exp(-pt)\,\mathrm{d}t=(\partial/\partial x)^2(c(x, p)) \quad (12)$$

If we substitute (11) and (12) into (5) we obtain

$$pc(x, p)=D(\mathrm{d}/\mathrm{d}x)^2(c(x, p)) \qquad (13)$$

One of the advantages of using Laplace transform to solve partial differential equations is that after transforming the partial differential equation we obtain an *ordinary* differential equation in the p domain and p can now be treated as a constant. The techniques for solving ordinary differential equations can then be applied. In equation (13) the derivative in relation to x is not a partial derivative any more since c is not now a function of t. If we rearrange (13) we obtain

$$(d/dx)^2(c(x, p)) - (p/D)c(x, p) = 0$$

Let us define q as

$$q = \sqrt{(p/D)}$$

then

$$(d/dx)^2(c(x, p)) - q^2 c(x, p) = 0 \tag{14}$$

The Laplace transform of (14) in relation to x is by definition

$$\int_0^\infty (d/dx)^2(c(x, p)) \exp(-sx)\, dx$$

$$-q^2 \int_0^\infty c(x, p) \exp(-sx)\, dx = 0 \tag{15}$$

The second term on the left-hand side of (15) is by definition $q^2 c(s, p)$. To find the Laplace transform of the first term we again integrate by parts. This term can be rewritten as

$$\int_0^\infty \exp(-sx)(d/dx)((d/dx)(c(x, p)))\, dx \tag{16}$$

If we define

$$u = \exp(-sx)$$
$$dv = (d/dx)((d/dx)(c(x, p))\, dx) \tag{17}$$

then

$$du = -s \exp(-sx)\, dx \tag{18}$$

and

$$v = (d/dx)(c(x, p)) \tag{19}$$

From (16), (17), (18), (19)

$$\int_0^\infty \exp(-sx)(d/dx)((d/dx)(c(x, p)))\, dx$$

$$= [\exp(-sx)(d/dx)(c(x, p))]_0^\infty$$

$$+ s \int_0^\infty \exp(-sx)(d/dx)(c(x, p))\, dx \tag{20}$$

The first term on the right-hand side of (20) is zero for $x \to \infty$, because of the exponential $\exp(-sx)$ and $c(x, p)$ is $c'(0, p)$ for $x = 0$. So

$$[\exp(-sx)(d/dx)(c(x, p))]_0^\infty = -c'(0, p) \tag{21}$$

The second term on the right-hand side of (20) can again be integrated by parts. If we define

$$u = \exp(-sx) \tag{22}$$
$$dv = (d/dx)(c(x, p)) \, dx \tag{23}$$

then

$$du = -s \exp(-sx) \, dx \tag{24}$$

and

$$v = c(x, p) \tag{25}$$

From (22), (23), (24) and (25)

$$\int_0^\infty \exp(-sx)(d/dx)(c(x, p)) \, dx$$

$$= [\exp(-sx)c(x, p)]_0^\infty + s \int_0^\infty c(x, p) \exp(-sx) \, dx \tag{26}$$

The first term on the right-hand side of (26) is zero for $t \to \infty$ because of the exponential $\exp(-sx)$ and $c(x, p)$ is $c(0, 0)$ for $t = 0$. The second term is the Laplace transform of $c(x, p)$ ($c(s, p)$). So

$$[\exp(-sx)c(x, p)]_0^\infty = -c(0, p) \tag{27}$$

and

$$\int_0^\infty c(x, p) \exp(-sx) \, dx = c(s, p) \tag{28}$$

From (20), (21), (27) and (28)

$$\int_0^\infty \exp(-sx)(d/dx)((d/dx)(c(x, p))) \, dx$$

$$= -c'(0, p) - sc(0, p) + s^2 c(s, p) \tag{29}$$

Equation (15) then becomes

$$-c'(0, p) - sc(0, p) + s^2 c(s, p) - q^2 c(s, p) = 0$$

or

$$c(s, p)(s^2 - q^2) = c'(0, p) + sc(0, p) \tag{30}$$

or

$$c(s, p) = (c'(0, p) + sc(0, p))/(s^2 - q^2) \tag{31}$$

The terms $c'(0, p)$ and $c(0, p)$ are independent of s so we can obtain the inverse transform of $c(s, p)$ in relation to s. In order to do this we expand $c(s, p)$ in partial fractions (see Appendix 8)

$$c(s, p) = (c'(0, p) + sc(0, p))/(s + q)(s - q)$$
$$= A/(s + q) + B/(s - q)$$

where

$$A = -(c'(0, p) - qc(0, p))/2q$$
$$= (qc(0, p) - c'(0, p))/2q \tag{32}$$

and

$$B=(qc(0, p)+c'(0, p))/2q$$

so

$$C(x, p)=A \exp(-qx)+B \exp(+qx)$$

This solution cannot apply both to positive and negative values of x, since for $x \to +\infty$ the second term on the right-hand side becomes infinite and for $x \to -\infty$ the first term becomes infinite. So for $x > 0$

$$c(x, p)=A \exp(-qx) \quad \text{applies}$$

and for $x < 0$ $\hspace{5cm}$ (33)

$$c(x, p)=B \exp(+qx) \quad \text{applies}$$

Since the solution must be symmetrical in relation x

$$A=B$$

and so $c'(0, p)$ must be zero. Then

$$c(x, p)=(c(0, p)/2) \exp(-qx) \hspace{3cm} (33a)$$

But this solution is only valid for positive values of x. For negative values of x the solution is

$$c(x, p)=(c(0, p)/2) \exp(qx)$$

For $x=0$ we have to use the whole solution, that is,

$$c(x, p)=c(0, p)/2(\exp(qx)+\exp(-qx))$$

At $x=0$,

$$\exp(qx)=\exp(-qx)=1$$

then

$$c(0, p)=(c(0, p)/2)(1+1)=c(0, p)$$

If we integrate (33) between zero and plus infinity we should obtain the Laplace transform in relation to t of *half* the total amount $(Q_0/2)$, which is, of course, a constant. Since the Laplace transform of a constant is the constant divided by p, on transformation we obtain $Q_0/2p$ (see Appendix 14). So

$$\int_0^\infty c(x, p)\, dx = \int_0^\infty (c(0, p)/2) \exp(-qx)\, dx$$

$$= (c(0, p)/2)(-1/q) \int_0^\infty \exp(-qx)\, dx$$

So

$$c(0, p)=(q/p)Q_0 \hspace{4cm} (34)$$

If we substitute (34) in (33a) we obtain

$$c(x, p)=(qQ_0/2p) \exp(-qx)$$

But

$$q=\sqrt{(p/D)}$$

so

$$q/p = \sqrt{p/(p\sqrt{D})} = 1/\sqrt{(pD)}$$

then

$$c(x, p) = (Q_0/2\sqrt{(Dp)}) \exp(-qx) \tag{35}$$

The inverse transform of (35) can be obtained directly from tables and is

$$c(x, t) = (Q_0/2\sqrt{(D\pi t)}) \exp(-(x/(2\sqrt{(Dt)}))^2) \tag{36}$$

As we are considering only half of the solution (that is, (36) is used to obtain $c(x, t)$ for either $x > 0$ or for $x < 0$), and as $c(x, t)$ is symmetrical in relation to $x = 0$, we have to divide equation (36) by 2.

(b) *Constant concentration at* $x = 0$

The concentration of the solution $(c(x, t))$ at $x = 0$ $(c(0, t))$ is constant and equal to c_0. When we solve the diffusion equation we use the same procedure as above up to equation (32a).

$$c(x, p) = A \exp(-qx) + B \exp(qx) \tag{37}$$

where A and B are defined in (32). Since the solution must be symmetrical around $x = 0$ then

$$A = B$$

and

$$c'(0, p)/2q = 0$$

the general solution will then be

$$c(x, p) = (c(0, p)/2)(\exp(-qx) + \exp(qx)) \tag{38}$$

Since for $X \to \infty$, $c(\infty, p)$ must be zero. For positive x we take only the exponential in $-qx$ and for negative x the exponential in qx. But at $x = 0$ the concentration is always c_0, that is,

$$c(0, t) = c_0$$

So (see Appendix 14)

$$c(0, p) = c_0/p \tag{39}$$

If we substitute (39) into (38) and we consider only the case when $x \geqslant 0$, then

$$c(x, p) = (c_0/2p) \exp(-qx) \tag{40}$$

The inverse transform can be obtained from the tables and is

$$c(x, t) = (c_0/2)(1 - \text{erf}(y)) \tag{41}$$

where

$$y = x/2\sqrt{(Dt)} \quad \text{and} \quad \text{erf}(y) = (2/\sqrt{\pi}) \int_0^y \exp(-y^2)\,dy \tag{42}$$

APPENDIX 20. Solution of the cable equation for different boundary conditions

The general solution

The cable equation, which is

$$\tau_m(\partial/\partial t)(V(x, t)) + V(x, t) = \lambda^2(\partial/\partial x)^2(V(x, t)) \tag{1}$$

is also a partial differential equation. If we define T as

$$T = t/\tau_m \tag{2}$$

then

$$\partial t = \tau_m \, \partial T$$

Also, if we define X as

$$X = x/\lambda \tag{3}$$

then

$$\lambda \, \partial X = \partial x$$

If we substitute (2) and (3) in (1) we obtain

$$(\tau_m/\tau_m)(\partial/\partial T)(V(X, T)) + V(X, T) = \lambda^2/\lambda^2(\partial/\partial X)^2(V(X, T)) \text{ or}$$
$$(\partial/\partial T)(V(X, T)) + V(X, T) = (\partial/\partial X)^2(V(X, T)) \tag{4}$$

Equation (4) can be simplified if we define V as

$$V = u \exp(-T) \tag{5}$$

where

$$u = f(X, T) = u(X, T)$$

so

$$(\partial/\partial T)(V(X, T)) = \exp(-T)(\partial/\partial T)(u) - u \exp(-T) \tag{6}$$

and

$$(\partial/\partial X)^2(V(X, T)) = \exp(-T)(\partial/\partial X)^2(u(X, T)) \tag{7}$$

If we substitute (5), (6) and (7) into (4) we obtain

$$\exp(-T)(\partial/\partial T)(u) - u \exp(-T) + u \exp(-T) = (\partial/\partial X)^2 u \exp(-T)$$

so

$$(\partial/\partial T)(u) = (\partial/\partial X)^2 u \tag{8}$$

If we Laplace transform (8) in relation to T we obtain

$$pu(X, p) - u(X, 0) = (d/dx)^2(u(X, p)) \tag{9}$$

But at time zero

$$V = u$$

and at time zero and $x > 0$

$$V = 0$$

so

$$u(X, 0) = V(X, 0) = 0$$

then

$$pu(X, p) = (d/dX)^2(u(X, p)) \tag{10}$$

If we Laplace transform (10) in relation to X we obtain

$$pu(s, p) = s^2 u(s, p) - u(0, p) - su(0, p)$$

Rearranging

$$u(s, p) = (u'(0, p) + su(0, p))/(s^2 - p) \tag{11}$$

The right-hand side of equation (11) can be expanded in partial fractions. So

$$u(s, p) = A/(s + \sqrt{p}) + B/(s - \sqrt{p}) \tag{12}$$

where

$$A = (\sqrt{p} u(0, p) - u'(0, p))/2\sqrt{p}$$

and

$$B = (\sqrt{p} u(0, p) + u'(0, p))/2\sqrt{p}$$

If we inverse transform (12), from tables we obtain

$$u(X, p) = A \exp(-\sqrt{p}X) + B \exp(+\sqrt{p}X) \tag{13}$$

In order to obtain the inverse transform of (13) in relation to p we have to define $u'(0, p)$ and $u(0, p)$ *so that we can define A.* We shall solve equation (13) for the special case where $X = 0$ is the middle of a nerve (or muscle) fibre which is of 'infinite length'. In this case solution (13) is symmetrical, so

$$A = B$$

or

$$(\sqrt{p} u(0, p) - u'(0, p))/2\sqrt{p} = (\sqrt{p} u(0, p) + u'(0, p))/2\sqrt{p}$$

so

$$u'(0, p)$$

must be equal to zero and

$$u(X, p) = (u(0, p)/2)[\exp(-\sqrt{p}X) + \exp(\sqrt{p}X)] \tag{14}$$

and for $x > 0$ the solution is

$$u(X, p) = (u(0, p)/2) \exp(-\sqrt{p}X) \tag{14a}$$

and for $x < 0$ the solution is

$$u(X, p) = (u(0, p)/2) \exp(\sqrt{p}X) \tag{14b}$$

But from (5)

$$V = u \exp(-T) \quad \text{or} \quad u = V \exp(T)$$

so

$$u(0, T) = V(0, T) \exp(T) \tag{15}$$

Voltage clamp under transient conditions

Voltage clamp at V_0 in the middle of an 'infinitely long' fibre
If the membrane voltage is clamped at V_0 when $x = 0$ then

$$V(0, T) = V_0$$

and

$$u(0, T) = V_0 \exp(T)$$

so

$$u(0, p) = \int_0^\infty u(0, T) \exp(-pT)\, dT = V_0 \int_0^\infty \exp(T) \exp(-pT)\, dt$$

$$= V_0 \int_0^\infty \exp(-(p-1)T)\, dt$$

or

$$\bar{u}(0, p) = V_0/(p-1) \tag{16}$$

If we substitute (16) into (14) we obtain

$$u(X, p) = (V_0/(p-1)2)[\exp(-\sqrt{p}X) + \exp(\sqrt{p}X)] \tag{17}$$

At $X = 0$ both exponentials are 1, so

$$u(0, p) = 2V_0/(p-1)2 = V_0/(p-1)$$

which is in agreement with (16).

For $X \to \infty$ the second term inside the exponential becomes infinite. Experimentally we know that the voltage decays, with distance, to zero so the solution must be

$$u(X, p) = (V_0/(p-1)) \exp(-\sqrt{p}X) \tag{18}$$

The right-hand side of (18) can be expanded in partial fractions. So

$$u(X, p) = (V_0/2) \exp(-\sqrt{p}X)(1/(\sqrt{p}-1) - 1/(\sqrt{p}+1)) =$$

$$(V_0/2) \exp(-\sqrt{p}X)(1/(\sqrt{p}-1)) - (V_0/2) \exp(\sqrt{p}X)(1/(\sqrt{p}+1)) \tag{19}$$

The inverse transforms (from tables) of the expressions on the right-hand side of (19) are

$$(V_0/2) \exp(-\sqrt{p}X)(1/(\sqrt{p}-1))$$

$$\Rightarrow (V_0/2)[(1/\sqrt{(\pi T)}) \exp(-X^2/4T)$$

$$+ \exp(-X) \exp(T) \operatorname{erfc}(-\sqrt{T} + X/2\sqrt{T})] \tag{20}$$

and

$$(V_0/2) \exp(-\sqrt{p}X)(1/(\sqrt{p}+1))$$

$$\Rightarrow (V_0/2)[(1/\sqrt{(\pi T)}) \exp(-X^2/4T)$$

$$- \exp(-X) \exp(T) \operatorname{erfc}(\sqrt{T} + X/2\sqrt{T})] \tag{21}$$

where erf is the error function and $\operatorname{erfc} = 1 - \operatorname{erf}$. So

$$u(X, T) = (V_0/2)[(1/\sqrt{(\pi T)}) \exp(-X^2/4T)$$

$$+ \exp(-X) \exp(T) \operatorname{erfc}(-\sqrt{T} + X/2\sqrt{T})$$

$$- (1/\sqrt{(\pi T)}) \exp(-X^2/4T)$$

$$+ \exp(X) \exp(T) \operatorname{erfc}(\sqrt{T} + X/2\sqrt{T})]$$

or

$$u(X, T) = (V_0/2) \exp(T)[\exp(-X) \operatorname{erfc}(-\sqrt{T} + X/2\sqrt{T})$$

$$+ \exp(X) \operatorname{erfc}(\sqrt{T} + X/2\sqrt{T})]$$

so

$$V(X, T) = u(XT)\exp(-T)$$
$$= (V_0/2)[\exp(-X)\operatorname{erfc}(-\sqrt{T}+X/2\sqrt{T})$$
$$+\exp(X)\operatorname{erfc}(\sqrt{T}+X/2\sqrt{T})] \tag{22}$$

Equation (22) is the final solution of the cable equation for $X \geq 0$, and the special case when the membrane voltage is clamped at V_0 when $x=0$ and when $T>0$.

Current clamp under transient conditions
Constant current injection (I_0) in the middle $(x=0)$ of an 'infinitely long' fibre

If the current injected at $x=0$ (in the middle of the fibre) is a constant current (I_0), then

$$(\partial V/\partial x)_{x=0} = -(r_iI_0/2)$$

the 2 in the denominator of the right-hand side is because the constant current I_0 divides equally between the two equal halves of the fibre. Since

$$V = u\exp(-T)\partial V/\partial x = (\partial u/\partial x)(\exp-T) \tag{23}$$

or

$$\partial u/\partial x = (\partial V/\partial x)\exp(T)$$

By definition

$$\lambda = \sqrt{(r_m/r_i)}$$

Since

$$\lambda\,\partial X = \partial x$$

then

$$\partial V/\partial X = (1/\lambda)\,\partial V/\partial X = -r_iI_0/2$$

or

$$\partial V/\partial X = -(I_0r_i\lambda)/2 = -(I_0/2)r_i\sqrt{(r_m/r_i)} = -(I_0/2)\sqrt{(r_ir_m)} \tag{24}$$

From (13) the general solution of the cable equation is of the form

$$u(X, p) = A\exp(-\sqrt{p}X) + B\exp(\sqrt{p}X)$$

where p is the Laplace variable. Since for $x \to \infty$ the second term of the right-hand side is infinite, then

$$B = 0$$

From (23) and (24)

$$\partial u/\partial = (\partial V/\partial X)\exp(T) = -(I_0/2)\sqrt{(r_ir_m)}\exp(T)$$

and

$$\int_0^\infty \partial u/\partial X \exp(-pT)\,dT = (-I_0/2)\sqrt{(r_i r_m)} \int_0^\infty \exp(T)\exp(-pT)\,dT$$

$$= -(I_0/2)\sqrt{(r_i r_m)}(1/(p-1))$$

$$= (\partial/\partial X)(u(X, p))$$

so

$$(\partial/\partial X)(u(X, p)) = (\partial/\partial X)(u(0, p)) = -(I_0/2)(\sqrt{(r_i r_m)}/(p-1)) \quad (25)$$

If we differentiate (13) with respect to X, we obtain

$$(\partial/\partial X)(u(X, p)) = -\sqrt{pA}\exp(-\sqrt{pX})$$

Also

$$(\partial/\partial X)(u(0, p)) = -\sqrt{pA} \quad (26)$$

From (25) and (26)

$$-\sqrt{pA} = -(I_0/2)\sqrt{(r_i r_m)}(1/(p-1))$$

so

$$A = (I_0/2)\sqrt{(r_i r_m)}(1/\sqrt{p}(p-1)) \quad (27)$$

If we substitute (27) and (13) and make $B=0$

$$u(X, p) = (I_0\sqrt{(r_i r_m)})(1/2)\exp(-\sqrt{pX})(1/\sqrt{p}(p-1))$$

Expanding in partial fractions

$$(1/\sqrt{p})(1/(p-1)) = (1/\sqrt{p})(1/(\sqrt{p}-1)) - (1/\sqrt{p})(1/(\sqrt{p}+1))$$

or

$$u(X, p) = (I_0\sqrt{(r_i r_m)})(1/2)[\exp(-\sqrt{pX})(1/\sqrt{p}(\sqrt{p}-1))$$
$$- \exp(-\sqrt{pX})(1/\sqrt{p}(\sqrt{p}+1))] \quad (28)$$

The inverse transform of (28) can be obtained from the tables and is

$$V(X, T) = u(X, T)\exp(-T)$$

$$= (I_0\sqrt{(r_i r_m)})(1/2)[\exp(-X)\,\mathrm{erfc}(X/2\sqrt{T} - \sqrt{T})$$
$$- \exp(X)\,\mathrm{erfc}(X/2\sqrt{T} + \sqrt{T})] \quad (29)$$

The steady-state solution of the cable equation (short and long cables)

At steady state

$$(\partial/\partial T)(V(X, T)) = 0$$

so

$$(d/dx)^2(V(x)) = V(x) \quad (30)$$

Let us consider the case where, as a result of the *injection of a current at* $x=0$ in the middle of the fibre, the local potential is constant and has the value V_0. So

$$V(0) = V_0$$

If we rearrange (30) we obtain

$$(d/dx)^2(V(x)) - V(x) = 0 \tag{31}$$

Let us apply the Laplace transform

$$s^2 V(s) - sV(0) - V'(0) - V(s) = 0$$

where $V'(0)$ is the derivative of $V(x)$ at $x = 0$; so, collecting terms

$$V(s)(s^2 - 1) = sV(0) + V'(0) \tag{32}$$

and

$$V(s) = (sV(0) + V'(0))/(s^2 - 1) \tag{33}$$

In order to obtain the inverse transform we expand the right-hand side in partial fractions (see Appendix 8). Then

$$V(s) = A/(s + 1) + B/(s - 1) \tag{34}$$

where

$$A = (-V_0 + V'(0))/(-2) = (V(0) - V'(0))/2$$

and

$$B = V_0 + V'(0)$$

The inverse transform of (34) is

$$V(x) = A \exp(-x) + B \exp(x) \tag{35}$$

Only one of the terms of the right-hand side has to be considered because for $x \to +\infty$ the second term is infinite, while for $x \to -\infty$ the first term is infinite. So

$$V(x) = A \exp(-x) \tag{35a}$$

But the system is symmetric in relation $x = 0$, so

$$A = B$$

then

$$V'(0) = 0$$

the final solution is thus

$$V(x) = V_0 \exp(-x) \tag{36}$$

The general solution (36) can be expressed in alternative forms. By definition

$$\cosh(X) = (\exp(X) + \exp(-X))/2 \tag{37}$$

and

$$\sinh(X) = (\exp(X) - \exp(-X))/2 \tag{38}$$

also

$$\cosh(L - X) = (\exp(L - X) + \exp(-L + X))/2 \tag{39}$$

and

$$\sinh(L - X) = (\exp(L - X) - \exp(-L + X))/2 \tag{40}$$

from (37), (38), (39) and (40)

$$\exp(X) + \exp(-X) = 2 \cosh(X) \tag{41}$$

and
$$\exp(X)-\exp(-X)=2\sinh(X) \tag{42}$$
also
$$\exp(L-X)+\exp(-L+X)=2\cosh(L-X) \tag{43}$$
and
$$\exp(L-X)-\exp(-L+X)=2\sinh(L-X) \tag{44}$$

If we add (41) and (42) we obtain
$$2\exp(X)=2\cosh(X)+2\sinh(X) \tag{45}$$
or
$$\exp(X)=\cosh(X)+\sinh(X)$$

If we subtract (42) from (41) we obtain
$$2\exp(-X)=2\cosh(X)-2\sinh(X)$$
or
$$\exp(-X)=\cosh(X)-\sinh(X)$$
so
$$A\exp(X)+B\exp(-X)=A\cosh(X)+A\sinh(X)+B\cosh(X)$$
$$-B\sinh(X)$$

The general solution becomes
$$V(X)=(A+B)\cosh(X)+(A-B)\sinh(X)$$
or
$$V(X)=c_1\cosh(X)+c_2\sinh(X) \tag{46}$$

If we add and subtract (43) and (44) we obtain
$$\exp(-X)=\exp(-L)\cosh(L-X)-\exp(-L)\sinh(L-X)$$
and
$$\exp(X)=\exp(L)\cosh(L-X)+\exp(L)\sinh(L-X)$$
so
$$V(X)=D_1\cosh(L-X)+D_2\sinh(L-X) \tag{47}$$
where
$$D_1=A(\exp(L)+\exp(-L))$$
and
$$D_2=B(\exp(L)-\exp(-L))$$

Equation (37) is used when the cable is 'infinite' $(X\to\infty)$, while equations (46) and (47) are used to solve 'finite' cable problems.

Instantaneous application of charge in the middle of an 'infinitely long' cable

This solution was used in Chapter 9 to describe an Ach-induced potential change across a membrane.

Let Q amount of charge be injected over an extremely short period of time, Δt, into a small annulus of membrane with a capacitance of δc. The charge is injected at $x=0$ as a current, I_t, into the middle of the fibre

$$(\partial/\partial x)(V(x, t)) = -r_i I_t/2$$

so

$$(\partial/\partial X)(V(X, T)) = -r_i I_t \lambda/2$$

where $X = x/\lambda$ and $T = t/\tau_m$ and λ and τ_m are defined above. The right-hand side has the dimensions of volts,

$$\Omega \cdot cm^{-1} \cdot amp \cdot cm = \Omega \cdot amp = V$$

Since I_t is very brief and short-lived it is a delta function of the general form $I_0 \, \delta(t)$, so

$$r_i I_t \lambda = r_i I_0 \lambda \, \delta(T)$$
$$\downarrow$$
$$= V_0 \, \delta(T)$$

This term is equivalent to a delta function of voltage. So

$$\partial V(X, T)/\partial x = -V_0 \, \delta(T)/2$$

for $X = 0$. We see that V_0, the voltage at $X = 0$, is, by definition:

$$V_0 = Q/\delta c$$

The cable equation is

$$(\partial/\partial T)(V(X, T)) + V(X, T) = (\partial/\partial X)^2 V(X, T)$$

If we Laplace transform in relation to T we obtain

$$sV(Xs) - V(X, 0) + V(X, T) = (d/dX)^2 V(Xs)$$

Since at time zero, $V(X, 0)$, the voltage along the axon is zero, except at $X = 0$

$$V(X, 0) = 0$$

so

$$sV(X, s) + V(X, s) = (d/dX)^2 V(X, s)$$

or, rearranging,

$$(d/dX)^2 V(X, s) - (s+1)V(X, s) = 0$$

This second-order differential equation in X has a general solution of the form

$$V(X, s) = A \exp(-\sqrt{(s+1)}X) + B \exp(\sqrt{(s+1)}X)$$

As $X \to \infty$ (equation (18)), $V(X, \infty)$ must be zero so

$$B = 0 \quad \text{and} \quad V(X, s) = A \exp(-\sqrt{(s+1)}X)$$

We have now to find A. But for $X = 0$

$$(\partial/\partial X)(V(X, T)) = -V_0 \, \delta(T)/2$$

Laplace transforming this equation:

$$(d/dX)(V(X, s)) = -V_0/2$$

If we now differentiate $V(X, s)$ we obtain

$$(d/dX)(V(X, s)) = -\sqrt{(s+1)}A \exp(-\sqrt{(s+1)}X)$$

and for $X = 0$

$$(d/dX)(V(X, s)) = -\sqrt{(s+1)}A$$

so

$$-V_0/2 = -\sqrt{(s+1)}A \quad \text{or} \quad A = V_0/2\sqrt{(s+1)}$$

Thus

$$V(X, s) = -V_0/2\sqrt{(s+1)}) \exp(-\sqrt{(s+1)}X)$$

From tables the inverse transform is

$$V(X, T) = (V_0/2)(1/\sqrt{(\pi T)}) \exp(-X^2/4T - T)$$

This solution is identical to the Hodgkin solution (see Fatt and Katz, 1951) that we used in Chapter 9, provided we make the following dimensional argument:

$$V_0 = Q/\delta c$$

$$= \text{coulomb/farad} \quad \text{(of an annulus)}$$

$$C \cdot F^{-1}$$

Now dimensionally $q_0/\lambda c_m$ is

$$= \text{coulomb/(cm} \cdot \text{farad} \cdot \text{cm}^{-1}) \quad \text{(note: } c_m \text{ is capacitance per unit length)}$$

$$= \text{coulomb/farad}$$

$$= C \cdot F^{-1}$$

so $V_0 \equiv q_0/\lambda c_m$.

APPENDIX 21. The Boltzmann factor

In the expression

$$n_1 = n_2 \exp(-(w_2 - w_1)/(kT)) \tag{1}$$

the term $\exp(-(w_2 - w_1)/(kT))$ is known as the Boltzmann factor. Equation (1) applies to a system in equilibrium and relates the number of particles (n_1) in an energy state w_1 to the number of particles (n_2) in energy state w_2. We shall first derive this relationship shown in equation (1) for a simple case and then show that it applies in general.

The barometric formula as an example of the Boltzmann factor

Imagine a gas in a gravitational field, such that the atmosphere is made up of a single gas species of molecular weight M. The difference in atmospheric pressure at x and $x + \Delta x$ is equal to the weight of the gas contained in the volume element Δv. This volume element is defined as

$$\Delta v = \Delta x \times 1 \quad (\text{cm}^3) \tag{2}$$

if we assume that the column of air described in Figure A21.1 has a cross-sectional area of 1 cm^2.

The weight ($\Delta\omega_g$) of the volume element of air is

$$\Delta\omega_g = \Delta x m \dot{g} N \tag{2a}$$

where N is the number of molecules per unit volume, $\dot{g}$ is the acceleration of the molecules due to the gravitational field (980 cm·s^{-2}), m is the mass of one molecule of the gas and $\Delta x \times 1$ is the volume element.

So dimensionally

$$cm^3 \cdot mass \cdot N^{-1} \cdot cm \cdot s^{-2} \cdot N \cdot cm^{-3}$$

$$= mass \cdot cm \cdot s^{-2}$$

$$\equiv force \equiv weight$$

Since pressure is *defined* as weight per unit area, equation (2a) divided by the

Fig.A21.1

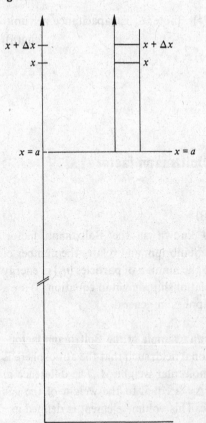

cross-sectional area (1 cm^2) becomes

$$\Delta P = -\Delta x m \dot{g} N \tag{3}$$

where ΔP is the change in pressure that occurs over distance Δx. The negative sign is used because P decreases as x increases. For an ideal gas at equilibrium

$$Pv = nRT \quad \text{or} \quad P = (n/v)RT \quad \text{or} \quad P = cRT \tag{4}$$

where n is the number of *moles* of gas contained in volume v at pressure P and absolute temperature T, and c is the concentration of gas in moles per unit volume. The ideal gas constant R is related to the Boltzmann's constant k by the expression

$$k = R/N_A \quad \text{or} \quad R = kN_A$$

where N_A is Avogadro's number. If we substitute for R in (4) we obtain

$$Pv = nN_A kT$$

or $\qquad P = (nN_A/v)kT$

The bracketed term is: (number of moles) × (number of molecules per mole/volume), and so has the dimensions of number of molecules per unit volume. It is thus the N of equation (2a). So

$$P = NkT \quad \text{or} \quad N = P/kT \tag{4a}$$

If we substitute (4a) in (3) we obtain

$$\Delta P = -\Delta x (m\dot{g}/kT)P$$

or $\qquad \Delta P/P = -(m\dot{g}/kT)\Delta x$

For small Δx ($\Delta x \to 0$)

$$dP/P = -(m\dot{g})/(kT)\,dx \tag{5}$$

we can now integrate (5)

$$\int (1/P)\,dP = -((m\dot{g})/(kT))\int dx$$

so

$$\ln(P) = -((m\dot{g})/(kT))x + A \tag{6}$$

where A is a constant of integration.

At

$$x = a, \quad P = P_a$$

so

$$\ln(P_a) = -((m\dot{g})/(kT))a + A \tag{7}$$

If we subtract (7) from (6) we obtain

$$\ln(P/P_a) = -((m\dot{g})/(kT))(x - a)$$

or

$$P/P_a = \exp(-m\dot{g}/(kT))(x - a) \tag{8}$$

If we rearrange (8) we obtain

$$P \exp((m\dot{g})/(kT)x) = P_a \exp(((m\dot{g})/(kT))a)$$

From (4)

$$RTc(x) \exp(((m\dot{g})/(kT))x) = RTc(a) \exp(((m\dot{g})/(kT))a)$$

or

$$c(x) \exp(((m\dot{g})/(kT))x) = c(a) \exp(((m\dot{g})/(kT))a) \qquad (9)$$

the exponents in (9) are of the form

$$\bar{W}_x/(kT)$$

where $\bar{W}_x$ is the potential energy of a molecule of gas. $m\dot{g}$ is the weight of a molecule of gas and thus is a force. $m\dot{g}x$ is the *work* (see Appendix 33) performed to raise a molecule of gas from 0 to x (since work = force times distance (Δx)). If we multiply top and bottom by N_A (Avogadro's number) we obtain

$$N_A \bar{W}_x / N_A kT = W_x/(RT)$$

where W_x is the potential energy per mole and R ($= N_A k$) is the ideal gas constant. Equation (9) can thus be rewritten as

$$c(x) = c(a) \exp(-(\bar{W}_x - \bar{W}_a)/(kT)) = c(a) \exp(-(W_x - W_a)/(RT)) \quad (10)$$

and relates the number of moles per unit volume (or concentration) at x, to the number of molecules per unit volume (concentration) at $x = a$. If we divide both sides of equation (10) by N_A (Avogadro's number) we obtain the Boltzmann factor.

The general derivation from mechanical statistics

For the more general case, let us imagine a system containing N particles. These particles can be in a discrete number of energy states, $e_1, e_2, \ldots, e_i$, and the numbers of particles in each energy state are

$$N_1, N_2, N_3, \ldots, N_i$$

Since we cannot distinguish between particles of the same energy state there are $N_i!$ possible ways in which each energy state can be obtained. For one particle there is one possible arrangement; for two particles there are two possible arrangements, that is, ab and ba; for three particles there are six arrangements, abc, bac, acb, bca, cba and cab. So we have

1	1
2	2·1
3	3·2·1
⋮	⋮
n	$n!$

The total number of ways (Ω) in which the system can be arranged is thus

$$\Omega = \frac{N!}{N_1! \, N_2! \ldots ! \, N_i!}$$

$$\times \frac{\text{Total number of arrangements disregarding energy levels}}{\text{Product of number of indistinguishable arrangements}}$$

If we apply logarithms,

$$\ln(\Omega) = \ln(N!) - \ln(N_1!) - \ln(N_2!) - \cdots - \ln(N_i!)$$

From Stirling's formula (see Appendix 10)

$$\ln(\Omega) = N \ln(N) - N - \sum_{i=1}^{n} (N_i \ln(N_i) - N_i)$$

If the energy of the system changes the distribution of the particles will also change. So

$$\ln(\Omega + \Delta\Omega) - \ln(\Omega)$$

$$= N \ln(N) - N - \sum_{i=1}^{n} \left[(N_i + \Delta N_i) \ln(N_i + \Delta N_i) - (N_i + \Delta N_i) \right]$$

$$- N \ln(N) + N + \sum_{i=1}^{n} \left[N_i \ln(N_i) - N_i \right]$$

or

$$\ln((\Omega + \Delta\Omega)/\Omega) = - \sum_{i=1}^{n} \left[(N_i + \Delta N_i) \ln(N_i + \Delta N_i) - N_i \ln(N_i) \right]$$

$$+ \sum_{i=1}^{n} (N_i + \Delta N_i - N_i)$$

But since the number of particles N is constant, $\Delta N_i = 0$ and the second term on the right-hand side is zero. The first term on the right-hand side can be expanded

$$(N_i + \Delta N_i) \ln(N_i + \Delta N_i) - N_i \ln(N_i)$$

$$= N_i \ln(N_i + \Delta N_i) + \Delta N_i \ln(N_i + \Delta N_i) - N_i \ln(N_i)$$

$$= N_i \ln((N_i + \Delta N_i)/N_i) + \Delta N_i \ln(N_i + \Delta N_i)$$

$$= N_i \ln((N_i + \Delta N_i)/N_i) + \Delta N_i \ln(((N_i + \Delta N_i)/N_i)N_i)$$

$$= N_i \ln((N_i + \Delta N_i)/N_i) + \Delta N_i \ln((N_i + \Delta N_i)/N_i) + \Delta N_i \ln(N_i)$$

$$= N_i \ln(1 + \Delta N_i/N_i) + \Delta N_i \ln(1 + \Delta N_i/N_i) + \Delta N_i \ln(N_i)$$

But around $x = 0$ the Taylor series for $\ln(1 + x)$ (see Appendix 4) is

$$\ln(1 + x) = x - x^3 + x^5 - \cdots$$

For small x

$$\ln(1 + x) \approx x$$

that is, when $\Delta N_i \ll N_i$

$$\ln(1 + \Delta N_i/N_i) \approx \Delta N_i/N_i$$

or

$$(N_i + \Delta N_i)\ln(N_i + \Delta N_i) - N_i \ln(N_i)$$
$$= N_i(\Delta N_i/N_i) + \Delta N_i(\Delta N_i/N_i) + \Delta N_i \ln(N_i)$$
$$= \Delta N_i + (\Delta N_i^2/N_i) + \Delta N_i \ln(N_i)$$

For small ΔN_i we can neglect the term $\Delta N_i^2/N_i$, so

$$(N_i + \Delta N_i)\ln(N_i + \Delta N_i) - N_i \ln(N_i) = \Delta N_i + \Delta N_i \ln(N_i)$$

then

$$\Delta\Omega/\Omega = -\sum_{i=1}^{n}(\Delta N_i + \Delta N_i \ln(N_i)) = -\sum_{i=1}^{n}\Delta N_i(1 + \ln(N_i))$$

If the system is at equilibrium it does not change, so $\Delta\Omega = 0$. (When a system is at equilibrium its macroscopic properties (Ω) do not change, but inside it may undergo compensatory changes (dynamic equilibrium).) So at equilibrium

$$0 = \sum_{i=1}^{n}\Delta N_i(1 + \ln(N_i))$$

But at equilibrium the total number of particles (N) is constant, so

$$\sum_{i=1}^{n}\Delta N_i = 0$$

and the total energy of the system is constant. The total energy of the system (E) is given by

$$E = \sum e_i N_i \quad \text{and} \quad \Delta E = \sum e_i \Delta N_i = 0$$

If $\sum \Delta N_i$ and $\sum e_i \Delta N_i$ are zero then

$$\alpha \sum \Delta N_i = \sum \alpha \Delta N_i = 0 \quad \text{and} \quad \beta \sum e_i \Delta N_i = \sum \beta e_i \Delta N_i = 0$$

so

$$0 = \sum_{i=1}^{n}(\alpha \Delta N_i + \beta e_i \Delta N_i + \Delta N_i(1 + \ln(N_i)))$$
$$= \sum_{i=1}^{n}\Delta N_i(\alpha + \beta e_i + 1 + \ln(N_i))$$
$$= \Delta N_i(\alpha + \beta e_i + 1 + \ln(N_i)) + \Delta N_2(\alpha + \beta e_2 + 1 + \ln(N_2)) + \cdots$$

since ΔN_i can have any value

$$\alpha + \beta e_i + 1 + \ln(N_i) = 0$$

so

$$\ln(N_i) = -(1 + \alpha) - \beta e_i$$

or

$$N_i = \exp(-(1 + \alpha))\exp(-\beta e_i)$$

If we define

$$A = \exp(-(1 + \alpha))$$

then

$$N_i = A \exp(-\beta e_i)$$

so

$$N = \sum N_i = A \sum \exp(-\beta e_i)$$

and

$$N_i/N = A \exp(-\beta e_i)/A \sum \exp(-\beta e_i) \tag{11}$$

Also for $i = a$ and $i = b$

$$N_a/N_b = A \exp(-\beta e_a)/A \exp(-\beta e_b) = \exp(-\beta e_a)/\exp(-\beta e_a)$$

or

$$N_a = N_b \exp(-\beta(e_a - e_b))$$

It was shown by Boltzmann that

$$\beta = 1/kT$$

then

$$N_a = N_b \exp(-(e_a - e_b)/kT)$$
$$= N_b \exp(-(\bar{W}_a - \bar{W}_b)/kT)$$

Equation (11) is called the partition function and $\exp(-(\bar{W}_a - \bar{W}_b)/kT)$ or $\exp(-(W_a - W_b)/(RT))$ is the Boltzmann factor, as defined as the beginning of this Appendix.

APPENDIX 22. The Poisson equation (also see Appendix 18)

The integration of the Poisson equation is similar to the integration of the steady-state diffusion equation or of the steady-state cable equation in that the particular solution depends upon the boundary conditions. In Appendix 18 we saw that the equation has the form (in one dimension)

$$(d/dx)^2(\psi) = -4\pi\rho/\varepsilon \tag{1}$$

where ε is the dielectric constant of the medium and ρ is the local charge density (coulomb $\cdot$ cm^{-3}). When the charge density is zero

$$(d/dx)^2(\psi) = 0 = (d/dx)(\text{constant})$$

or

$$(d/dx)(\psi) = \text{constant}$$

this means that

$$E = -\text{constant} \tag{2}$$

so the field is constant. Such a case is assumed in the G–H–K integration of the Nernst–Planck equation.

If $\rho \neq 0$, then

$$(d/dx)(\psi) = -E = 4\pi\rho(1/\varepsilon)x + c$$

If ρ is sufficiently small so that $4\pi\rho x/\varepsilon$ is negligible when compared with c we can write

$$(d/dx)(\psi) = -E \approx c \tag{3}$$

where c is a constant (the approximate field intensity).

Biological membranes are mostly lipid and the partition of ions into lipids is very small; this means that the concentration of ions in the lipid core of the membrane will be low and so ρ in (1) will be small. Thus, from (3), the assumption often made, that the voltage profile across a lipid bilayer is linear, is reasonably valid. For a more detailed discussion of this point the reader is referred to Finkelstein and Mauro (see further reading for Appendix 22). One application of Poisson's equation is to examine the distribution of ions in solution in the presence of an electrical field.

From the Nernst–Planck equation (see Chapter 4)

$$j_i = -u_i[RT(d/dx)(c_i) + ZFc_i(d/dx)(\psi)] \tag{4}$$

where j_i is the local flux density of ion i, u_i is the ion mobility and c_i and ψ are the local concentration and electrical potential respectively. At equilibrium $j_i = 0$, so

$$RT(d/dx)(c_i) = -ZFc_i(d/dx)\psi \tag{5}$$

If we rearrange (5) by dividing both sides by c_i and multiplying by dx, we obtain

$$RT(d/dc_i)(c_i) = -ZF\,d\psi \tag{6}$$

If we integrate both sides then

$$RT\int(1/c_i)\,dc_i = -ZF\int d\psi$$

or

$$RT\ln(c_i) = -ZF\psi + A$$

where A is constant of integration. Let us assume that at x in the solution near the membrane the concentration c_i is $c_i(x)$ and the potential here is $\psi(x)$. Then

$$RT\ln(c_i(x)) = -ZF\psi(x) + A \tag{7}$$

Let us also assume that when x is far away from the membrane ($x \rightarrow \infty$), that is, in the bulk solution, c_i is just c_i and ψ is $\psi(\infty)$. So

$$RT\ln(c_i) = -ZF\psi(\infty) + A \tag{8}$$

If we subtract (7) from (8) we obtain

$$RT\ln(c_i/c_i(x)) = -ZF(\psi(\infty) - \psi(x)) \tag{9}$$

Let us now define V as the electrical potential at point x and refer it to $x \rightarrow$

∞, then

$$V = \psi(x) - \psi(\infty) \tag{10}$$

From (9) and (10)

$$RT \ln(c_i/c_i(x)) = ZFV$$

on rearranging

$$c_i/c_i(x) = \exp(ZFV/(RT))$$

then

$$c_i(x) = c_i \exp(-ZFV/(RT)) \tag{11}$$

Boltzmann relationship

Equation (11) is a form of the *Boltzmann* relationship, and for sodium ions is

$$c_{Na}(x) = c_{Na} \exp(-FV/(RT)) \tag{11a}$$

For chloride ions it is

$$c_{Cl}(x) = c_{Cl} \exp(FV/(RT)) \tag{11b}$$

We may also have other ions present (at a concentration c_x) to which the membrane is impermeable, but, for the moment, we shall neglect them. So

$$\rho = F(c_{Na}(x) - c_{Cl}(x))$$
$$= F(c_{Na} \exp(-FV/(RT)) - c_{Cl} \exp(-FV/(RT)))$$

At $x \to \infty$, $V \to 0$, so from electroneutrality

$$c_{Na}(x) \to c_{Na} = c_{Cl} \leftarrow c_{Cl}(x)$$

and

$$\rho = c_{NaCl}F(\exp(-FV/(RT)) - \exp(FV/(RT))) \tag{12}$$
$$= -2c_{NaCl}F \sinh(FV/(RT))$$

From (10)

$$dV/dx = (d/dx)(\psi(x)) - (d/dx)(\psi(\infty)) = (d/dx)(\psi(x))$$

So from (1) and (12)

$$(d/dx)^2(V) = 8c_{NaCl}\pi F \sinh(FV/(RT))/\varepsilon \tag{13}$$

In order to find V and thus $c_{Na}(x)$ and $c(x)$ equation (12) has to be solved for the appropriate boundary conditions.

The first conclusion to be drawn is that if $V \neq 0$, ρ will be a function of x. In other words, there will be either a net positive or negative charge near the membrane. If we define Y as

$$Y = FV/(RT) \tag{13a}$$

then

$$dY = (F/(RT)) \, dV$$

or

$$dV = ((RT)/F) \, dY$$

so

$$(dV)^2 = ((RT)/F)\, dY^2$$

and then (13) becomes

$$(d/dx)^2(Y) = \underbrace{8c_{NaCl}\pi F(1/\varepsilon)(F/(RT))}_{A} \sinh(Y) \tag{14}$$

Constant A can be written dimensionally as

$$c_{NaCl} = mol \cdot cm^{-3}$$

$$ZF = (coul \cdot gr\text{-}eq^{-1})(gr\text{-}eq \cdot mol^{-1}) = coul \cdot mol^{-1} = C \cdot mol^{-1}$$

There is a missing constant (Z, the valence) because it was 1 for sodium and -1 for chloride. As

$$R = joule \cdot mol^{-1} \cdot deg^{-1}$$

$$T = degrees$$

and

$$\varepsilon = coul^2 \cdot joule^{-1} \cdot m^{-1} \quad or \quad coul^2 \cdot joule^{-1} \cdot (cm \times 100)^{-1}$$

so

$$\frac{mol \cdot cm^{-3} \cdot coul \cdot mol^{-1} \cdot coul \cdot mol \cdot deg \cdot mol^{-1} \cdot joule^{-1} \cdot deg^{-1}}{coul^2 \cdot joule^{-1} \cdot cm^{-1}} = cm$$

this means that

$$\sqrt{(1/A)} = cm = L_D \tag{15}$$

Debye length

L_D is called the Debye length of the solution and is a measure of the length over which there is a charge unbalance ($\rho \neq 0$). So (14) becomes

$$(d/dx)^2(Y) = (1/L_D^2) \sinh(Y) \tag{16}$$

Equations (14), (15) and (16) include Poisson's equation and Boltzmann's relationship. They are sometimes known as Poisson–Boltzmann's equations. Integration of these equations needs to take into account specific boundary conditions. However, equation (16) is zero only when x approaches infinity, that is, when y is zero (see equations (10) and (13a)). Near the membrane–solution interphase (x near 0) it has a non-zero value so $\rho \neq 0$.

Since this takes place on both sides of the membrane there is a separation of charge. This means that when there is a potential across a membrane there is an accumulation (or depletion) of positive charge on one side and an accumulation (or depletion) of negative charge on the other side. For a more detailed treatment of this subject see Finkelstein and Mauro who are referred to in the further reading of Appendix 22. This Appendix is similar to their approach.

APPENDIX 23. Coulomb's Law and the dielectric constant

It is possible to charge a sphere so that on bringing it closer to another charged sphere there is either repulsion or attraction between the two spheres. The degrees of repulsion or attraction depend upon the distances between the two spheres and Coulomb was able to measure (with a torsion balance) these forces. Since these forces are experienced without the spheres touching, it must be said that the space around each sphere has special properties. These properties are the result of an electric field which is associated with every charged body. In order to quantify this field we imagine the force on a unit charge that is attached to a torsion balance and then placed in the electric field. We call the size of this force the *field strength* (E) and the greater the deflection of the torsion balance the greater the *field strength* (E). Large field strengths are due to large charges (Q). We can then relate the field strength (E) at any point in space to the associated charge by the relationship

$$E \propto Q \tag{1}$$

As the unit charge is moved away from Q the deflections of the torsion balance become smaller, that is, E becomes weaker. The relationship between the field strength E and the distance from the associated charge Q was experimentally derived by Coulomb (later on, confirmed by Cavendish) and can be derived as follows. Charge Q is shown in Figure A23.1 with the associated field. The field is represented as lines of force emanating from the charge which is at the centre of a sphere or radius a.

If we move the unit charge along the spherical surface of radius a we find that the field is uniform over the whole surface. For any small area element dA (Figure A23.2), the field strength can be assumed to be proportional to the local density of lines of force dN/dA. Thus

$$\varepsilon E = dN/dA \tag{2}$$

where ε is a proportionality constant. However, the local field strength is also proportional to Q, if we define N in such a way that

$$N = Q$$

We can now write

$$E\varepsilon = dQ/dA \tag{3}$$

Since the field is uniform (constant) across the whole surface area of the sphere

$$dQ/dA = \text{constant} = \overbrace{Q}^{\text{total charge}} \Big/ \overbrace{\text{surface area of sphere}}^{4\pi a^2} \tag{4}$$

If we substitute (4) into (3) we obtain

$$\varepsilon E = Q/4\pi a^2 \tag{4a}$$

or

$$E = (1/\varepsilon)(Q/4\pi a^2) = (1/4\pi\varepsilon)(Q/a^2) \tag{5}$$

If, instead of examining the field with a unit test charge, we had used a charge Q_1 the force felt (F) would have been Q_1 times bigger. That is,

$$F = (1/4\pi\varepsilon)(QQ_1/a^2) \tag{6}$$

Equation (6) is known as Coulomb's Law and states that two charges (Q and Q_1) attract or repel each other with a force (F) which is proportional to their product (QQ_1) and inversely proportional to the square of the distance (a) between them ($1/a^2$). The proportionality constant ε is also called the *dielectric constant* and has a value which depends on the medium surrounding charges Q and Q_1. For the same charges (Q and Q_1) the force of attraction and repulsion is smaller the larger the value of ε. The values of ε are usually tabulated as dielectric coefficients. The dielectric coefficient of a material is the ratio between its dielectric constant and the dielectric

Fig.A23.1

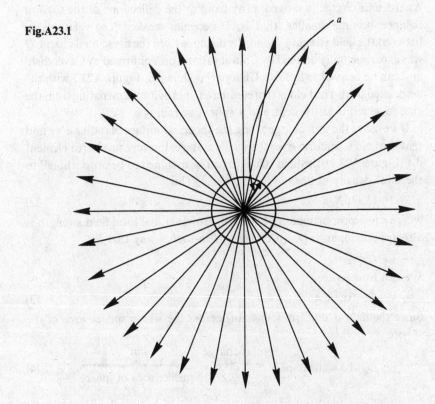

constant of a vacuum (ε_0), which by convention is set at unity. The dielectric coefficient K is then given by

$$K = \varepsilon/\varepsilon_0 \tag{7}$$

from which we obtain the value of

$$\varepsilon = K\varepsilon_0 \tag{8}$$

If we substitute (8) in equation (6) we obtain

$$F = (1/4\pi K\varepsilon_0)(QQ_1/a^2) \tag{9}$$

Since by convention ε_0 is assumed to be one

$$F = (1/4\pi K)(QQ_1/a^2) \tag{10}$$

The value of K for water at 25 °C is 78.5 and for membrane lipids is around 2–5.

If we used a similar approach to derive the equation relating the force of attraction or repulsion between two magnetic poles of strength P and P' we would obtain

$$F = (1/4\pi m)(PP'/a^2)$$

where m is the *magnetic permeability*.

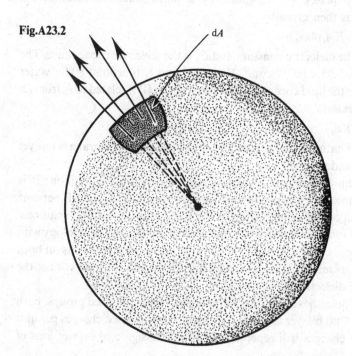

Fig.A23.2

dA

APPENDIX 24. Membrane capacitance and charge movements

A capacitor can be defined as being made up of two conductors in the vicinity of each other and charged with equal charges (q) of opposite sign. In Chapters 4 and 6 we showed that when a constant current is injected across a biological membrane the membrane potential V does not change instantaneously because the membrane has a certain capacitance which has to be charged (or discharged) so that the potential can change.

In Appendix 15 we also showed that the voltage across a capacitor is given by the expression

$$V_c = Q/(4\pi\varepsilon C) \tag{1}$$

where ε is the dielectric constant, Q the charge in the plates of the capacitor and C its capacitance. A conventional capacitor is made up of two plates of metal of area A and separated by a distance l. When the two plates are in the vacuum the capacitance is given by

$$C_g = A/(4\pi\varepsilon_0 l) \tag{2}$$

where ε_0 is the permittivity of the vacuum and C_g is known as the *geometrical* capacitance.

If the two plates are separated by a non-conducting medium the capacitance is then given by

$$C_d = KA/(4\pi\varepsilon_0 l) \tag{3}$$

where K is the dielectric constant and C_d is the *dielectric* capacitance. The value of ε_0 is 8.85×10^{-12} coul$^2 \cdot$ N$^{-1} \cdot$ m^{-2} and K is around 80 for water and 2 to 5 for the lipid core of lipid bilayers. ε from (1) is related to ε_0 from (2) by the expression

$$\varepsilon = K\varepsilon_0 \tag{4}$$

The physical nature of the capacitance of a biological membrane is not yet completely understood.

When a lipid bilayer (BLM) separates two electrolyte solutions it is possible to measure a capacitance that ranges from 0.3 to 1.3 μF per cm^2 depending upon the composition of the BLM and the bathing solutions. This capacitance is independent of the applied voltage. So, by analogy with a conventional capacitor, it is assumed that the bathing solutions on both sides of the membrane are the conducting plates and the lipid core of the BLM is the dielectric.

Since the polar heads of the phospholipids contain ionized groups, both faces of the lipid bilayer contain a certain number of fixed charges per unit area. These charges will repel ions of the same sign and attract ions of opposite sign in the adjacent layers of solution. As a result of these electrostatic interactions there is an adjacent electric double layer on both sides of the BLM and an associated electrical potential field ($V(x)$). The net charge density in this double layer is related to the local potential by the Poisson–Boltzmann equation (see Appendix 22) which on integration gives the expression

$$((d/dx)y)^2 = (2/L_D^2)\cosh y + A \tag{5}$$

where L_D is the Debye layer, y is defined as $y = FV(x)/RT$ and A is the constant of integration.

Since for $x \to \infty$ (see Appendix 22)

$$V(x) = 0 \quad \text{and} \quad y(x) = 0$$

then

$$(d/dx)(y) = 0 \quad \text{or} \quad (2/L_D^2)\cosh y = 0$$

so

$$((d/dx)(y))^2 = (2/L_D^2)(\cosh y - 1) \tag{6}$$

Equation (6) can be reduced to a first-order differential equation by taking the square root of both sides. So

$$(d/dx)(y) = (\sqrt{2}/L_D)\sqrt{(\cosh y - 1)}$$

which can be integrated easily.

If we integrate equation (6) with the appropriate boundary conditions, the net charge ρ can be computed from Poisson's equation, that is,

$$(d/dx)^2(V) = -4\pi\rho/\varepsilon$$

But, since $y = FV(x)/RT$, we obtain

$$(d/dx)^2 V = (RT/F)(d/dx)^2(y) = -4\pi\rho/\varepsilon$$

When a current is injected through the BLM an additional accumulation of charge will take place in the adjacent solution on both sides of the membrane. This charge accumulation is diffuse, that is, the charge density changes with x. It is, however, concentrated in the solution near the membrane faces. The charge accumulation is the result of the migration of negative and positive ions from the bulk of the solution towards the vicinity of the membrane and into the negative and positive sides respectively. Since the migration of ions in solution (Chapter 3) is a current, this current which does *not* cross the membrane is called a capacitative current.

The capacitative current measured in biological membranes is not entirely due to ion accumulation in the Debye Layers. Another source of capacitative currents is the displacement of charges inside the dielectric (the lipid core) resulting from the attraction of positive charges to the negative side and of negative charges to the positive side. Through this mechanism induced dipoles are produced in the dielectric. (These dipoles are called *induced* because they are not permanent, that is, they are produced by the electrical field across the membrane.) Because the formation of induced dipoles entails a displacement of charges inside the membrane there is a corresponding movement of ions in the bathing solution. The overall result is that for the same transmembrane voltages more ions have to accumulate as net charges in the Debye Layers.

Finally, the membrane may contain polar molecules, that is, molecules that are neutral but in which the charges are not distributed symmetrically. Such molecules constitute permanent dipoles which, in the absence of an applied transmembrane potential, may be randomly oriented. When an electrical potential is applied across the membrane these dipoles will orient themselves in the field. Since the orientation involves a displacement of the dipole charges inside the membrane there is again a corresponding movement of ions in the surrounding solution similar to that described for the induced dipoles.

This orientation of permanent dipoles has two specific characteristics. One is that the dipoles only re-orientate themselves when the transmembrane potential (and thus the local field intensity) is large enough to overcome the local electrostatic interactions. The greater the transmembrane potential, the greater the number of dipoles that move. Since there is a limited number of permanent dipoles per unit area, there will be a voltage above which no further re-orientation occurs and thus dipole re-orientation exhibits saturation.

The study of charge displacements inside biological membranes, which relies on the measurement of capacitative currents, is a means of studying the biophysical properties of biological membranes. To this end a number of attempts have been made to relate these charge displacements to opening or closing of ion gates, or to a key role in the process of excitation–contraction coupling in skeletal muscle.

APPENDIX 25. Free energy

The concept of free energy is one of the fundamentals of thermodynamics since it allows us to predict the direction of the natural evolution of a given process. In order to understand the concept of free energy we have first to introduce the concept of *Entropy*.

First Law of thermodynamics

When we bring together two blocks of metal at different temperatures energy will flow from one of the blocks to the other. If the amount of energy lost by the first block is ΔE_1 and the energy gained by the second block is ΔE_2, the *First Law of thermodynamics* tells us that, provided that these two blocks are unable to exchange energy with anything else,

$$\Delta E_1 + \Delta E_2 = 0 \qquad (1)$$

This means that energy is *conserved*.

Universe of an event

When we have a system (like the two blocks of metal), which does not interact with anything else we can say that the system is an *isolated* one. If we say that the only event that can take place within this isolated system is the exchange of energy between two blocks of metal, this set of conditions under which the interaction between the two blocks takes place is now called the *universe* of that *event*.

The universe of an event means that the system is now completely defined. However, equation (1) is not a complete description of the event which involves the transfer of energy between two blocks. It does not tell us, for example, whether the hotter block of metal will get hotter or cooler as a result of the exchange of energy.

However, from our experience of the world we know that the two blocks will share energy until eventually they will reach the same temperature. This means that if we know the temperatures of the two blocks we can predict which one will lose energy (get cooler) and which one will gain energy (get hotter).

Although temperature can help us in predicting how the two blocks of metal can exchange their energy, it cannot be used in making predictions about many other processes. For example, if we suddenly increase the volume of a reservoir containing a gas we know that eventually the gas will fill the new volume uniformly, and yet it is possible that this process could take place at a constant temperature.

Concept of equilibrium

The exchange of energy between two blocks of metal and the expansion of a gas are two processes that share a number of common characteristics with all natural processes that take place in isolated systems. That is, all of them evolve in only one direction and all of them will run to a final situation where the properties of the system do not change any more. This situation when the properties do not change is called *equilibrium*.

Entropy

The behaviour of isolated systems can be adequately discussed by introducing the concept of entropy. To understand entropy, let us consider our derivation of the Boltzmann factor in Appendix 21.

Here, we considered a system with N particles (a gas, for example) and these particles may have energies $E_0, E_1, E_2, \ldots, E_i$. If there are n_0 particles with energy E_0, n_1 particles with energy E_1, and so on, the energy (E_σ) of the system (σ) is given by

$$E_\sigma = \sum_{i=1}^{i=i} n_i E_i \tag{2}$$

and the number of ways (Ω) in which energy E_σ can be distributed among the N particles, so that the system remains the same, is given by

$$\Omega = N!/(n_0! \, n_1! \ldots n_i!) \quad \text{(see Appendix 21)} \tag{3}$$

The *entropy* of the system (S) was *defined* by Boltzmann as being given by the relationship

$$S = k \ln(\Omega) = k \ln(N!/n_0! \, n_1! \ldots n_i!) \tag{4}$$

where k is the Boltzmann constant.

Boltzmann's constant (k) has the value

$$k = 1.380\,54 \times 10^{-23} \text{ joule} \cdot \text{deg}^{-1}$$

Ω is said to measure the *disorder* of a system; that is, the larger the number of ways in which a system can be rearranged 'inside' while still looking the same outside, the larger the disorder of the system. For example, if we heat a certain amount of gas (1 mole) in a closed container the value of Ω will increase, that is, at the new temperature and pressure it will be possible to distribute the total energy of the gas in a larger number of ways. This means that at the new constant temperature and pressure the disorder of the system has increased when compared with the gas before heating. We shall now derive an expression for the entropy of an homogeneous system such as a given amount of a gas or of a liquid (such as water) or of a pure solid metal.

Let us assume that we place the system in contact with a slightly hotter body and that we allow the system to gain a small amount of energy (dE), but that the amount of energy is so small that the temperature of the system does not change (we can imagine this as if the system is a large volume of water into which we dip a very small piece of metal at a slightly higher temperature). We call such a system a thermal reservoir. As a result of the gain in energy some molecules of the system will jump from energy state E_0 to energy state E_1 or E_2, and from energy state E_1 to energy state E_2, etc. The total change in energy of the system is then given by

$$dE = \sum_{i=0}^{i=i} E_i \, dn_i \tag{5}$$

As a result of these changes, the entropy of the system will also change by an amount dS; and

$$S + ds = k \ln(N!/(n_0 + \Delta n_0)!(n_1 + \Delta n_1)! \ldots (n_i + \Delta n_i)!) \qquad (6)$$

$\Delta n_0, \Delta n_1, \ldots, \Delta n_i$ can be positive or negative and

$$\sum_{i=1}^{i=i} \Delta n_i = 0 \qquad (6a)$$

since the total number of molecules of the system (N) does not change. If we expand the right-hand side of both (4) and (6) we obtain

$$S = k \ln(N!) - k(\ln(n_0!) + \ln(n_1!) + \cdots + \ln(n_i!)) \qquad (4a)$$

$$S + dS = k \ln(N!) - k(\ln(n_0 + dn_0)! + \ln(n_1 + dn_1)! + \cdots$$
$$+ \ln(n_i + dn_i)!) \quad (6b)$$

If we subtract (4a) from (6b)

$$dS = -k[\ln(n_0 + dn_0)! - \ln(n_0)! + \ln(n_1 + dn_1)! - (n(n_1)! + \cdots)] \quad (6c)$$

From Stirling's formula (see Appendix 5)

$$\ln(n_0 + dn_0)! = (n_0 + dn_0) \ln(n_0 + dn_0) - (n_0 + dn_0)$$
$$= n_0 \ln(n_0 + dn_0) + dn_0 \ln(n_0 + dn_0) - (n_0 + dn_0) \qquad (7)$$

and

$$\ln(n_0)! = n_0 \ln(n_0) - n_0 \qquad (8)$$

The other terms can be treated in a similar way.

For a small dn

$$n_0 + dn_0 \approx n_0$$

So (7) becomes

$$\ln(n_0 + dn_0)! = n_0 \ln(n_0) + dn_0 \ln(n_0) - n_0 \qquad (7a)$$

If we subtract (8) from (7a) we obtain

$$\ln(n_0 + dn_0)! - \ln(n_0)! = dn_0 \ln(n_0) \qquad (9)$$

In a similar way we obtain

$$\left. \begin{array}{l} \ln(n_1 + dn_1)! - \ln(n_1) = dn_1 \ln(n_1) \\ \ln(n_i + dn_i)! - \ln(n_i) = dn_i \ln(n_i) \end{array} \right\} \qquad (10)$$

and from (6c), (9) and (10)

$$dS = -k \sum_{i=0}^{i=1} dn_i \ln(n_i) \qquad (11)$$

But from Boltzmann's factor

$$n_i = n_0 \exp(-E_i/k)$$

so

$$\ln(n_i) = \ln(n_0) - (E_i/(kT)) \qquad (12)$$

If we substitute (12) in (11)

$$dS = -k\left[\sum_{i=0}^{i=i} dn_i \ln(n_0) - \sum_{i=0}^{i=i} dn_i E_i/(kT)\right]$$

$$= -k\left[\ln(n_0)\sum_{i=0}^{i=i} dn_i - \sum_{i=0}^{i=i} dn_i E_i/(kT)\right]$$

but from (6a)

$$\sum_{i=0}^{i=i} dn_i = 0$$

and from (5)

$$\sum_{i=0}^{i=i} dn_i E_i = dE$$

So

$$dS = k\, dE/(kT) \tag{13}$$

that is

$$dS = dE/T \tag{14}$$

Equation (14) implies that dE is absorbed at a constant temperature. In reality there will be a slight increase in temperature. This can be shown in the following way. Let us assume that ΔE is absorbed while the temperature of the thermal reservoir increases from $T - \Delta T$ to $T + \Delta T$. We can assume that $\Delta E/3$ is absorbed over three steps $T - \Delta T$, T and $T + \Delta T$. So

$$\Delta S = \Delta E/3(T - \Delta T) + \Delta E/3T + \Delta E/3(T + \Delta T)$$

$$= (\Delta E/3)[1/(T - \Delta T) + 1/T + 1/(T + \Delta T)]$$

$$= (\Delta E/3)((T^2 + T\,\Delta T + T^2 - \Delta T^2 + T^2 - T\,\Delta T)/(T^3 - T\,\Delta T^2))$$

If we divide top and bottom by T^2 we obtain

$$\Delta S = (\Delta E/3)[(3 - (\Delta T/T)^2)/(T - (\Delta T^2/T))]$$

for very small ΔT, T is assumed to be constant and so

$$\Delta S = \Delta E/T$$

Equation (14) tells us that when a thermal reservoir absorbs a small amount of energy, dE, its entropy increases by dE/T.

Third Law of thermodynamics

Physicists have shown that entropy of a perfect crystal, regardless of its chemical composition, is zero at zero Kelvin ($-273.15\,°C$) (this is the Third Law of thermodynamics). If we want to measure the entropy of a given mass of substance we start with a crystal at zero K and warm it very slightly changing its entropy. Δs becomes $\Delta E/T_1$ where ΔE_1 is the amount of energy absorbed and T_1 is the average temperature during the absorption of ΔE_1. If we keep warming the crystal very slowly its entropy will keep increasing and its entropy at temperature T will be

$$S = \sum_{i=1}^{n} \Delta E_i/T_i = (\Delta E_1/T_1) + (\Delta E_2/T_2) + \cdots + (\Delta E_n/T_n)$$

$$\text{in the limit } S = \int_0^T (1/T)\,dE \quad (14a)$$

The entropy (S) is thus a function of T and because the method of measuring S is based on the Third Law it is called a third law entropy. In fact, the integral of (14a)

$$S = \int_0^T (1/T)\,dE$$

is

$$S = S(T) - S(0)$$

where $S(T)$ is the entropy at T Kelvin and $S(0)$ is the entropy at zero K which is zero from the third law.

Properties of entropy

Entropy (S), like energy (E), is called a thermodynamic function and has the following properties:

(a) It measures microscopic disorder (Ω). The larger Ω the larger is S (from equation (4)).

(b) It can be shown that it never decreases in a spontaneous process and that when a system reaches equilibrium it becomes constant, this is the **Second Law** of thermodynamics.

(c) It is zero for a perfect crystal at zero K (**Third Law**).

(d) It can also be shown that it is additive. If a certain amount of substance (M_1) has entropy S_1 and another amount of substance M_2 has entropy S_2 then $M_1 + M_2$ has entropy $S_1 + S_2$.

(e) Finally, it can be shown that S increases when the energy of the system (E) increases.

Free energy

In order to introduce the concept of *free energy* let us consider a Universe consisting of a thermal reservoir and a chemical system (the chemical system σ may be a solution of reacting substances) in contact with the atmosphere (P_{atm}). Let us also assume that the system contains a machine which raises a weight (W_g) and does some electrical work (W_{cl}) (it may charge membrane capacitance, for example). In order to have a feel for the concept of free energy let us consider an event that takes place in a living system. When a skeletal muscle contracts and lifts a weight, it contracts and does work (W_{mech}). The energy for this work is provided by adenosine triphosphate (ATP) which breaks down to give adenosine diphosphate (ADP), inorganic phosphate (Pi) and energy.

$$\text{ATP} \rightleftharpoons \text{ADP} + \text{Pi} + \text{energy}$$

The energy of ATP can also be used to transfer charges (ions) from one side of a membrane to another. If charge is transferred against an electrical potential, electrical work (W_{el}) is done. During muscle contraction many other processes take place which could be included in our analysis. For the sake of simplicity we shall limit our considerations to a few of these processes.

In mammalian cells these processes take place at constant temperature and at atmospheric pressure. We can think of the chemical system (σ) as being effectively surrounded by a thermal reservoir so these processes take place at constant temperature. The thermal reservoir is defined on page 442 and can be compared with a thermostatically controlled waterbath. This waterbath surrounds the system and the temperature-regulated body of the mammal is equivalent to a waterbath. In addition, the system is at a constant atmospheric pressure. This means that if as a result of the chemical reactions there is a change in volume (Δv) the system will perform pressure–volume work ($P \Delta v$) against the atmosphere. The product $P \Delta v$ has the dimensions of work (see Appendix 33) since pressure is force per unit area, so

$$P \Delta v = \frac{\text{force}}{\text{distance}^2} \times \text{distance}^3 = \text{force} \times \text{distance} = \text{work}$$

From the First Law of thermodynamics (conservation of energy), the total change in energy (ΔE total) is due to changes in different types of energy.

Let us assume, for the sake of simplicity, that there are only five processes, which are: (i) the chemical reaction, (ii) pressure-related work, (iii) mechanical work, (iv) electrical work, and (v) absorption of energy by the thermal reservoir. The energy terms are the changes in energy in the system (ΔE_σ) as a result of the chemical reactions (hydrolysis of ATP), the pressure–volume relationship ($P \Delta v_\sigma$), the mechanical work (W_{mech}) done by the system, the electrical work (W_{el}) done by the system, and the absorption of energy by the thermal reservoir (ΔE_θ).

$$\Delta E_{\text{total}} = \Delta E_\sigma + P \Delta v_\sigma + W_{\text{mech}} + W_{\text{el}} + \Delta E_\theta \tag{15}$$

By the first law, work (W_{el}, W_{mech}) and internal energy (such as ΔE_σ) are all measured in the same units. The first two terms on the right-hand side of equation (15) represent the energy gained or lost by the system (σ). We assume that we are at constant temperature and pressure (the pressure is constant because the displacements, corresponding to the Δv_σ term, are very small when compared with the height of the atmosphere). The sum of ΔE_σ and Pv_σ is called the change in enthalpy (ΔH_σ) of the system. At constant pressure enthalpy (H_σ) is thus defined by

$$H_\sigma = E_\sigma + Pv_\sigma$$

and therefore the change in enthalpy (ΔH_σ) is given by

$$\Delta H_\sigma = \Delta E_\sigma + P\,\Delta v_\sigma \tag{16}$$

The two work (W) terms do not refer to the system although the *universe* of this event (the contraction of a muscle resulting in a weight being lifted) includes the five terms.

If we substitute (16) in (15) and rearrange, assuming that the total energy change is zero, we obtain

$$\Delta E_\theta = -(\Delta H_\sigma + W_{mech} + W_{el}) \tag{17}$$

In order to derive an expression for the change in free energy of the system (ΔG_σ) let us first define free energy (G_σ).

$$G_\sigma = H_\sigma - TS_\sigma$$

So the change in free energy (ΔG_σ) is given by

$$\Delta G_\sigma = \Delta H_\sigma - T\,\Delta S_\sigma \tag{17a}$$

where T is the absolute temperature and ΔS_σ is the change in entropy of the system.

From the properties of entropy the total change in entropy of a universe (ΔS_{total}) is the sum of the changes in entropy in the different parts of that universe (property d) and this change in entropy can never be negative (property b). So for our contracting muscle the change in entropy (ΔS_{total}) is the sum of the five terms

$$\Delta S_{total} = \Delta S_\theta + \Delta S_\sigma + \Delta S_{atm} + \Delta S_{mech} + \Delta S_{el} \geqslant 0 \tag{18}$$

The ΔS_{mech} term is the change in entropy associated with the raising of the weight and is zero. This is because there is no increase in disorder of the universe of the event by the change of position of the weight. The term ΔS_{el} associated with the electrical work is also zero because the charge that was shifted is still available for doing work, and so the charge movement does not increase the disorder of the system. The term ΔS_{atm} associated with pressure–volume work can be likened to the ΔS_{mech} term. This is because the pressure–volume work is like lifting a weight, the weight of the atmosphere, and so this term is also zero.

Rewriting equation (18)

$$\Delta S_{total} = \Delta S_\theta + \Delta S_\sigma \geqslant 0 \tag{19}$$

But by definition (equation (14)) the change in entropy of the thermal reservoir (ΔS_0) is given by

$$\Delta S_0 = \Delta E/T \tag{20}$$

where T is the absolute temperature.

If we substitute (17) in (20) we obtain

$$\Delta S_0 = -(\Delta H_\sigma + W_{mech} + W_{el})/T \tag{21}$$

Substituting (21) in (19)

$$\Delta S_{total} = \Delta S_\sigma - (\Delta H_\sigma + W_{mech} + W_{el})/T \geqslant 0 \tag{22}$$

If we multiply (22) by T we obtain

$$T \Delta S_{total} = T \Delta S_\sigma - \Delta H_\sigma - (W_{mech} + W_{el}) \tag{23}$$

But from (17a)

$$\Delta G_\sigma = -(T \Delta S_\sigma - \Delta H_\sigma)$$

so

$$T \Delta S_{total} = -\Delta G_\sigma - (W_{mech} + W_{el}) \geqslant 0 \tag{24}$$

If we rearrange equation (24) we obtain

$$-\Delta G_\sigma = +T \Delta S_{total} + W_{mech} + W_{el} \tag{25}$$

Equation (25) means that the decrease in free energy of the system ($-\Delta G_\sigma$) accounts for (i) the *increase of entropy* of the universe of the event at temperature T ($T \Delta S_{total}$), and (ii) the mechanical and electrical work (useful work) performed by the system. In order for the decrease in free energy of the system to be completely converted into work (mechanical and electrical) the increase in the entropy of the universe of the event must be zero. From property (b) of the entropy function (because there is no change in S_{total}), ΔS_{total} is zero for an equilibrium process. This means that under equilibrium conditions the chemical system (σ) can perform a maximal amount of work for a given change in its free energy. So at equilibrium

$$-\Delta G_\sigma = W_{mech} + W_{el} = W_{max} \tag{26}$$

But the change in free energy of the chemical system is due to the chemical transformations involved in the hydrolysis of ATP. This hydrolysis involves the breakdown of ATP and the generation of ADP and Pi and these three compounds make up the chemical system. In order to quantify their contribution to the change in free energy of the system (ΔG_σ) thermodynamicists have defined the *chemical potential* (μ_i) function of component i (ATP, or ADP or Pi) as

$$\mu_i = (\partial G_\sigma / \partial n_i) T, P, j \tag{27}$$

where n_i is the number of moles of component i, and the partial derivative is at constant pressure (P), constant temperature T and the concentrations of the other components (j) are fixed. This definition means that the chemical potential of component i of the chemical system (σ) is the change in free energy of this system per mole of component i. In order to understand the meaning of this definition the change in free energy (∂G_σ) is assumed to occur when a very small amount of the component i (∂n_i) is added to a very large chemical system; so that adding ∂n_i moles of component i will not affect the concentrations of the other components.

So the total change in free energy (ΔG_σ) of a chemical system in in the course of a chemical reaction is the sum of the contributions of the changes in free energy of the individual components. From (27) we can write

$$\Delta G_i \approx (\partial G_\sigma / \partial n_i) \, \Delta n_i = \mu_i \, \Delta n_i \tag{28}$$

Since one molecule of ATP yields one molecule of ADP and one of Pi when Δn molecules of ADP and Pi are produced, Δn molecules of ATP are used. So, for the ATP reaction

$$\Delta G_\sigma = - \mu_{ATP} \, \Delta n + \mu_{ADP} \, \Delta n + \mu_{Pi} \, \Delta n$$

$$= \Delta n (\mu_{ADP} + \mu_{Pi} - \mu_{ATP}) \tag{29}$$

Thus the change in free energy of the chemical system depends upon the chemical potentials of the three components (ATP, ADP, Pi). In Chapter 2 we derived (from the Boltzmann factor) an expression for the chemical potential. For a component i it is

$$\mu = \mu_i^0 + RT \ln c_i + Z_i F V \tag{30}$$

With expressions (29) and (30) we can thus calculate the change in free energy of a chemical reaction.

APPENDIX 26. The temperature dependence of rate constants

This temperature dependence is usually expressed as Q_{10}. This Q_{10} can be defined as the ratio of the *rate constants* of a process measured at two temperatures that differ by $10\,°C$.

The relationship between the rate constant of a process and the absolute temperature was discovered *empirically* by Arrhenius and is

$$\ln(k) = \ln A - B(1/T)$$

where $\ln(A)$ is the intercept and B the gradient of the line, where A and B are empirical constants whose values are dependent on the nature of the process (see Figure A26.1).

Constant A is generally known as the *frequency factor* and B is often expressed as a ratio of two constants

$$B = E/R$$

where R is the gas constant and E is known as the *activation energy* of the process. Because the slope of a straight line is constant we can write

$$(\ln(k_3) - \ln(k_1))/(1/T_3 - 1/T_1) = (\ln(k_2) - \ln(k_1))/(1/T_2 - 1/T_1)$$

If

$$T_3 - T_1 = 10\,^{\circ}\text{C}$$

then by the definition of Q_{10}

$$Q_{10} = k_3/k_1$$

since $T_3 \times T_1 \approx T_2 \times T_1$

$$\ln(k_3) - \ln(k_1) = \ln(k_3/k_1) = \ln(Q_{10})$$

then

$$\ln Q_{10}/10 \approx \ln(k_2/k_1)/(T_2 - T_1)$$

On rearranging one obtains

$$\ln Q_{10} = \ln(k_2/k_1)(10/(T_2 - T_1))$$

The relationship between activation energy and Q_{10} can be derived from the original equation of Arrhenius. At two temperatures that differ by $10\,^{\circ}\text{C}$

$$\ln(k_1) = \ln(A) - B(1/T_1)$$
$$\ln(k_2) = \ln(A) - B(1/(T_1 + 10))$$

The difference between these two equations is

$$\ln(k_2) - \ln(k_1) = \ln(k_2/k_1) = -B(1/(T_1 + 10) - 1/T_1)$$

Fig.A26.1

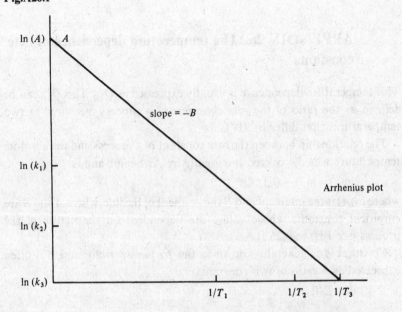

Arrhenius plot

From the definition of Q_{10}

$$\ln(Q_{10}) = -B(1/(T_1 + 10) - 1/T_1)$$

since

$$B = E/R$$

$$\ln(Q_{10}) = (-E/R)(1/(T_1 + 10) - 1/T_1)$$

This equation shows that, if the Arrhenius holds, the value of the activation energy E can be obtained from the Q_{10} value.

APPENDIX 27. Junction potentials

In Chapter 4, equation (4.42) enabled us to compute the potential across a membrane that separates two different ion solutions when the net current is zero. It is also possible to compute the potential (V) between two different ionic solutions which meet at a liquid–liquid boundary (liquid junction potential). To do this our starting point is the set of equations (4.36), from Chapter 4, and the standard procedure is to assume that the zone where the two solutions meet (the liquid junction) is composed of a series of slabs which are made up of a mixture of the two bulk solutions (see Figure A27.1a). For a slab of width Δx at position x, for example, the volume of the slab for a unit cross-sectional area of liquid junction is given by

$$\Delta v = 1 \, \Delta x \quad \text{cm}^3$$

If we let this volume (Δv) be a mixture of a cm^3 of solution (1) and b cm^3 of solution (2) we can write

$$a + b = \Delta v$$

and the fraction (Y) of Δv due to b is

$$Y = b/\Delta v$$

so that the concentration of ion (i) in the slab is then given by

$$c_i(x) = (c_{i,1}a + c_{i,2}b)/\Delta v$$
$$= (c_{i,1}a/\Delta v) + (c_{i,2}b/\Delta v)$$

But

$$(a/\Delta v) + (b/\Delta v) = 1$$

or

$$a/\Delta v = 1 - (b/\Delta v) = 1 - Y$$

So Y varies between 0 (in solution (1)) and 1 (in solution (2)).

$$c_i(x) = c_{i,1}(1 - Y) + c_{i,2}Y$$
$$= c_{i,1} + (c_{i,2} - c_{i,1})Y \tag{1}$$

Equation (1) can now be written for the three ions

$$c_{Na}(x) = c_{Na.1} + (c_{Na.2} - c_{Na.1})Y$$
$$c_K(x) = c_{K.1} + (c_{K.2} - c_{K.1})Y \quad\quad\quad (2)$$
$$c_{Cl}(x) = c_{Cl.1} + (c_{Cl.1} - c_{Cl.2})Y$$

If we return to the set of equations (4.36), when there is no net current flowing through the liquid junction we can write

$$\bar{I}_{Na} + \bar{I}_K + \bar{I}_{Cl} = 0$$

or substituting (4.36), and V now is the junction potential:

$$0 = -FD_{Na}[(d/dx)(c_{Na}) + (F/(RT))c_{Na}(d/dx)(V)]$$
$$- FD_K[(d/dx)(c_K) + (F/(RT))c_K(d/dx)(V)]$$
$$+ FD_{Cl}[(d/dx)(c_{Cl}) - (F/(RT))c_{Cl}(d/dx)(V)]$$

By dividing the three terms by F and rearranging, we obtain

$$- D_{Na}(d/dx)(c_{Na}) - D_K(d/dx)(c_K) + D_{Cl}(d/dx)(c_{Cl})$$
$$= [(D_{Na}F/RT)c_{Na} + (D_KF/RT)c_K + (D_{Cl}F/RT)c_{Cl}](d/dx)(V)$$

Fig.A27.1

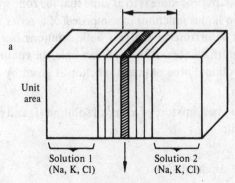

Liquid junction of
thickness δ

a

Unit
area

Solution 1   Solution 2
(Na, K, Cl)   (Na, K, Cl)

Slab of thickness Δx
of liquid junction

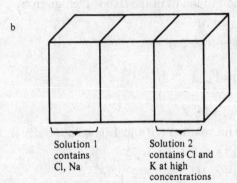

b

Solution 1   Solution 2
contains   contains Cl and
Cl, Na   K at high
                     concentrations

or

$$(d/dx)(V) = \frac{-D_{Na}(d/dx)(c_{Na}) - D_K(d/dx)(c_K) + D_{Cl}(d/dx)(c_{Cl})}{(D_{Na}F/RT)c_{Na} + (D_K F/RT)c_K + (D_{Cl}F/RT)c_{Cl}}$$

so

$$(d/dx)(V) = (RT/F)$$
$$\times \left\{ \frac{-D_{Na}(d/dx)(c_{Na}) - D_K(d/dx)(c_K) + D_{Cl}(d/dx)(c_{Cl})}{D_{Na}c_{Na} + D_K c_K + D_{Cl}c_{Cl}} \right\}$$

This equation can be rewritten as

$$(d/dx)(V) = (-(RT)/F)\{(1/(D_{Na}c_{Na} + D_K c_K + D_{Cl}c_{Cl}))$$
$$\times (d/dx)(D_{Na}c_{Na} + D_K c_K - D_{Cl}c_{Cl})\} \quad (3)$$

If we substitute (2) into (3) we obtain

$$(d/dx)(V) = (-RT/F)$$
$$\times \{1/[(D_{Na}c_{Na.1} + D_K c_{K.1} + D_{Cl}c_{Cl.1}) + Y(D_{Na}(c_{Na.2} - c_{Na.1})$$
$$+ D_K(c_{K.2} - c_{K.1}) + D_{Cl}(c_{Cl.2} - c_{Cl.1}))]\}$$
$$\times (d/dx)\{(D_{Na}c_{Na.1} + D_K c_{K.1} - D_{Cl}c_{Cl.1}) + \{D_{Na}(c_{Na.2} - c_{Na.1})$$
$$+ D_K(c_{K.2} - c_{K.1}) - D_{Cl}(c_{Cl.1} - c_{Cl.2})\} Y\} \quad (4)$$

If we define

$$D_{Na}c_{Na.1} + D_K c_{K.1} + D_{Cl}c_{Cl.1} = A$$
$$D_{Na}(c_{Na.2} - c_{Na.1}) + D_K(c_{K.2} - c_{K.1}) + D_{Cl}(c_{Cl.2} - c_{Cl.1}) = B$$
$$D_{Na}c_{Na.1} + D_K c_{K.1} - D_{Cl}c_{Cl.1} = C$$
$$D_{Na}(c_{Na.2} - c_{Na.1}) + D_K(c_{K.2} - c_{K.1}) - D_{Cl}(c_{Cl.2} - c_{Cl.1}) = D$$
$$(5)$$

Then, on substitution of (5) into (4) we obtain

$$(d/dx)(V) = -(RT/F)(1/(A + BY))(d/dx)(C + DY)$$

where A, B, C and D are constants.

But

$$(d/dx)(C + DY) = D(d/dx)(Y)$$

so

$$(d/dx)(V) = -(RT/F)(D/(A + BY))(d/dx)(Y) \quad (6)$$

In order to integrate equation (6) we first multiply both sides by dx

$$dV = -(RT/F)(D/(A + BY))\,dY \quad (7)$$

On integration across the width of the junction (see Appendix 2 on integration between limits) we obtain

$$\int_0^\delta dV \approx V$$

the potential difference across the junction where δ is the thickness of the junction. So

$$V = V(2) - V(1) \quad (8)$$

where V is the difference between the electrical potentials of solution (2) ($V(2)$) and solution (1) ($V(1)$).

In order to integrate the right-hand side we can use the substitution

$$Z = A + BY$$

so

$$dZ = B\,dY \quad \text{and} \quad dY = dZ/B \tag{9}$$

If we substitute (9) into (7) we obtain, for the integration between 0 and 1,

$$\int_0^1 -(RT/F)(D/(A+BY))\,dY = -(RT/F)D\int_{Z_1}^{Z_2} dZ/(BZ)$$

$$= -(RT/F)(D/B)\int_{Z_1}^{Z_2} dZ/Z \tag{10}$$

where Z_2 and Z_1 are the values of Z when Y is 0 ($x=0$) and 1 ($x=\delta$) respectively, that is,

$$Z_1 = A \quad \text{and} \quad Z_2 = A + B$$

On integration the term $(1/B)\int_{Z_1}^{Z_2}$ becomes

$$\int_{Z_1}^{Z_2} dZ/Z = \ln(Z_2) - \ln(Z_1) = \ln(Z_2/Z_1) \tag{10a}$$

If we substitute all of (10a) into (10) we obtain

$$-((RTD)/(FB))\int_{Z_1}^{Z_2} dZ/Z = -((RTD)/(FB))\ln((A+B)/A)$$

Since on integration of both sides of equation (7) we obtain

$$\int_0^\delta dV = -(RTD/F)\int_0^1 (1/(A+BY))\,dY$$

Then

$$V = -(RTD/FB)\ln((A+B)/A) \tag{10b}$$

We can now substitute A, B and D from equations (5) into equation (10b), so

$$V = -(RT/F)\left[\frac{D_{Na}(c_{Na.2}-c_{Na.1}) + D_K(c_{K.2}-c_{K.1}) - D_{Cl}(c_{Cl.2}-c_{Cl.1})}{D_{Na}(c_{Na.2}-c_{Na.1}) + D_K(c_{K.2}-c_{K.1}) - D_{Cl}(c_{Cl.2}-c_{Cl.1})}\right]$$

$$\times \ln\left(\frac{D_{Na}c_{Na.2} + D_K c_{K.2} + D_{Cl}c_{Cl.2}}{D_{Na}c_{Na.1} + D_K c_{K.1} + D_{Cl}c_{Cl.1}}\right) \tag{11}$$

Equation (11) can be written using mobilities instead of *diffusion constants*. From Chapter 3 we know that

$$D_i = u_i RT$$

If we divide top and bottom of both fractions of equation (11) we obtain

$$V = -(RT/F)\left[\frac{u_{Na}(c_{Na.2}-c_{Na.1}) + u_K(c_{K.2}-c_{K.1}) - u_{Cl}(c_{Cl.2}-c_{Cl.1})}{u_{Na}(c_{Na.2}-c_{Na.1}) + u_K(c_{K.2}-c_{K.1}) - u_{Cl}(c_{Cl.2}-c_{Cl.1})}\right]$$

$$\times \ln\left(\frac{u_{Na}c_{Na.2} + u_K c_{K.2} + u_{Cl}c_{Cl.2}}{u_{Na}c_{Na.1} + u_K c_{K.1} + u_{Cl}c_{Cl.1}}\right) \tag{12}$$

where u_{Na}, u_K and u_{Cl} are the mobilities of sodium, potassium and chloride respectively.

In the case of liquid junctions commonly found in electrophysiology (see Figure A27.1b) one side of the junction is made up of a dilute poly-electrolyte solution containing Na, K and Cl, while the other side is a salt bridge that contains a concentrated KCl solution (see Chapter 4). The potassium concentration of extracellular biological fluids is generally low so, in order to simplify the calculation of the liquid junction potential, we will assume it to be zero. Since the anionic concentration must be equal to the cationic concentration in solutions (1) and (2) (electroneutrality) we can say that

$$c_{Na.1} = c_{Cl.1} = c_1 \quad \text{and} \quad c_{K.2} = c_{Cl.2} = c_2 \tag{13}$$

As solution (2) does not contain sodium, and we assume that there is no potassium in solution (1), then (see Figure A27.1b)

$$c_{Na.2} = 0 \quad \text{and} \quad c_{K.1} = 0 \tag{14}$$

These assumptions mean that equation (12) becomes

$$V = (RT/F) \left[\frac{-u_{Na}c_1 + u_K(c_2 - c_1) - u_{Cl}(c_2 - c_1)}{-u_{Na}c_1 + u_K(c_2 - c_1) + u_{Cl}(c_2 - c_1)} \right] \ln\left(\frac{c_2(u_K + u_{Cl})}{c_1(u_{Na} + u_{Cl})} \right) \tag{15}$$

If we rearrange equation (15) we obtain

$$V = -(RT/F) \left[\frac{(c_2 - c_1)(u_K - u_{Cl}) - (u_{Na}c_1)}{(c_2 - c_1)(u_K + u_{Cl}) - (u_{Na}c_1)} \right] \ln\left(\frac{c_2(u_K + u_{Cl})}{c_1(u_{Na} + u_{Cl})} \right) \tag{16}$$

Since electrophysiologists normally use $3M$ KCl solutions in their salt bridges (see Chapter 4), c_2 is much greater than c_1 or

$$c_2 - c_1 \approx c_2$$

If c_1 is small, equation (16) becomes

$$V = -(RT/F) \left[\frac{c_2(u_K - u_{Cl})}{c_2(u_K + u_{Cl})} \right] \ln\left(\frac{c_2(u_K + u_{Cl})}{c_1(u_{Na} + u_{Cl})} \right) \tag{17}$$

Since the value of u_K is very similar to u_{Cl}, then the term $(u_K - u_{Cl})$ is very small and V, the junction potential, is small.

APPENDIX 28. Competitive inhibition kinetics

In this Appendix we consider the competition of acetylcholine (Ach) and curare for the same binding site (see Chapter 9). If both Ach (A) and curare (C) can be bound at the same site (S) the following binding reactions can take place

$$A+S \rightleftharpoons AS$$
$$C+S \rightleftharpoons CS \tag{1}$$

By the law of mass action the velocities of the backward reactions are given by

$$v_{A_{-1}} = k_{A_{-1}}[AS]$$
$$v_{C_{-1}} = k_{C_{-1}}[CS] \tag{2}$$

where the brackets refer to molar concentrations. The velocities of the forward reactions are similarly given by

$$v_{A_1} = k_{A_1}[A][S]$$

and

$$v_{C_1} = k_{C_1}[C][S] \tag{3}$$

At equilibrium

$$v_{A_1} = v_{A_{-1}} \quad \text{and} \quad v_{C_1} = v_{C_{-1}} \tag{4}$$

so

$$\left. \begin{array}{l} k_{A_1}[A][S] = k_{A_{-1}}[AS] \\ k_{C_1}[C][S] = k_{C_{-1}}[CS] \end{array} \right\} \tag{5}$$

The response to Ach is assumed to be proportional to the concentration of sites bound to Ach, that is, to $[AS]$. Thus

$$[AS] = (k_{A_1}/k_{A_{-1}})[A][S]$$

Also

$$[CS] = (k_{C_1}/k_{C_{-1}})[C][S] \tag{5a}$$

$[AS]$ is then given by

$$[AS] = [S_t]/(1 + (K_C[C]+1)/(K_A[A])) \tag{6}$$

where

$$[S_t] = [AS] + [CS] + [S]$$

In the absence of the inhibitor ($[C]=0$) the value of $[AS]$ is

$$[AS] = [S_t]/(1 + 1/(K_A[A])) \tag{7}$$

We can now select the concentration of Ach ($[A]$) in such a way that in the presence of the inhibitor (C) it will have the same effect (that is, will achieve the same concentration of $[AS]$) as the concentration $[A']$ in the absence of curare. If we equate (6) and (7)

$$[S_T]/(1 + (K_C[C]+1)/(K_A[A])) = [S_t]/(1 + 1/(K_A[A'])) \tag{8}$$

After simplification equation (8) becomes

$$(K_C[C]+1)/(K_A[A]) = 1/(K_A[A'])$$

or

$$K_C[C]+1 = [A]/[A']$$

or

$$[A]/[A'] - 1 = K_C[C] \qquad (9)$$

If we do several experiments at different values of $[C]$ and $[A]$ and we plot the left-hand side of equation (9) against $[C]$ we obtain a straight line (of slope K_C). Under these conditions obtaining a straight line is a demonstration of competitive inhibition.

APPENDIX 29. Acetylcholine–receptor interaction

The number of molecules of Ach that bind to a single receptor can be estimated in the following way: If n molecules of transmitter (T) interact with the receptor (R) the interaction will result in the formation of a receptor–transmitter complex (T_nR). This interaction is described by

$$nT + R \underset{k_{-1}}{\overset{k_1}{\rightleftharpoons}} T_nR$$

The rate of formation of the complex $((d/dt)[T_nR])$ is the difference between the velocity (v_1) at which it is formed

$$v_1 = k_1[T]^n[R]$$

and the velocity (v_{-1}) at which it dissociates

$$v_{-1} = k_{-1}[T_nR]$$

So

$$(d/dt)[T_nR] = v_1 - v_{-1}$$
$$(d/dt)[T_nR] = k_1[R][T]^n - k_{-1}[T_nR] \qquad (1)$$

If the total concentration of receptor ($[R_t]$) is constant, or

$$[R_t] = [T_nR] + [R] = \text{constant}$$

so

$$[R] = [R_t] - [T_nR] \qquad (2)$$

If we substitute (2) into (1) we obtain

$$(d/dt)([T_nR]) = k_1[T]^n([R_t] - [T_nR]) - k_{-1}[T_nR] \qquad (3)$$

At steady-state the concentrations of the complex ($[T_nR]$), of the receptor ($[R]$) and of the transmitter ($[T]$) are constant so the velocity of formation is equal to the velocity of breakdown and thus

$$(d/dt)([T_nR]) = 0$$

Equation (3) then becomes

$$0 = k_1[T]^n([R_t] - [T_nR]) - k_{-1}[T_nR] \qquad (4)$$

If we rearrange equation (4) we obtain

$$[T_nR] = (k_1[T]^n[R_t])/(k_1[T]^n + k_{-1}) \qquad (5)$$

Equation (5) can be rearranged in order to obtain a linearized relationship by calculating the reciprocals of both sides.

$$1/[T_nR] = 1/[R_t] + (k_{-1}/(k_1[R_t]))(1/[T])^n \tag{6}$$

If we assume that the postsynaptic membrane conductance (G_s) is proportional to the concentration of the complex $([T_nR])$, we can write

$$G_s = B[T_nR] \tag{7}$$

where B is the proportionality constant. So

$$1/G_s = 1/[R_t]B + ((k_{-1})/(k_1B[R_t]))(1/[T])^n$$

This is the equation of a straight line of the form

$$Y = a + b$$

where

$$Y = 1/G_s$$
$$a = 1/[R_t]B$$

and

$$b = k_{-1}/(k_1B[R_t])$$

With a proper choice of n a plot of $1/G_s$ versus $(1/[T])^n$ will give a straight line. In the frog neuromuscular junction $(1/G_s)$ is linearly related to the first power of $(1/[T])$ which means that one Ach molecule switches on one channel.

APPENDIX 30. Measurement of membrane permeability with radioisotopes

Definition of radioisotopes

Radioisotopes are chemical elements which differ by the number of neutrons in their nuclei. Different radioisotopes of the same element have different stabilities. For example, of all the radioisotopes of sodium (^{22}Na, ^{23}Na and ^{24}Na), ^{22}Na and ^{24}Na are unstable. ^{22}Na disintegrates with a half-life which is years while ^{24}Na has a half-life of approximately half a day. When they disintegrate, both these isotopes of sodium emit γ radiation which can be detected by appropriate detectors. Other radioisotopes (^{14}C and tritium) will emit electrons (β particles) on disintegration which can also be detected by appropriate detectors. The methods of measuring the radiation are extremely sensitive and enable us to measure minute amounts of radioisotopes. Although different radioisotopes of the same element can be distinguished by their physical properties (mass, type of radiation that they emit) they have the *same* chemical properties. For example, a protein will bind several radioisotopes of calcium with the same affinity. Also the sodium pump is activated in the same way by all the isotopes of Na. This is the basis for the use of radioisotopes in that chemical, biochemical or biological processes in general do not distinguish between several isotopes of the same element. With this assumption we can trace a given element or compound in a compartment by adding to the compartment a small amount of a radioisotope. In the case of an element, ^{23}Na for example, we add a small amount of ^{22}Na or ^{24}Na. In the case of a compound, glucose for example, we add a small amount of labelled glucose in which one of the carbons has been replaced by ^{14}C.

In order to explain this tracer technique we shall show how we measure the flux of an ion across a membrane separating two compartments (1 and 2).

Specific activity

Let us assume that we have a certain amount of radioisotope (Q_i^*) of an element i which produces a certain number of disintegrations per minute or counts per minute (c.p.m.). We can express Q_i^* in c.p.m. If compartment (1) has a volume v_1 when we add the amount Q_i^* to compartment v_1 it will be at concentration c_i^* (c.p.m./cm^3). If the compartment contains Q_i moles of the element at a concentration c_i (moles/cm^3) then there will be a_i^* c.p.m./mole of the radioisotope. a_i^* is called the *specific activity* and can be expressed as

$$a^* = Q_i^*/Q_i = c_i^* v_1/c_i v_1 = c_i^*/c_i \tag{1}$$

If we rearrange (1) we obtain

$$Q_i = Q_i^*/a_i^* \tag{2}$$

Equation (2) means that in a compartment in which a radioisotope is homogeneously distributed, if we can measure Q_i^* and a_i^* we are able to compute Q_i.

Let us now add an amount Q_{Na} of radioactive sodium to compartment 1 and allow sufficient time for the radioisotope to distribute itself homogeneously in this compartment. Let us assume also that we can measure Q_{Na}, that is, the total amount of sodium in the compartments. From (1) we can compute the specific activity $a_{Na_1}^*$.

If the membrane separating compartment 1 from 2 is permeable to sodium there will be a continuous movement of sodium ions from 1 to 2 (J_{12}) and from 2 to 1 (J_{21}). The net flux (J) from 1 to 2 will then be

$$J = J_{12} - J_{21} \tag{3}$$

At steady-state J_{12} and J_{21} will be constant. The net flux of radioactive isotope J^* from 1 to 2 will then be given by

$$J^* = J_{12}a^*_{Na_1} - J_{21}a^*_{Na_2} \qquad (4)$$

where $a^*_{Na_1}$ and $a^*_{Na_2}$ are the specific activities in compartments 1 and 2. Equation (4) is based on the assumption that the flux of sodium from 1 to 2 contains the radioisotope at the same specific activity $(a^*_{Na_1})$ as the compartment (1) from which it comes. In other words, if, in compartment 1, for every 1000 non-radioactive sodiums there is one sodium ion that is radioactive, since the membrane does not distinguish between the radioactive and non-radioactive element, for every 1000 sodiums from compartment 1 that collide with the membrane, one is radioactive.

As a result of the fluxes across the membrane the radioactivity in compartments 1 $(Q^*_{Na_1})$ and 2 $(Q^*_{Na_2})$ will be changing continuously with time. For compartment 1

$$(d/dt)(Q^*_{Na_1}) = J_{21}a^*_{Na_2} - J_{12}a^*_{Na_1} \qquad (5)$$

rate of change of total amount of radioisotope in compartment 1	flux of radioisotope into compart- ment 1	amount of radioisotope leaving compartment 1 per unit time (outflux)

At time zero all the radioisotope was in compartment 1 $(Q^{*(0)}_{Na_1})$ so at any time, assuming that the duration of the experiment was very short compared with the half-life of the isotope, we can write

$$Q^{*(0)}_{Na_1} = Q^*_{Na_1} + Q^*_{Na_2}$$

or

$$Q^*_{Na_2} = Q^{*(0)}_{Na_1} - Q^*_{Na_1} \qquad (6)$$

From the definition of specific activity

$$a^*_{Na_2} = Q^*_{Na_2}/Q_{Na_2}$$

and

$$a^*_{Na_1} = Q^*_{Na_1}/Q_{Na_1} \qquad (7)$$

where Q_{Na_1} and Q_{Na_2} are the total amounts of sodium in compartments 1 and 2. Substituting (6) and (7) in (5) we obtain

$$(d/dt)(Q^*_{Na_1}) = J_{21}((Q^{*(0)}_{Na_1} - Q^*_{Na_1})/Q_{Na_2}) - J_{12}(Q^*_{Na_1}/Q_{Na_1}) \qquad (8)$$

At steady state Q_{Na_1}, Q_{Na_2}, J_{21} and J_{12} are constant.

Experiments are normally designed in such a way that equation (8) is simplified.

Let us assume that compartment 1 refers to the intracellular compartment of a nerve cell and compartment 2 is the extracellular bath, which is very large. In this experiment the cell is preloaded first with radioactive sodium, so that when we start the measurement the cell contains $Q^{*(0)}_{Na}$ c.p.m. of radioactive sodium.

Since Q_{Na_2} is very large

$$J_{21}((Q_{Na_1}^{*(0)} - Q_{Na_1}^*)/Q_{Na_2}) \ll Q_{Na_1}^*/Q_{Na_1}$$

Equation (8) becomes

$$(d/dt)(Q_{Na_1}^*) \approx -J_{12}(Q_{Na_1}^*/Q_{Na_1}) = J_{12}a_{Na_1}^* \tag{9}$$

By measuring $Q_{Na_1}^*$ and Q_{Na_1} we obtain J_{12}, that is, the unidirectional efflux of sodium, since

$$Q_{Na_1}^* = v_1 a_{Na_1}^*$$

Permeability

If the efflux of sodium is diffusional (see Chapter 3)

$$J = (J_{12} - J_{21}) = P(c_1 - c_2) = Pc_1 - Pc_2$$

where P is the membrane permeability, so

$$J_{12} = Pc_1 \quad \text{and} \quad J_{21} = Pc_2 \tag{10}$$

If we multiply both sides of (10) by $a_{Na_1}^*$ we obtain

$$J_{12}a_{Na_1}^* = Pc_{Na_1}a_{Na_1}^* = Pc_{Na_1}^* \tag{11}$$

The left-hand side of the equation is the efflux of radioactivity which we may call J_{12}^* while $c_{Na_1}a_{Na_1}^*$ is the concentration of radioactivity ($c_{Na_1}^*$) in the cell compartment.

Dimensionally

$$J_{12}^* = J_{12}a_{Na_1}^* = (\text{mol} \cdot \text{cm}^{-2} \cdot \text{s}^{-1})(\text{c.p.m.} \cdot \text{mol}^{-1})$$
$$= \text{c.p.m.} \cdot \text{cm}^{-2} \cdot \text{s}^{-1} \tag{11a}$$

and

$$c_{Na_1}^* = c_{Na_1}a_{Na_1}^* = (\text{mol} \cdot \text{cm}^{-3})(\text{c.p.m.} \cdot \text{mol}^{-1})$$
$$= \text{c.p.m.} \cdot \text{cm}^{-3} \tag{12}$$

so

$$J_{12}^*/c_{Na_1}^* = P = (\text{c.p.m.} \cdot \text{cm}^{-2} \cdot \text{s}^{-1})/(\text{c.p.m.} \cdot \text{cm}^{-3})$$
$$= \text{cm} \cdot \text{s}^{-1} \tag{13}$$

It should be noted that J_{12}^* and $c_{Na_1}^*$ are expressed in radioactive units. So by measuring the concentration of radioactivity and the flux of radioactivity we can measure the permeability P.

APPENDIX 31. Voltage- and current-clamp techniques

Current clamp

A *current clamp* is an electronic device which injects a constant current across a load (a biological membrane, for example), regardless of variations in the impedance of the load. The simplest current clamp is a voltage source (E_S) in series with a resistance (R_S). If the resistance of the load is R_L then the injected current (I) is, from Ohm's law:

$$I = E_S/(R_S + R_L) = E_S/R_S(1/(1 + R_L/R_S))$$

If R_S is so large that

$$R_S \gg R_L$$

then

$$1 \gg R_L/R_S$$

and

$$I \approx E_S/R_S \quad \text{(independent of } R_L)$$

A more complicated current-clamp source is based upon the use of *electronic feedback*. The simplest example of this type is shown in Figure A31.1. Here C_m and R_m are the membrane capacitance and resistance respectively, A is an amplifier with a very large gain and very large input impedance. E_R is the voltage of an external generator (a battery, or a pulse generator).

From simple circuit theory we can write

(i) $e_0 = A(E_R - e_1)$ (this is the basic definition of an amplifier)

where e_0 is the output voltage, and e_1 the voltage at the negative input

Fig.A31.1

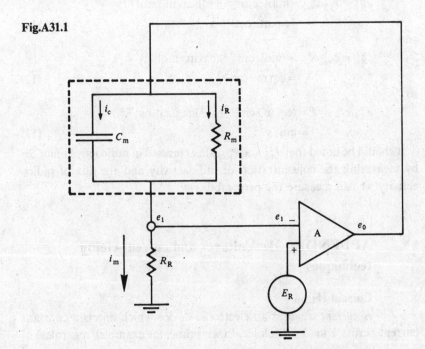

terminal of the amplifier

(ii) $e_1 = i_m R_R$ Ohm's law

(iii) $i_m = i_c + i_R$ Kirchhoff's law for the currents

Since

$$i_c = C_m((d/dt)(e_0 - e_1))$$

$$i_R = (e_0 - e_1)/R_m$$

So

$$i_m = C_m((d/dt)(e_0 - e_1)) + (e_0 - e_1)/R_m$$

$$= C_m((d/dt)(A(E_R - e_1) - e_1)) + (A(E_R - e_1) - e_1)/R_m$$

then

$$i_m = C_m((d/dt)(AE_R - e_1(1 + A))) + (AE_R - e_1(1 + A))/R_m \tag{1}$$

for $A \gg 1$

$$A + 1 \approx A$$

and equation (1) simplifies to

$$i_m = AC_m(d/dt)(E_R - e_1) + (A/R_m)(E_R - e_1)$$

or

$$i_m = (A/R_m)[\tau_m(d/dt)(E_R - e_1) + (E_R - e_1)] \tag{2}$$

where $\tau_m = R_m C_m$.

If we make the substitution

$$t = \tau_m T \quad \text{and} \quad dt = \tau_m \, dT \tag{3}$$

Substituting (3) in (2)

$$i_m = (A/R_m)[(d/dT)(E_R - e_1) + (E_R - e_1)] \tag{4}$$

But

$$e_1 = i_m R_R \tag{5}$$

Substituting (5) in (4) and rearranging

$$i_m + (A/R_m)(d/dT)(i_m R_R) + (AR_R i_m)/R_m$$
$$= [A/R_m]((d/dT)(E_R) + E_R) \tag{6}$$

If A is sufficiently large so that

$$(AR_R)/R_m \gg 1$$

then $(AR_R i_m)/R_m \gg i_m$ and so we ignore the first i_m term and write

$$(A/R_m)((d/dT)(i_m R_R) + i_m R_R) = (A/R_m)((d/dT)(E_R)EE_R) \tag{7}$$

In order for the equation to be true

$$E_m \text{ must be equal to } i_m R_R$$

or

$$E_R = i_m R_R \quad \text{and} \quad i_m = E_R/R_R \tag{8}$$

Equation (8) means that i_m is independent of R_m and C_m and is effectively *clamped* at E_R/R_R.

Voltage clamp

In a voltage-clamp system the voltage is maintained across a load regardless of the value of the load. If we have a generator (E_S), of output resistance R_S, and apply this generator across a load (R_L), the voltage across the load (V_L) will be given by (see Appendix 15, section III).

$$V_L = E_S R_L/(R_L + R_S) = E_S/(1 + R_S/R_L)$$

If

$$R_S \ll R_L$$

then

$$V_L = E_S$$

that is, the simplest voltage-clamp system is an *ideal* voltage source (zero output impedance). In electrophysiology currents are injected through salt bridges, microelectrodes or other conductors which are part of R_S and are not small, and so for this reason we have to use feedback electronic circuits based on the following principle.

Figure A31.2 shows the arrangement in a voltage-clamp set up. The symbols in this diagram have the same meaning as in Figure A31.1. We can then write

$$e_0 = A(E_R - e_1) \tag{9}$$
$$e_1 = e_0 \tag{10}$$

so

$$e_0 = AE_R - Ae_0$$

or

$$e_0(1 + A) = AE_R$$

Fig. A31.2

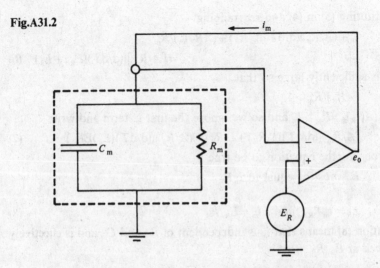

So

$$e_0 = (A/(1+A))E_R \tag{11}$$

If

$$A \gg 1$$

then

$$1 + A \approx A$$

and

$$e_0 = E_R \tag{12}$$

Equation (12) means that the voltage applied across the membrane (10) is independent of R_m and almost equals (*clamped* at) E_R.

APPENDIX 32. Tables of constants for axons and muscles

In this Appendix we include the equations that are usually used by electrophysiologists to compute action potentials.

Table 1. *Rate constant equations for axons*
(*after Hodgkin and Huxley, 1952; from Adrian, Chandler and Hodgkin, 1970*)

$$\alpha_n = \frac{\bar{\alpha}_n(V - \bar{V}_n)}{1 - \exp{-\dfrac{(V - \bar{V}_n)}{10}}}$$

$$\beta_n = \bar{\beta}_n \exp{-\frac{(V - \bar{V}_n)}{80}}$$

$$\alpha_m = \frac{\bar{\alpha}_m(V - \bar{V}_m)}{1 - \exp{-\dfrac{(V - \bar{V}_m)}{10}}}$$

$$\beta_m = \bar{\beta}_m \exp{-\frac{(V - \bar{V}_m)}{18}}$$

$$\alpha_h = \bar{\alpha}_h \exp{-\frac{(V - \bar{V}_h)}{20}}$$

$$\beta_h = \bar{\beta}_h \left[1 + \exp{-\frac{(V - \bar{V}_h)}{10}} \right]^{-1}$$

Table 2. *Values of constants for axons (after Hodgkin and Huxley, 1952) (6.3 °C)*

$\bar{\alpha}_m$	0.100 msec^{-1}
$\bar{\beta}_m$	0.996 msec^{-1}
$\bar{V}_m$	-37 mV
$\bar{G}_{Na}$	120 mmho/cm^2
E_{Na}	$+53$ mV
$\bar{\alpha}_h$	0.016 msec^{-1}
$\bar{\beta}_h$	1.0 msec^{-1}
$\bar{V}_h$	-32 mV
$\bar{\alpha}_n$	0.01 msec^{-1}
$\bar{\beta}_n$	0.11 msec^{-1}
$\bar{V}_n$	-52 mV
$\bar{G}_K$	34 mmho/cm^2
E_K	-74 mV
$\bar{G}_L$	0.3 mmho/cm^2
E_L	-51 mV

Similar equations exist for muscle fibres, thus for frog skeletal muscle the constants are shown in Tables 3 and 4.

Table 3. *Rate constant equations for frog sartorius muscle (after Adrian, Chandler and Hodgkin, 1970)*

$$\alpha_n = \frac{\bar{\alpha}_n(V - \bar{V}_n)}{1 - \exp -\dfrac{(V - \bar{V}_n)}{7}}$$

$$\beta_n = \bar{\beta}_n \exp -\frac{(V - \bar{V}_n)}{40}$$

$$\alpha_m = \frac{\bar{\alpha}_m(V - \bar{V}_m)}{1 - \exp -\dfrac{(V - \bar{V}_m)}{10}}$$

$$\beta_m = \bar{\beta}_m \exp -\frac{(V - \bar{V}_m)}{18}$$

$$\alpha_h = \bar{\alpha}_h \exp -\frac{(V - \bar{V}_h)}{14.7}$$

$$\beta_h = \bar{\beta}_h \left[1 + \exp -\frac{(V - \bar{V}_h)}{7.6} \right]^{-1}$$

Table 4. *Values of constants for frog muscle* (1–3 °C)

$\bar{\alpha}_m$	0.016, 0.042 msec^{-1}
$\bar{\beta}_m$	0.16, 0.42 msec^{-1}
$\bar{V}_m$	−40 to −48 mV
$\bar{G}_{Na}$	55 to 70 mmho/cm^2
E_{Na}	+15 to +22 mV
α_h	0.003 msec^{-1}
$\bar{\beta}_h$	0.65 msec^{-1}
$\bar{V}_h$	−41 mV
$\bar{\alpha}_n$	0.0021 to 0.0044 msec^{-1}
$\bar{\beta}_n$	0.009 to 0.0185 msec^{-1}
$\bar{V}_n$	−40 to −45 mV
$\bar{G}_K$	8.5 to 20 mmho/cm^3
E_K	−70 to −85 mV
$\bar{G}_L$	0.5 to 1.0 mmho/cm^2
E_L	−95 mV

APPENDIX 33. Work, energy and potential energy

A force is an influence acting on a body which modifies or tends to modify (i) its form, (ii) its state of rest, or (iii) its movement in a straight line at a constant velocity. (The units of force were discussed in Appendix 1.)

A force is a *vector* quantity since it is defined by both magnitude and direction. If a force F displaces its point of application along its direction by a distance dl, it performs an amount of work (dw) which is given by the relationship

$$dw = F \, dl \tag{1}$$

The work (Δw) performed in raising a mass M_L from $l = 0$ to $l = L$ is given by

$$\Delta w = \int_0^L F \, dl$$

where

$$F = Mg$$

and g is the acceleration due to gravity, then

$$\Delta w = \int_0^L F \, dl = F \int_0^L dl = F(L-0) = Fl$$

Since, when the body is released, it returns to position $l = 0$ we say that the body has increased its internal energy (E) or *potential energy* by Δw. In other words, by raising the body to position L, Δw units of work, or energy, are stored in the body.

Potential energy may be stored in a number of ways. When several elements combine to form a compound, for example when carbon, hydrogen and oxygen combine to form glucose, energy is stored as chemical energy in the bonds between C, H and O of the glucose molecule. When we compress a spring which behaves according to Hook's law

$$F = -kl$$

where l is the length of the spring from l_1 to l_2

$$\Delta w = -\int_{l_1}^{l_2} kl \, \mathrm{d}l$$

$$= -k[l^2/2]_{l_1}^{l_2} = k\left[\frac{l_2^2}{2} - \frac{l_1^2}{2}\right]$$

In all these cases we talk of *potential* energy because by reversing the process which leads to the storage of energy we can *release* this energy.

SUGGESTED FURTHER READING

CHAPTER 2

Bent, H. A. (1965). *The Second Law*, chapters 1 and 4. New York, Oxford University Press.

Dickenson, R. E. & Geis, I. (1979). *Chemistry, Matter and the Universe*, chapter 17. Menlo Park, California, Benjamin/Cummings Publishing Company.

Eisenberg, D. & Crothers, D. (1979). *Physical Chemistry*, chapters 8 and 9. Menlo Alto, California, Benjamin/Cummings Publishing Company.

Glasstone, S. (1942). *An Introduction to Electrochemistry*, chapters 2–5. Princeton, D. Van Nostrand Company Inc.

Laidler, K. J. (1980). *Physical Chemistry with Biological Applications*, chapters 6–8. Menlo Park, Benjamin/Cummings Publishing Company.

Robinson, R. A. & Stokes, R. H. (1959). *Electrolyte Solutions*, chapters 1–9. London, Butterworths.

CHAPTER 3

Crank, J. (1970). *The Mathematics of Diffusion*, chapters 1–6. London, Oxford University Press.

Eisenberg, D. & Crothers, D. (1979). *Physical Chemistry*, chapter 15. Menlo Park, California, Benjamin/Cummings Publishing Company.

Finkelstein, A. & Mauro, A. (1963). Equivalent circuits as related to ionic systems. *Biophysical Journal* 3:215–37.

Robinson, R. A. & Stokes, R. H. (1959). *Electrolyte Solutions*, chapter 11. London, Butterworths.

Weast, R. C. (ed.). (1983). *CRG Handbook of Chemistry and Physics*. Boca Raton, Florida, CRG Press.

CHAPTER 4

Arndt, R. A. & Roper, L. David. (1972). *Simple Membrane Electrodiffusion Theory*. Blacksburg, Virginia, Physical Biological Sciences Miscellaneous.

Finkelstein, A. & Mauro, A. (1977). Physical principles and formalisms of electrical excitability. In *Handbook of Physiology, The Nervous System*, section 1, vol. 1, chapter 6. Bethesda, American Physiological Society.

Goldman, D. E. (1943). Potential, impedance and rectification in membranes. *Journal of General Physiology* 27:37–60.

Hodgkin, A. L. & Katz, B. (1949). The effect of sodium ions on the electrical activity of the giant axon of the squid. *Journal of Physiology* (London) 108:37–77.

Jack, J. J. B., Noble, D. & Tsein, R. W. (1975). *Electric Current Flow in Excitable Cells.* Oxford, Clarendon Press.

CHAPTER 5

Adersen, O. S. (1978). Permeability properties of unmodified lipid bilayer membranes. In *Membrane Transport in Biology*, vol. 1, ed. D. C. Tosteson, pp. 369–446. Berlin, Springer-Verlag.

Caldwell, P. C. (1969). Energy relationships and the active transport of ions. *Current Topics in Bioenergetics* 3:251–78.

Cass, A., Finkelstein, A. & Krespi, V. (1970). The ion permeability induced in thin lipid membranes by the Polyene Antibiotics Nystatin and Amphotericin B. *Journal of General Physiology* 56:100–24.

Finkelstein, A. & Mauro, A. (1977). Physical principles and formalisms of electrical excitability. In *Handbook of Physiology, The Nervous System*, section 1, vol. 1, chapter 6. Bethesda, American Physiological Society.

Glynn, I. M. & Karlish, S. J. D. (1975). The sodium pump. *Annual Review of Physiology* 37:13–56.

Hadley, S. B. & Hayton, A. (1972). Ion transfer across lipid membranes in the presence of Gramicidin A. 1 – Studies on the unit conductance channel. *Biochimica Biophysica Acta* 374:194–312.

Marty, A. & Finkelstein, A. (1975). Pores formed in lipid bilayer membranes by Nystatin. *Journal of General Physiology* 65:515–28.

Mullins, L. J. & Noda, K. (1963). The influence of sodium free solutions on the membrane potential of frog muscle fibres. *Journal of General Physiology* 47:117–32.

Rosenberg, P. A. & Finkelstein, A. (1978). Interaction of ions and water in Gramicidin A channels. *Journal of General Physiology* 73:327–40.

Tanford, C. (1973). *The Hydrophobic Effect.* New York, Wiley.

CHAPTER 6

Finkelstein, A. & Mauro, A. (1963). Equivalent circuits as related to ionic systems. *Biophysical Journal* 3:215–37.

Finkelstein, A. & Mauro, A. (1977). Physical principles and formalisms of electrical excitability. In *Handbook of Physiology, The Nervous System*, section 1, vol. 1, chapter 6. Bethesda, American Physiological Society.

Hille, B. (1977). Ionic basis of resting and action potentials. In *Handbook of Physiology, The Nervous System*, section 1, vol. 1, chapter 4. Bethesda, American Physiological Society.

Hodgkin, A. L. (1964). *The Conduction of the Nervous Impulse.* Springfield, Ill., Thomas.

Katz, B. (1966). *Nerve, Muscle and Synapse*, chapters 2–4. New York, McGraw-Hill Book Company.

CHAPTER 7

Hille, B. (1977). Ionic basis of resting and action potentials. In *Handbook of Physiology, The Nervous System*, section 1, vol. 1, chapter 4. Bethesda, American Physiological Society.

Hodgkin, A. L. & Katz, B. (1949). The effect of sodium ions in the electrical activity of the giant squid axon. *Journal of Physiology* (London) **108**:37–77.

Hodgkin, A. L., Huxley, A. F. & Katz, B. (1952). Measurement of current–voltage relations in the membrane of the giant axon of *Loligo*. *Journal of Physiology* (London) **116**:424–48.

Hodgkin, A. L. & Huxley, A. F. (1952). Currents carried by sodium and potassium ions through the membrane of the giant axon of *Loligo*. *Journal of Physiology* (London) **116**:449–72.

Hodgkin, A. L. & Huxley, A. F. (1952). The components of membrane conductance in the giant axon of *Loligo*. *Journal of Physiology* (London) **116**:473–96.

Hodgkin, A. L. & Huxley, A. F. (1952). The dual effect of membrane potential on sodium conductance in the giant axon of *Loligo*. *Journal of Physiology* (London) **116**:497–506.

Hodgkin, A. L. & Huxley, A. F. (1952). A quantitative description of membrane current and its application to conduction and excitation in nerve. *Journal of Physiology* (London) **117**:500–44.

Hodgkin, A. L. (1964). *The Conduction of the Nervous Impulse*. Springfield, Ill., Thomas.

Jack, J. J. B., Noble, D. & Tsein, R. W. (1975). *Electric Current Flow in Excitable Cells*, chapters 7 and 8. Oxford, Clarendon Press.

CHAPTER 8

Adrian, R. H., Chandler, W. K. & Hodgkin, A. L. (1970). Voltage clamp experiments in striated muscle fibres. *Journal of Physiology* (London) **208**:607–44.

Adrian, R. H. & Marshall, M. W. (1977). Sodium currents in mammalian muscle. *Journal of Physiology* (London) **268**:223–50.

Hodgkin, A. L. & Rushton, W. A. H. (1946). The electrical constants of a crustacean nerve fibre. *Proceedings of the Royal Society*, Series B **133**:444–79.

Hodgkin, A. & Huxley, A. F. (1952). A quantitative description of membrane current and its application to conductance and excitation in nerve. *Journal of Physiology* (London) **117**:500–44.

Hodgkin, A. (1964). *The Conduction of the Nervous Impulse*. Springfield, Ill., Thomas.

Huxley, A. F. & Stämffli, R. (1949). Evidence for saltatory conduction in peripheral myelinated nerve fibres. *Journal of Physiology* (London) **108**:315–39.

Jack, J. J. B., Noble, D. & Tsein, R. W. (1975). *Electric Current Flow in Excitable Cells*, chapters 7 and 8. Oxford, Clarendon Press.

Rall, W. (1977). Core conductance theory and cable properties of neurons. In *Handbook of Physiology, The Nervous System*, section 1, vol. 1, chapter 3. Bethesda, American Physiological Society.

CHAPTER 9

Anderson, C. R. & Stevens, C. F. (1973). Voltage clamp analysis of acetylcholine produced end-plate current fluctuations of frog neuromuscular junction. *Journal of Physiology* (London) **235**:655–91.

Bennett, M. V. L. (1977). Electrical transmission: a functional analysis and comparison to chemical transmission. In *Handbook of Physiology, The Nervous System*, section 1, vol. 1. Bethesda, American Physiological Society.

Boyd, I. A. & Martin, A. R. (1956). The end-plate potential in mammalian muscle. *Journal of Physiology* (London) **132**:79–91.

Coombs, J. S., Eccles, J. C. & Fatt, P. (1955). The specific ionic conductances and ionic movements across the motorneuronal membrane that produce the inhibitory post-synaptic potential. *Journal of Physiology* (London) **130**:291–326.

Dale, H. H., Feldberg, W. & Vogt, M. (1936). Release of acetylcholine at voluntary motor nerve endings. *Journal of Physiology* (London) **86**:353–80.

Del Castillo, J. & Katz, B. (1954). Quantal components of the end-plate potential. *Journal of Physiology* (London) **124**:560–73.

Del Castillo, J. & Katz, B. (1954). Statistical factors involved in neuromuscular facilitation and depression. *Journal of Physiology* (London) **124**574–85.

Fatt, P. & Katz, B. (1951). An analysis of the end-plate potential recorded with an intracellular electrode. *Journal of Physiology* (London) **115**:320–70.

Fatt, P. & Katz, B. (1952). Spontaneous subthreshold activity at motor nerve endings. *Journal of Physiology* (London) **117**:109–28.

Henser, J. E. & Reese, T. S. (1977). Structure of the synapse. In *Handbook of Physiology, The Nervous System*, section 1, vol. 1, chapter 8. Bethesda, American Physiological Society.

Jack, J. J. B. & Redman, G. J. (1971). An electrical description of the motorneurone and its application to the analysis of synaptic potentials. *Journal of Physiology* (London) **215**:321–52.

Katz, B. (1966). *Nerve Muscle and Synapse*, chapters 7–10. New York, McGraw-Hill Book Company.

Katz, B. & Miledi, R. (1967). The release of acetylcholine from nerve endings by graded electrical pulses. *Proceedings of the Royal Society*, Series B **167**:23–38.

Katz, B. & Miledi, R. (1967). The timing of calcium action during neuro-muscular transmission. *Journal of Physiology* (London) **189**:535–44.

Katz, B. & Miledi, R. (1973). The characteristics of 'end-plate noise' produced by different depolarizing drugs. *Journal of Physiology* (London) **230**:707–17.

Martin, A. R. (1977). Junctional transmission II. Presynaptic mechanisms. In *Handbook of Physiology, The Nervous System*, section 1, vol. 1. Bethesda, American Physiological Society.

Mountcastle, V. B. (1980). Sensory receptors and neural encoding: introduction to sensory processes. In *Medical Physiology*, ed. V. Mountcastle, chapter 11. St Louis, C. V. Mosby Company.

Patton, H. D. (1982). *Receptor Mechanisms in Physiology and Biophysics*, ed. T. Ruch and H. D. Patton, vol. IV, chapter 5. Philadelphia, W. B. Saunders Company.

Takeuchi, A. (1977). Functional transmission I. Postsynaptic mechanisms. In *Receptor Mechanisms in Physiology and Biophysics*, ed. T. Ruch and H. D. Patton, vol. IV, chapter 9. Philadelphia, W. B. Saunders Company.

CHAPTER 10

Anderson, C. R. & Stevens, C. F. (1972). Voltage clamp analysis of acetylcholine produced end-plate current fluctuations of frog neuromuscular junction. *Journal of Physiology* (London) **235**:655–91.

Colquhoun, D. & Hawkes, A-G. (1983). The principles of the stochastic interpretation of ion-channel mechanisms. In *Single Channel Recording*, ed. B. Sakmann and E. Neher, chapter 9. New York, Plenum Press.

Conti, F., De Felice, L. J. & Wanke, F. (1975). Potassium and sodium ion current noise in the membrane of the squid giant axons. *Journal of Physiology* (London) **248**:45–82.

Katz, B. & Miledi, R. (1973). The characteristics of end-plate noise produced by different depolarizing drugs. *Journal of Physiology* (London) **230**:707–17.

Stevens, C. F. (1972). Inferences about membrane properties from electrical noise measurements. *Biophysical Journal* **12**:1028–47.

Steinbach, J. H. & Stevens, C. F. (1976). Neuromuscular transmission. In *Frog Neurobiology*, ed. D. Llinas and W. Precht, chapter 2. Berlin, Springer-Verlag.

APPENDIX 1

Riggs, D. S. (1963). *The Mathematical Approach to Physiological Problems*, chapters 1 and 2. Baltimore, Williams and Wilkins Company.
Zuckerman, M. M. (1980). *Algebra and Trigonometry*, chapter 10. New York, W. W. Norton & Company.

APPENDIX 2

Anton, H. (1981). *Calculus, Brief Edition*. New York, John Wiley & Sons.
Zuckerman, M. M. (1980). *Algebra and Trigonometry*. New York, W. W. Norton & Company.

APPENDIX 3

Zuckerman, M. M. (1980). *Algebra and Trigonometry*, chapters 8–10. New York, W. W. Norton & Company.

APPENDIX 4

Anton, H. (1981). *Calculus, Brief Edition*, chapter 11. New York, John Wiley & Sons.

APPENDIX 5

Courant, R. (1958). *Differential and Integral Calculus*, page 361. London, Blackie & Son.

APPENDIX 6

Courant, R. (1958). *Differential and Integral Calculus*, page 223. London, Blackie & Son.

APPENDIX 7

Boas, M. L. (1966). *Mathematical Methods in the Physical Sciences*, chapter 15. New York, John Wiley & Sons.
Hald, A. (1960). *Statistical Theory with Engineering Applications*, chapters 2, 6, 21 and 22. New York, John Wiley & Sons.
Lee, Y. W. (1961). *Statistical Theory of Communication*, chapter 3. New York, John Wiley & Sons.

APPENDIX 8

Cheng, D. K. (1959). *Analysis of Linear Systems*, page 187. Reading, Mass., Addison-Wesley Publishing Company.
Hodgman, C. D. (ed.). (1962). *Handbook of Mathematical Tables*, page 388. Cleveland, Chemical Rubber Publishing Company.

APPENDIX 9

Fagg, S. V. (1962). *Differential Equations*, chapter 1. London, English Universities Press Ltd.

APPENDIX 10

Cheng, D. K. (1959). *Analysis of Linear Systems*, chapter 2. Reading, Mass., Addison-Wesley Publishing Company.
Fagg, S. V. (1962). *Differential Equations*, chapter 2. London, English Universities Press Ltd.

APPENDIX 11

Cheng, D. K. (1959). *Analysis of Linear Systems*, chapter 5. Reading, Mass., Addison-Wesley Publishing Company.
Papoulis, A. (1962). *The Fourier Integral and Its Applications*. New York, McGraw-Hill Book Company.

APPENDIX 12

Cheng, D. K. (1959). *Analysis of Linear Systems*, chapter 5. Reading, Mass., Addison-Wesley Publishing Company.
Papoulis, A. (1962). *The Fourier Integral and Its Applications*. New York, McGraw-Hill Book Company.

APPENDIX 13

Lee, Y. W. (1960). *Statistical Theory of Communication*, chapters 2–4. New York, John Wiley & Sons.
Papoulis, A. (1977). *Signal Analysis*, chapters 3, 9, 11 and 12. New York, McGraw-Hill Book Company.

APPENDIX 14

Boas, M. L. (1966). *Mathematical Methods in the Physical Sciences*, chapter 13. New York, John Wiley & Sons.
Cheng, D. K. (1959). *Analysis of Linear Systems*, chapters 6–8. Reading, Mass., Addison-Wesley Publishing Company.

APPENDIX 15

Gillie, A. C. (1961). *Electrical Principles of Electronics*. New York, McGraw-Hill Book Company.
Skilling, H. H. (1961). *Electrical Engineering Circuits*, chapters 1–12. New York, John Wiley & Sons.

APPENDIX 16

Cheng, D. K. (1959). *Analysis of Linear Systems*, chapters 6–8. Reading, Mass., Addison-Wesley Publishing Company.

Skilling, H. H. (1961). *Electrical Engineering Circuits*, chapter 17. New York, John Wiley & Sons.

APPENDIX 17

Cheng, D. K. (1959). *Analysis of Linear Systems*, chapter 7. Reading, Mass., Addison-Wesley Publishing Company.

Skilling, H. H. (1961). *Electrical Engineering Circuits*, chapter 3. New York, John Wiley & Sons.

APPENDIX 18

Boas, M. L. (1966). *Mathematical Methods in the Physical Sciences*, chapter 5. New York, John Wiley & Sons.

Purcell, E. M. (1965). *Electricity and Magnetism, Berkeley Physics Course*, vol. 2, chapter 2. New York, McGraw-Hill Book Company.

APPENDIX 19

Crank, F. (1970). *The Mathematics of Diffusion*, chapters 1–6. London, Oxford University Press.

APPENDIX 20

Cheng, D. K. (1959). *Analysis of Linear Systems*, chapter 11. Reading, Mass., Addison-Wesley Publishing Company.

Hodgkin, A. L. In Fatt, P. & Katz, B. (1951). An analysis of the end-plate potential recorded with an intracellular electrode. *Journal of Physiology* (London) 115:320–70.

Jack, J. J. B., Noble, D. & Tsein, R. W. (1975). *Electric Current Flow in Excitable Cells*, chapters 2 and 3. London, Clarendon Press.

Rall, W. (1977). Core conductor theory and cable properties of neurons. In *Handbook of Physiology, The Nervous System*, section 1, vol. 1, pages 39–98. Bethesda, American Physiological Society.

APPENDIX 21

Bent, H. A. (1965). *The Second Law*, chapters 20–23. New York, Oxford University Press.

Moore, W. J. (1957). *Physical Chemistry*, page 182. London, Longmans Owen & Co.

Reif, F. (1967). Statistical physics. In *Berkeley Physics Course*, vol. 5, chapter 4. New York, McGraw-Hill Book Company.

APPENDIX 22

Finkelstein, A. and Mauro, A. (1977). Physical principles and formalisms of electrical excitability. In *Handbook of Physiology, The Nervous System*, section 1, vol. 1, pages 161–214. Bethesda, American Physiological Society.
Purcell, E. M. (1965). Electricity and magnetism. In *Berkeley Physics Course*, vol. 2, chapter 2. New York, McGraw-Hill Book, Company.

APPENDIX 23

Purcell, E. M. (1965). Electricity and magnetism. In *Berkeley Physics Course*, vol. 2, chapters 1, 2 and 9. New York, McGraw-Hill Book Company.

APPENDIX 24

Armstrong, C. M. & Bezanilla, F. (1973). Currents related to movement of the gating particles of the sodium channels. *Nature* (London) **242**:459–61.
Schneider, M. F. & Chandler, W. K. (1973). Voltage-dependent charge movement in skeletal muscle: a possible step in excitation–contraction coupling. *Nature* (London) **242**:244–6.

APPENDIX 25

Bent, H. A. (1965). *The Second Law*. New York, Oxford University Press.

APPENDIX 26

Eisenberg, D. & Crothers, D. (1979). *Physical Chemistry*, chapter 6. Menlo Park, California, Benjamin/Cummings Publishing Company.
Laidler, K. J. (1980). *Physical Chemistry with Biological Applications*, chapter 9. Menlo Park, California, Benjamin/Cummings Publishing Company.

APPENDIX 27

MacInnes, D. A. (1961). *The Principles of Electrochemistry*, chapter 13. New York, Dover Publications.

APPENDIX 28

Jenkinson, D. H. (1960). The antagonism between tubocurarine and substances which depolarize the motor end-plate. *Journal of Physiology* (London) **152**:309–24.

APPENDIX 30

Sheppard, C. W. (1962). *Basic Principles of the Tracer Method*. New York, John Wiley & Sons.

APPENDIX 31

Moore, J. W. & Cole, K. S. (1963). Voltage clamp techniques. In *Physical Techniques in Biological Research*, ed. W. L. Nastuk, pp. 263–322. New York, Academic Press.
Schanne, O. F. & Ceretti, E. R. (1978). *Impedance Measurements in Biological Cells*, chapter 1. New York, John Wiley & Sons.

APPENDIX 32

Adrian, R. H., Chandler, W. K. & Hodgkin, A. L. (1970). Voltage clamp experiments in striated muscle. *Journal of Physiology* (London) **208**:607–44. (Note: Table 6A, p. 637; for *axon* read *muscle* and vice versa.)
Hodgkin, A. L. & Huxley, A. F. (1952). A quantitative description of membrane current and its application to conduction and excitation in nerve. *Journal of Physiology* (London) **117**:500–54.

APPENDIX 33

Kittel, C., Knight, W. D. & Rudermann, M. A. (1965). *Mechanics, Berkeley Physics Course*, vol. 1, chapter 5. New York, McGraw-Hill Book Company.

INDEX

acetylcholine (Ach), 200
  receptor interaction, 202
  release, 200
  containing vesicles, 202
  depolarization, 202
Ach, 200
Ach–receptor interaction, 457
activation energy, 450
activity, 17
  conductivity and ion, 30
  EMF and ion, 30
  of ions, 17
admittance, 401
Adrian, 225
affinity electron, 6
aliasing, 375
aliphatic chains, 72
ammeters, 397
amino acids, 213
amphiphilic molecules, 71
Amphotericin B, 82
analysis fluctuation, 204
angiotensin II, 213
angle, 307
anions, 22
anode, 22
Argand diagram, 265
aspartate, 213
ATP, 88
autocorrelation, 380
  function, 382
autocovariance, 386
  of channel current, 254
average
  ensemble, 377
  of a periodic function, 356
  statistical, 336
axon at rest, 179

barometric formula, 425

barrier porous, 6
bibliography, 469
bilayer, 73
  undoped lipid, 122
binomial distribution, 340, 343
  mean of, 342
binomial expansion, 273
biogenic amines, 213
BLMs, 75
Boltzmann's constant, 261
Boltzmann's factor, 425
bombesin, 213
bond
  covalent, 5
  ionic, 5
Boyd, 229
bradykinin, 213
bridge salt, 13, 50

cable equation, 417, 421
calcium
  and synaptic transmission, 198
  and synaptic vesicles, 201
capacitance, 393
  membrane, 108, 438
  per unit length, 175
carnosin, 213
cartesian coordinates, 265
cathode, 22
cations, 22
CGS system, 260
chain rule, 291
channel(s), 134
  Ach-gated, 204
  conductance at end plate, 251
  ohmic potassium, 143
  ohmic sodium, 156
  potassium, 134
  selectivity, 167
  sodium, 155

channel(s) (*continued*)
  voltage dependent, 85, 117
charge
  electronic, 261
  movements inside membranes, 138
  separation across a membrane, 108
  total ionic, in a cell, 110
cholecystokinin, 213
cholesterol, 71
circuit
  analysis, 400
  equivalent, 44, 47, 100, 120
  equivalent (axon), 172
  equivalent (synapse), 204
  fundamental, equations, 390
  lumped and non-lumped, 48
  membrane equivalent, 107, 99
  RC, 350
clamp
  current, 119
  voltage, 119
coefficient, 270
  activity, 29
  dielectric, 5
  differential, 294
  diffusion, 32, 35
  partition, 54, 56
complex
  exponential, 361
  impedance, 400
conceptual random experiment, 333
condition(s)
  boundary, 39
  initial, 39
conductance, 248
  and mobility of ions, 26
  and permeability, 82
  at infinite dilution, 27
  blocking, 128
  changes in excitation, 125
  changes in receptor, 224
  chord, 63, 66, 106
  fluctuations, 84
  in parallel, 394
  in series, 395
  ionic, 24, 35
  leakage, 157
  linear (ohmic), 57
  maximum potassium, 135
  measurement of ionic, 28
  molar, 21, 22
  non-linear, 57
  of a solution, 20
  of end plate channel, 251
  per unit length, 175
  pore, 83
  postsynaptic changes, 203
  potassium, 133, 134
  slope, 63, 64, 65, 106

conductance (*continued*)
  sodium, 145
  specific, 392
  transient (synapse), 221
  unit, 164, 204
  voltage dependent, 85
conductivity, 20
conjugate complex, 267
constant, 270
  Boltzmann's, 261, 442
  dielectric, 391, 435, 436
  Faraday's, 261
  field assumptions, 53, 55
  field equation, 60, 61, 66
  field I/V curve, 57
  field rectification, 57
  integration, 303
  membrane time, 183
  molar gas, 261
  of integration, 302
  permeability, 37
  rate, 449
  space, 180, 181
  time, 180, 276
convention current sign, 121
cosecant, 311
cosine, 309
  derivative of, 317
  of the sum, 314
cotangent, 311
Coulomb's law, 435
coulomb (C), 391
coulombic attraction, 5
curare, 200
current (I), 391
  capacitative, 110, 111, 130
  clamp, 420, 461
  density of, 23, 24
  diffusional, 44
  displacement, 138
  distribution, 168
  end plate, 203, 221, 249
  flow (synapse), 214
  injection, 184
  ionic, 22
  leakage, 132
  noise, 249
  per unit length, 171
  removal of capacitative, 114, 130
  sodium, 145
  step, 110
curve I/V, 18, 128
  instantaneous, 144
  linear, 18
  non-linear, 18
cycles per second, 354

De Moivre's theorem, 361
Debye, 29

Debye length, 434
degree (trigonometry), 308
delta function, 247
density
  current, 44
  flux, 44
depolarization
  postsynaptic, 199
  presynaptic, 199
depolarizing blockers, 201
derivative, 287
  of a constant, 287
  of a power of x, 288
  of a product, 290
  of a quotient, 292
  of a sum, 289
  of ax, 289
  of an implicit function, 293
  of an inverse function, 286
  of $\ln(x)$, 286
differential, 297
differential equations, 399
differentiation
  partial, 402
  rules of, 285
diffusion, 31
  across a slab, 35
  coefficient, 32
  Fick's first law of, 31
  in free solution, 31
  of electrolytes, 43
  of non-electrolytes, 31
  over synaptic cleft, 202
  speed of, 39
  times, 42
  within a membrane, 51
digital data processing, 368
dimensions, 259
dissociation, 22
distributed model of an axon, 192
distribution
  amplitude of EPPs, 198
  passive, 94
  Poisson, 198
divergence, 402, 405
domain time, 365
dopamine, 213
downhill transport, 88
drag, 88

effect sieve, 82
Einstein equation, 34
electrode, 6
  silver/silver chloride, 14
  copper, 10
  hydrogen, 11
  standard reference, 11
  zinc, 10
electrolyte, 20

encephalins, 213
energy, 467
  activation, 167, 450
  free, 440, 445
  potential, 467
ensemble, 377
  average, 379
  variance, 377, 379
enthalpy, 447
entropy, 441
  properties of, 445
epc, 221
EPP, 196
EPPs, 199
EPSPs, 213, 214
equation
  cable, 180, 181
  derivation of cable, 178
  derivation of wave, 189
  differential, 350
  dimensional, 262
  Einstein, 34
  flux, 32
  Goldman, 51
  Goldman–Hodgkin–Katz, 55, 58, 62, 99
  Nernst, 14, 17
  Nernst–Planck, 34, 43, 51, 53, 100
  one-dimensional wave, 191
  Poisson, 16
  solution of cable, 417
  solution of wave, 192
equilibrium, 8, 441
  electrode/solution, 7
error function, 347
event
  certain, 339
  compound, 334
  impossible, 339
  simple, 334
expected value, 336

factor, Boltzmann, 7
factorial, 271
Faraday's constant, 261
Fick, 31
  second law of, 36
  solution of second law of, 39
field
  electrical, 24, 25, 31
  strength, 435
fluctuation analysis, 204
flux
  coupling, 88
  density, 32
force
  driving, 26, 32
  electrical, 25
  frictional, 25
  per mole, 33

Fourier, 354
Fourier expansion, 354
Fourier integral, 365, 367
frequency, 333
  coding in receptors, 224
  domain, 365
  factor, 449
Frey and Edidin's experiment, 76
function, 269, 355
  argument of a, 277
  autocorrelation, 380
  average value of a, 320
  cumulative distribution, 338, 347
  delta, 219, 371
  discontinuous, 284
  exponential, 276
  integrating, 212
  inverse, 278, 286
  probability distribution, 338
  pulse, 366
  sampling, 371
  transcendental, 277
fundamental rule of calculus, 299, 300

gama-aminobutyric acid (GABA), 213
Gauss's theorem, 408
glucagon, 213
glutamate, 213
glycine, 213
Goldman equation, 51
Goldman–Hodgkin–Katz equation, 55, 58, 62, 99
Gorter and Grandel's experiment, 73
gradient, 402
  concentration, 15, 31, 32
  electrical potential, 25
  local chemical potential, 33
  local electrical, 26

harmonic analysis, 375
head groups, phosphate-containing, 71
histamine, 213
Hodgkin, 54, 127, 210
Hodgkin cycle, 158
Hodgkin–Huxley model, 136
Huckel, 29
Huxley, 127
hydrophobic, 71
hypothalamic releasing hormones, 213
Hz, 354

inactivation, sodium, 147, 148, 150
independence of membrane conductances, 126
indetermination, 284
inhibition
  competitive, 201, 455
  of Ach release, 201
  postsynaptic, 201

inhibitors, 126
insulin, 213
integral, 298
  computation of definite, 304
  definite, 299
  indefinite, 300
  of a constant, 300
  of the sum, 302
  of x, 300
integration
  by parts, 305
  by recurrence, 329
  by substitution, 306
  of differential equations, 350, 353
interphase metal/solution, 7
ion(s)
  activity of, 17, 29
  flux densities of, 22
  formation of, 5
  independent migration of, 27
  mobile, 6
  mobility of, 25
  movement, 18
  substitutions, 126
  velocities of, 22, 24
ionophores, 81
IPSPs, 213, 214
isothionate, 128

Joule (J), 391
junction
  gap, 225
  potential, 451

Katz, 54, 201, 235, 236, 240
Kirchhoff, laws of, 45, 103, 207
Kohlraush, 27

Langmuir trough, 73
law of mass action, 134
Lee, 379, 386
limit, 284
lipid, 71
  bilayers, 76
  bilayers cholesterol in, 77
  bilayers flip-flopping in, 77
  bilayers fluidity of, 76
  bilayers permeability of, 76, 80
liposomes, 73, 75
literal quantities, 268
local flux, 43
local gradient, 43
logarithm, 279
  decimal, 280

m, voltage and time-dependence of, 152
magnetic permeability, 437
Martin, 227

membrane
  conductance, 103
  resistance, 103
MEPP, 197
MEPPs amplitude, 234
micelles, 73
microelectrode, 119
microsomes, 73
Miledi, 235, 236, 240
MKS system, 259
mobility, 33
  and conductance of ions, 26
  at infinite dilution, 27
  concentration and ion, 28
model
  cable (synapse), 205
  Hodgkin–Huxley, 136
  lumped (synapse), 206
  of quantal release, 232
  of sodium channel, 154
  of synaptic transmission, 217, 218
  partition diffusion, 78
modulus of complex numbers, 267
molal solution, 260
mole, 260
monolayers, 72
Mullins and Noda, 97

Na–glucose co-transport, 71
Na/Ca exchange, 71
natural membranes, 87
  carriers in, 87
  pores in, 87
Nernst–Planck equation, 14, 17, 34, 43, 51,
    53, 100
Nernst potential, 204
neuroactive peptides, 213
  of gut and brain, 213
neuromuscular junction, 195
neurotensin, 213
neutral exchange, 82
noise, 163
  Ach voltage, 236
  analysis, 239, 243
  current at end plate, 249
  measurement of synaptic, 236
  membrane, 84, 163, 227
  postsynaptic membrane, 235, 239
  reduction, 238
  synaptic, 240, 257
non-infinite cables, 183
norepinephrine, 213
normal distribution, 234, 346
  mean of, distribution, 347
  variance of, distribution, 348
number e, 273
numbers, 259
  complex, 264
  integers, 263

numbers (*continued*)
  irrational, 263
  rational, 263
  real, 263
Nystatin, 82

Ohm's law, 207, 392
orthogonal relationships, 322
orthogonality, 357
osmotic pressure, 88
ouabain, 98
oxytocin, 213

partial fractions, 348
particle
  inactive, 136
  active, 136
Pascal's triangle, 273, 342
patch-clamp, 163
period, 313
periodicity, 313
permeability, 55
  conductance and, 82
  measurement of, 458
  membrane, 55, 68
  of lipid bilayers, 80, 78
permittivity, 391
phase transitions, 73
  and temperature, 75
phospholipid, 71
  aggregation, 72
physical constants, 261
pituitary peptides, 213
plasmalogens, 71
point voltage clamp, 186
Poisson distribution, 198, 235, 344, 345
Poisson's equation, 16, 410, 431
Poisson–Boltzmann's equation, 434
polar coordinates, 265
polynomials, 270, 323
pore, 83
  conductance, 83
  diameter, 165
  formation (kinetics of), 83
  selectivity, 84
potential, 8, 9
  biological, 12
  chemical, 8
  definition of chemical, 448
  difference (V), 391
  diffusion, 15, 49
  due to Na/K pump, 95
  electrical, 9
  electrochemical, 9
  electrode, 11
  end plate (EPP), 196, 210
  equilibrium, 17, 99
  generation of action, 158
  generator, 223

potential (*continued*)
  graded, 223
  junction, 10, 50, 451
  local action, 117
  membrane, 94, 95
  membrane action, 160
  membrane equilibrium, 105
  miniature end plate (MEPP), 197
  Nernst, 204
  non-propagated, 223
  open circuit, 107
  postsynaptic reversal, 204
  potassium equilibrium, 144
  propagated action, 117, 189, 192
  receptor, 223
  resting membrane, 62
  standard electrochemical, 9
  standard electrode, 11
  stationary, 223
  transients, 120
pressure, osmotic, 88
principle independence, 61, 67
probability, 333
  addition, 334
  conditional, 335
  multiplication, 335
profile of concentration, 31
proteins, 71
pump, 88
  electrogenicity, 98
  Na/K, 92
  operation, 89
  stoichiometry, 97

quantal release, 227
quantities, 259

radian, 309, 354
radians per second, 354
random walk, 40
rate constants, voltage dependence of, 141,
  157
receptor
  phasic, 224
  sensory, 223
  tonic, 224
  transmitter, 215
rectification
  anomalous, 57
  constant field, 57, 58, 59
  delayed, 128
resistance
  input, 182
  per unit length, 175
  specific, 392
  slope, 45
  in parallel, 394
  in series, 395
resistivity, 20, 101

Runge–Kutta, 162

saltatory conduction, 194
sampling frequency, 369
sampling theorem, 375
secant, 311
series, 271
  coefficients of, Fourier, 355
  expansion, 277
  exponential, Fourier, 360
  Fourier, 354
  Taylor, 323
  power, 271
serotonin, 213
Shannon's theorem, 369
sign conventions for currents, 57
signal
  averaging, 238
  non-periodic, 376
  non-stationary, 376
  stationary, 376
  time average of, 236
  variance of a, 236
sine, 309, 312
  derivative of, 316
  of the sum, 314
sinusoid, parameters of a, 355
sodium pumping and membrane potential,
  96
source
  current, 396
  voltage, 396
space clamping, 185
spectral density, 368
spectrum
  power, 359, 383
  power density, 257, 383, 384
standard deviation, 339
  error of the mean, 339
steady state, 37
Stirling's formula, 324
substance P, 213
succinylcholine, 201
sulphate, 128
summation
  spatial, 211
  temporal, 212
surface pressure, 73
symbols, 261
sympathetic ganglia, 214
synapse, 195
  electrical, 224
synaptic delay, 200, 202
synaptic potential, 195
synaptic vesicles, 201

Takeuchi, 203, 221
tangent, 311
Taylor series, 323

temperature, absolute, 261
tetraethylammonium (TEA), 127, 199, 204
tetrodotoxin (TTX), 127, 199, 204
thermal reservoir, 442
thermodynamics
   first law of, 440
   second law of, 445
   third law of, 444
thought experiment, 333
time constant of a membrane, 112
transducer biological, 224
transfer number, 28
transform, Laplace, 219, 220, 386, 387, 388, 389, 390
transient conditions, 35
   solution, 36
transitions in membrane particles, 141
transmitter, 213
   receptor complex, 243
   receptor interaction, 214
   depolarizing, 213
   hyperpolarizing, 213
transport
   downhill, 88
   number, 28, 108

transport (*continued*)
   uphill, 70, 87
trigonometric function, 307

units, 259
universe of an event, 441
uphill transport, 70, 87

Valinomycin, 81
variables, 270
variance, 338
   ensemble, 379
   time, 379
vasoactive intestinal peptide (VIP), 213
vasopressin, 213
velocity conduction, 194
voltage clamp, 114, 131, 187, 188, 418, 464
   double pulse, 148
   of postsynaptic membrane, 203
voltage distribution, 168
voltage transients, 130
voltmeters, 397

Walli's formula, 329
work, 467